FUNDAMENTAL FAULT IN HYPERTENSION

DEVELOPMENTS IN
CARDIOVASCULAR MEDICINE

Lancée CT, ed: Echocardiology, 1979. ISBN 90-247-2209-8.

Baan J, Arntzenius AC, Yellin EL, eds: Cardiac dynamics. 1980. ISBN 90-247-2212-8.

Thalen HJT, Meere CC, eds: Fundamentals of cardiac pacing. 1970. ISBN 90-247-2245-4.

Kulbertus HE, Wellens HJJ, eds: Sudden death. 1980. ISBN 90-247-2290-X.

Dreifus LS, Brest AN, eds: Clinical applications of cardiovascular drugs. 1980. ISBN 90-247-2295-0.

Spencer MP, Reid JM, eds: Cerebrovascular evaluation with Doppler ultrasound. 1981. ISBN 90-247-2348-1.

Zipes DP, Bailey JC, Elharrar V, eds: The slow inward current and cardiac arrhythmias. 1980. ISBN 90-247-2380-9.

Kesteloot H, Joossens JV, eds: Epidemiology of arterial blood pressure. 1980. ISBN 90-247-2386-8.

Wackers FJT, ed: Thallium-201 and technetium-99m-pyrophosphate myocardial imaging in the coronary care unit. 1980. ISBN 90-247-2396-5.

Maseri A, Marchesi C, Chierchia S, Trivella MG, eds: Coronary care units. 1981. ISBN 90-247-2456-2.

Morganroth J, Moore EN, Dreifus LS, Michelson EL, eds: The evaluation of new antiarrhythmic drugs. 1981. ISBN 90-247-2474-0.

Alboni P: Intraventricular conduction disturbances. 1981. ISBN 90-247-2484-X.

Rijsterborgh H, ed: Echocardiology. 1981. ISBN 90-247-2491-0.

Wagner GS, ed: Myocardial infarction: Measurement and intervention. 1982. ISBN 90-247-2513-5.

Meltzer RS, Roelandt J, eds: Contrast echocardiography. 1982. ISBN 90-247-2531-3.

Amery A, Fagard R, Lijnen R, Staessen J, eds: Hypertensive cardiovascular disease; pathophysiology and treatment. 1982. ISBN 90-247-2534-8.

Bouman LN, Jongsma HJ, eds: Cardiac rate and rhythm. 1982. ISBN 90-247-2626-3.

Morganroth J, Moore EN, eds: The evaluation of beta blocker and calcium antagonist drugs. 1982. ISBN 90-247-2642-5.

Rosenbaum MB, ed: Frontiers of cardiac electrophysiology. 1982. ISBN 90-247-2663-8.

Roelandt J, Hugenholtz PG, eds: Long-term ambulatory electrocardiography. 1982. ISBN 90-247-2664-8.

Adgey AAJ, ed: Acute phase of ischemic heart disease and myocardial infarction. 1982. ISBN 90-247-2675-1.

Hanrath P, Bleifeld W, Souquet, J. eds: Cardiovascular diagnosis by ultrasound. Transesophageal, computerized, contrast, Doppler echocardiography. 1982. ISBN 90-247-2692-1.

Roelandt J, ed: The practice of M-mode and two-dimensional echocardiography. 1983. ISBN 90-247-2745-6.

Meyer J, Schweizer P, Erbel R, eds: Advances in noninvasive cardiology. 1983. ISBN 0-89838-576-8.

Morganroth J, Moore EN, eds: Sudden cardiac death and congestive heart failure: Diagnosis and treatment. 1983. ISBN 0-89838-580-6.

Perry HM, ed: Lifelong management of hypertension. 1983. ISBN 0-89838-582-2.

Jaffe EA, ed: Biology of endothelial cells. 1984. ISBN 0-89838-587-3.

Surawicz B, Reddy CP, Prystowsky EN, eds: Tachycardias. ISBN 0-89838-588-1.

Spencer MP, ed: Cardiac Doppler diagnosis. 1983. ISBN 0-89838-591-1.

Villarreal H, Sambhi MP, eds: Topics in pathophysiology of hypertension. 1984. ISBN 0-89838-595-4.

Messerli FH, ed: Cardiovascular disease in the elderly. 1984. ISBN 0-89838-596-2.

Simoons ML, Reiber JHC, eds: Nuclear imaging in clinical cardiology. 1984. ISBN 0-89838-599-7.

Ter Keurs HEDJ, Schipperheyn JJ, eds: Cardiac left ventricular hypertrophy. 1983. ISBN 0-89838-612-8.

Sperelakis N, ed: Physiology and pathophysiology of the heart. ISBN 0-89838-612-2.

Messerli FH, ed: Kidney in essential hypertension. ISBN 0-89838-616-0.

Sambhi MP, ed: Fundamental fault in hypertension. ISBN 0-89838-638-1.

Marchesi C, ed: Ambulatory monitoring: Cardiovascular system and allied applications. ISBN 0-89838-642-X.

Kupper W, MacAlpin RN, Bleifeld W, eds: Coronary tone in ischemic heart disease. ISBN 0-89838-646-2.

Sperelakis N, Caulfield JB, eds: Calcium antagonists: Mechanisms of action on cardiac muscle and vascular smooth muscle. ISBN 0-89838-655-1.

Godfraind T, Herman AS, Wellens D, eds: Calcium entry blockers in cardiovascular and cerebral dysfunctions. ISBN 0-89838-658-1.

Morganroth J, Moore EN, eds: Interventions in the acute phase of myocardial infarction. ISBN 0-89838-659-4.

FUNDAMENTAL FAULT IN HYPERTENSION

edited by

MOHINDER P. SAMBHI, MD, PhD

Professor and Chief, Division of Hypertension, Department of Medicine, UCLA,
San Fernando Valley Medical Program, Veterans Administration Medical Center, Sepulveda CA

SPRINGER-SCIENCE+BUSINESS MEDIA, B.V.

Library of Congress Cataloging in Publication Data

Main entry under title:

Fundamental fault in hypertension.

   (Developments in cardiovascular medicine)
   Includes index.
   1. Hypertension. I. Sambhi, Mohinder P. II. Series.
[DNLM: 1. Hypertension--Etiology. W1 DE997VME / WG 340
F481]
RC685.H8F86 1984   616.1'32   84--1554
ISBN 978-94-010-9006-3   ISBN 978-94-009-5678-0 (eBook)
DOI 10.1007/978-94-009-5678-0

Copyright

CONTENTS

IV. A DEFECT IN CELL MEMBRANE PERMEABILITY

V. THE ANTIHYPERTENSIVE HORMONES OF THE KIDNEY

VI. THE ROLE OF THE CENTRAL NERVOUS SYSTEM: MEDIATION OR INITIATION?

VII. ALTERED HEMODYNAMICS: A CAUSE OR A CONSEQUENCE?

VIII. HOW IS THE RENIN SYSTEM INVOLVED?

PREFACE

The fundamental fault in hypertension is unknown. Calling it a fundamental fault, indeed, tacitly begs the question: Is there one fundamental fault, or are there several that are interlinked or interdependent? A simple yes or no answer cannot be offered. This volume is not designed to survey the up-to-date recent advances in research on hypertension, nor intended to provide provisional answers to the so many unknowns in this topic. It is, in fact, an attempt to articulate questions that are worth asking, given the license of an unhibited, albeit disciplined, inquiry. The range of expression varies from dogmatic opinion to a declared speculation.

Is the primary abnormality an excessive sodium and reduced potassium intake over generations? Or is it hormonal excess, deficiency, imbalance or altered synthesis of abnormal forms? Does the nervous system play a role of active initiation or only of passive maintenance in the genesis of hypertension? Is the heart only a pump acting in concert with the happenings to the vasculature trying to provide adequate flow in the face of vasconstriction induced by neural or humoral factors, or does it sometimes become the culprit by pumping blood flow in excess of demand and thus initiating hypertrophic changes in blood vessels, or by assuming the role of an endocrine organ and being the source of a hormone with influence on cellular transport of sodium and on vasomotor tone? Is an elusive and mysterious fault in the kidney, the primary basis of all of the above factors, or does that circumstance pertain only to hypertension secondary to renal disease? Or is hypertension marked by a generalized membrane abnormality leading to altered ionic transport?

The answers to these questions have to be reconciled with several general recognized characteristics of the disease. The potential hypertensives in the population display a genetic tendency toward developing the disease. The tendency in its mildest forms may be almost averted by a radical behavioral change in lifestyle. In most others it leads to mosaic expression of the disease (Page) that may end up almost randomly distributed in the general population (Pickering). The mode of expression may depend not only on the variance in environmental factors, but also on the organ specific inherited genetic tendency. Thus the multiple initiating modes may eventually merge into a common pathway, expressing itself as a disregulation of overall circulatory control with faulty feedback mechanisms (Guyton). Once initiated, the phenomenon leads to a snow-balling effect, a positive feedback in causing structural changes in the vasculature (Folkow).

The preceeding remarks of this writer do not represent accurate quotes from interspersed distinguished names that are given as identification of the general area of thought.

My sincere thanks are due to all contributors, to Mr Boudewijn F. Commandeur, Martinus Nijhoff Publishers, and Kurt R. Hoffmann, M.D., Vice President, Professional Relations, Boehringer Ingelheim Ltd. for making this publication possible.

MOHINDER P. SAMBHI

LIST OF CONTRIBUTORS

Bevan, Rosemarie D., Department of pharmacology, School of Medicine and Brain Research Institute, Center for the Health Sciences, University of California, Los Angeles CA 90024, USA
    co-authors: John A. Bevan
Birkenhäger, William H., Department of Internal Medicine, Zuiderziekenhuis, Groene Hilledijk 315, 3075 EA Rotterdam, The Netherlands
    co-author: P.W. de Leeuw
Bohr, David F., Department of Physiology, University of Michigan, Ann Arbor, Michigan 48109, USA
Carretero, Oscar A., Hypertension Research Division, Department of Medicine, Henry Ford Hospital, Detroit MI 48202, USA
    co-author: A.G. Scicli
Doyle, Austin E., Department of Medicine, University of Melbourne, Austin Hospital, Heidelburg, Victoria, Australia
Fasciolo, Juan Carlos, Departamento de Fisiología, Facultad de Ciencias Médicas, Universidad Nacional de Cuyo, Mendoza, Argentina
Guyton, Arthur C., Department of Physiology and Biophysics, University of Mississippi Medical Center, Jackson, MS 39216, USA
    co-authors: Thomas E. Lohmeier, John E. Hall, Manis J. Smith, and Philip R. Kastner
Haddy, Francis J., Department of Physiology, Uniformed Services University, Bethesda, MD 20014, USA
    co-authors: M.B. Pamnani, D.L. Clough
Imai, Yutaki, Monash University, Department of Medicine, Prince Henry's Hospital, St. Kilda Road, Melbourne, Australia 3004
    co-authors: Peter L. Nolan, Colin I. Johnston
de Jong, Wybren, Rudolf Magnus Institute for Pharmacology, Medical Faculty, University of Utrecht, Catharijnesingel 101, 3511 CV Utrecht, The Netherlands
    co-author: Dirk H.G. Versteeg
Julius, Stevo, Division of Hypertension, University of Michigan Medical School, Ann Arbor MI 48109, USA
Lovenberg, Walter, National Heart, Lung and Blood Institute, Section on Biochemical Pharmacology, National Institute of Health, Bethesda MD 20205, USA
    co-authors: Donald Kuhn, Judith Juskevich
Lijnen, P., Hypertension and Cardiovascular Rehabilitation Unit, Department of Pathophysiology, University of Leuven, Belgium
    co-authors: R. Fagard, J. Staessen, L. Verschueren, A. Amery
Mahoney, L.T., Departments of Pediatrics, Pharmacology, Psychology and Surgery and Cardiovascular Center, University of Iowa, Iowa City IA 52242
    co-authors: J.R. Haywood, R. Correy, N.P. Patel, A.K. Johnson, M.J. Brody
Mancia, Guiseppe, Istituto Clinica Media IV, Università di Milano, and Centro Fisiologia Clinica e

XII

Ipertensione, Ospetale Maggire, Milano, Italy
co-author: Alberto Zanchetti

Mason, P., MCR Blood Pressure Unit, Western Infirmary, Glasgow G11, 6NT, United Kingdom
co-authors: D.G. Beevers, Dudley Road Hospital, Birmingham; C. Beretta-Piccoli, see Mason; J.J. Brown, see Mason; A.M.M. Cumming, see Mason; D.L. Davies, Department of Medicine, see Mason; R. Fraser, see Mason; A.F. Lever, see Mason; J.J. Morton, see Mason; P.L. Padfield, Western General Hospital, Edinburgh; Y. Young, see Mason

Muirhead, Eric E., University of Tennessee Center for the Health Sciences, and Baptist Memorial Hospital, Memphis, TN 38146, USA
co-authors: J.A. Pitcock, W.A. Rightsel, P.S. Brown, M.F. Hall, B. Brooks

Page, Irvine H., Research Division, Cleveland Clinic Foundation, Cleveland, OH 44106, USA

Page, Lot B., Newton-Wellesley Hospital, Tufts University School of Medicine, Boston MA, USA

Pickering, Thomas G., The New York Hospital – Cornell Medical Center, 525 68th Street, New York, NY 10021, USA

Sambhi, Mohinder P., Department of Medicine, UCLA, San Fernando Valley Medical Program, V.A. Medical Center, 16111 Plummer Street, Sepulveda CA 91343, USA

Swales, John D., Department of Medicine, Clinical Sciences Building, Leicester Royal Infirmary, P.O. Box 65, Leicester LE2 7LX, United Kingdom

Tarazi, Robert C., Research Division, Cleveland Clinic Foundation, 9500 Euclid Avenue, Cleveland OH 44106, USA

Walker, Gordon W., Department of Medicine, John Hopkins University School of Medicine, The John Hopkins Hospital and The O'Neill Laboratories of the Good Samaritan Hospital, Baltimore MD, USA

Yamori, Yukio, Japan Stroke Prevention Center and Department of Pathology, Shimane Medical University, Izumo, Japan 693
co-authors: Yasuo Nara, see Yamori; Hiroshi Imafuku, Department of Pathology; Masahiro Kihara, see Yamori; Ryoichi Horie, see Yamori, also Department of Neurosurgery; Ahira Ooshima, see Yamori

I. THE PREAMBLE

1. THE LONG SLOW ROAD TO PROGRESS: A LESSON IN HUMILITY

IRVINE H. PAGE

It is generally not known, or forgotten, by modern investigators that in the second and third decades of this century there were less than a dozen serious researchers in hypertension in the world. Hypertension was held in low esteem by the public, physicians, and researchers alike. It should not be surprising then that serious thinking about the cause of essential hypertension is a recent preoccupation. Nevertheless, several concepts have already been advanced, none of which is totally convincing.

Many workers used to believe that most hypertension was relatively harmless. Just the terms, 'essential' and 'malignant' seemed to satisfy their curiosity. As knowledge accumulated, however, so did confusion and argument. As you know, almost every conceivable mechanism has been enlisted to explain hypertension, and each to the exclusion of the others. Angiotensin, for example, was 'ruled in' or 'out' so many times, I lost track!

Confrontation was the order of the day, and those who currently do not believe this did not know Frederick Allen, Harry Goldblatt, Henry Schroeder, Reginald Smithwick, Max Peet, or Walter Kempner, among others.

Let me now briefly review most of the widely debated theses on the genesis of hypertension.

Perhaps the most common failing of the several theories of pathogenesis is the ignoring of evidence clearly at variance with the proposed concept or purpose – rather like the newspaper ad that stated, 'Now Delta Flies Nonstop to Jacksonville and Back'.

The second most common characteristic is not saying precisely what is meant. I am reminded of a church bulletin in which it was stated, with a gentle diuretic nudge, 'The service will close with "Little Drops of Water," which one of the ladies will start quietly and the rest of the congregation will join in'.

THE GENETIC-ENVIRONMENTAL CONCEPT

One of the most widely accepted concepts of pathogenesis is the one superbly presented by Pickering (1968). With consummate stylistic skill, he argued that essential hypertension is a disease only in the sense that it is a quantitative

Sambhi, M.P. (ed.) Fundamental fault in hypertension
© *1984, Martinus Nijhoff Publishers. Boston/The Hague/Dordrecht/Lancaster.*
ISBN 978-94-010-9006-3

extreme of a normal function. This is in contrast with the theory that essential hypertension is a *specific* disease, due to a single gene with a unique cardiovascular fault, as argued by Platt.

Pickering and his associates found nothing in the literature of hypertension that convinced them of a specific fault leading to essential hypertension. With this in mind, he examined the problems of the dividing line between normal and abnormal blood pressure, the genetic and environmental factors, and the clinical manifestations, all of which convinced him that, '. . . we cannot, in my view, escape calling essential hypertension a disease. But at the same time we must not, in so doing, imply that this disease represents the manifestation of a specific and unique fault of a qualitative kind'. He accepted, then, the ancient concept that disease may include a quantitative deviation from the normal, as well as qualitative one.

The breeding of pure strains of spontaneously hypertensive rats has done much to strengthen the concept of genetically induced hypertension. Many believe that the mechanisms of the clinical manifestations of these animals resemble essential hypertension closely.

The environmental aspects have been most cogently presented by Lot Page, who has tirelessly, and persuasively, presented the case for the effects of acculturation on various racial groups. Western civilization seems to increase the risk factors of cardiovascular disease. Low sodium, reduced psychosocial stress, maintenance of lean body weight, and physical activity seem to protect entire populations. A low-salt, high-potassium diet may be a critical facet.

SALT

The oldest concept, beginning at the turn of the century, is that excess salt is responsible for hypertension. There are several ideas as to the cause. Some accept a genetic predisposition as proposed by Dahl; others, such as Freis, derive support from clinical observations.

Tobian limited his speculation to the mechanisms possibly involved in the Dahl-S rats, or the Kyoto SHR, with heavy emphasis on the metabolism of salt.

The most cogent argument is the therapeutic effect of diuretics and low-salt intake.

NEURAL

About as old as the concept of the etiologic significance of salt is that of autonomic neural pathogenesis. It is not surprising that early serious attempts to reduce blood pressure were by surgical sympathectomy, followed some years later by the chemical blocking agents, tetraethylammonium chloride, phentolamine, beta-receptor blocking agents, and clonidine. Subsequent work on the development of spontaneously hypertensive rat strains further strengthened the neurogenic concept. Several of the now widely used neurotransmitter blocking agents, such as clonidine, are effective in treating hypertension.

Derived from clinical observation, the idea that chronic hypertension resulted from repeated neural-instigated acute rises in arterial pressure became prevalent. Later, when it was shown that, due to resetting of the buffer nerve, hypertension tended to be maintained, the idea was even more appealing. With the passage of time, the notion of resetting of the renal receptors has become popular.

Wilhelm Raab (1952) was the most ardent proponent of the neural concept, though he added little experimental evidence in its support.

Brown et al.'s case rests on the assumption of a stepwise interaction of sympathetic overactivity and the kidneys' ability to sustain hypertension of non-renal origin, neither of which is capable itself of producing severe hypertension. It depends upon the hypertension-producing changes of renal resistance and compensating for its sodium-retaining effect (i.e., resetting of pressure).

THE RENAL CONCEPT

Goldblatt was deeply committed to the renal concept. Ischemia of the kidney was its keystone.

The most recent important contribution has been that of Guyton and his associates. They make a formidable case.

Guyton et al. (1974) presented a comprehensive and carefully reasoned theoretical analysis of the role of the kidney in the genesis of hypertension; this is a sophisticated, quantitative expression of the mosaic concept, to be discussed later. The authors considered the kidney to be the servocontroller of arterial blood pressure, and the key determinant in long-range blood pressure control. They emphasized pressure natriuresis, arguing that preoccupation with acute changes in blood pressure, cardiac output, and total peripheral resistance, have misled investigators into believing they can predict from these data the ultimate steady-state level of arterial pressure control. The most superficial study of the literature on hemodynamics confirms this preoccupation – but whether the preoccupation is misleading is for current investigators to prove.

Both Borst and Ledingham in 1963 proposed independently that hypertension develops '. . . when some aspect of renal function is disturbed'. Salt and water are retained transiently along with rise in venous pressure, resulting in increased cardiac work ('performance' or 'contractility'). Autoregulation is the mechanism for the increase in peripheral resistance. Ledingham emphasized that when cardiac work is increased through increased filling pressure or enhanced contractility, there is a rise in cardiac output greater than the metabolic need. The increase in output raises both pressure and peripheral flow, and the resistance vessels respond by constriction (autoregulation), which further raises blood pressure. When blood pressure attains a level that restores to normal the 'disturbed aspect of renal function' the process reaches a new equilibrium in which all changes revert to the normal range.

Bianchi et al. (1979) suggested that 'the renal abnormality which causes hypertension in the Milan strain of hypertensive rats disappears as hypertension develops'. From this they proposed, by analogy but without evidence, that a 'primary kidney abnormality causes' essential hypertension.

A renal abnormality was also postulated by Brown, Lever, Robertson and Schalekamp (1974) in a slight modification of Guyton's concept. They proposed that plasma renin activity decreases in some essential hypertensives and sodium status remains normal because the pressure-natriuresis mechanism is reset by an increased filtration fraction. Essential hypertension would become renal in origin when the increased filtration fraction fails to reverse upon removal of a hypothetical neurogenic component.

Sambhi and Wiedeman (1972) took an entirely different view. They believed they have shown that the generation rate of angiotensin is much higher in renal venous plasma from a clipped kidney. In hypertensives, circulating levels of angiotensin may, or may not, be elevated. They proposed that some function of the increased angiotensin turnover, directly or through aldosterone, leads to suppression of renin secretion in essential hypertension. This feedback mechanism would fail to operate in advanced stages of the disease when renin is high.

Arthur Grollman postulated more than 30 years ago a 'renal deficiency theory', according to which essential hypertension would result from a primary deficit in the incretory function of the kidney, resulting in failure to secrete adequate amounts of vasodepressor material. This idea has been greatly developed by Muirhead, who concluded that strong evidence favors the elaboration of a vasodepressor material by the interstitial cells of the renal medulla. He is about to announce the chemical nature of this substance, which is said to differ from the prostaglandins that are also believed to be synthesized by those cells.

CARDIOGENIC HYPERTENSION

Although it has been hinted at, chronic cardiogenic hypertension has not been produced in animals nor observed in man. A cardiac factor has repeatedly been noted and has recently been emphasized by Tarazi et al. (1974) in hypertensive patients. Whether the slight rise in cardiac output during the initial phase of experimental renal hypertension is of sufficient magnitude to play a critical role remains moot.

HUMORAL CONCEPTS

The primacy of some humoral agents has been repeatedly suggested. There is, however, difficulty in differentiating cause and effect. Thus, norepinephrine is an integral part of the mechanism of hypertension in pheochromocytoma – but it also acts as a critical neurotransmitter, independently of catecholamine-producing tumors.

Angiotensin has been widely suspected of being critically involved. It seems to originate from more than one source, and to have multiple, subtle actions, many of which relate to hypertension.

The immense literature on angiotensin supports the concept that, whether produced in the brain or body, it functions to modulate arterial pressure in its broadest connotation.

The kinins are suspect but their function is undefined. How much the prostaglandins and serotonin are involved also remains for study.

As pointed out above, one of the most important contributions has been made by Muirhead and Grollman, especially by the former, who over many years has developed cogent evidence that an anti-hypertensive agent is produced by the interstitial cells of the renal medulla. Elucidation of the chemical structure of this agent seems imminent.

ANGIOGENIC CONCEPT

Here, again, whether the heart and blood vessels themselves can play a *primary* role remains problematic. Evidence is accumulating that vessel walls are able to synthesize vasoactive agents such as angiotensin and norepinephrine, and are able to change their reactivity to agonists; both qualities make them potentially able to modulate blood pressure. Changes in reactivity due to alteration of receptor affinity or population are coming to be recognized. Primacy of the heart remains speculative.

Blaustein (1977) put the matter as succinctly as currently possible. Because there is resting tone in resistance vessels, the $[Ca^{2+}]_i$ in the smooth muscle cells must be maintained above the contractile threshold. Presumably, the Na^+-Ca^{2+} exchange mechanismis set to hold the $[Ca^{2+}]$ at this level. Any change in sodium gradient will be reflected in $[Ca^{2+}]_i$. The correlation between sodium metabolism and arterial pressure could then be accounted for if a circulating natriuretic hormone affected the sodium gradient across the sarcolema, hence the $[Ca^{2+}]_i$ and tone.

Bohr, Haddy, and Overbeck have all given important testimony concerning the Na-K pump and ouabain inhibition. This aspect seems to be rapidly approaching fruition.

Understanding of vessel wall participation will depend chiefly on:

(a) quantitation of ion flux through plasma membranes and its regulation;

(b) quantitation of receptor regulation of cardiovascular architecture and function;

(c) structural elasticity of vessel walls and its regulation;

(d) humoral and renal mechanisms maintaining prolonged increased tone.

Hermsmeyer (1976) is pursuing the interesting possibility that the vascular wall might contribute to the development of essential hypertension by being more responsive to norepinephrine because of an inherently lower membrane potential. Arterial muscle from SHR rats was shown to be less negative than that of normotensive controls. Ventricular myocardium and portal venous myovascular cells do not show the hyperreactivity to norepinephrine or the altered membrane potential. It appears that a trophic influence of sympathetic nerves causes the membrane alteration that produces the hypersensitivity of arterial muscle in hypertension.

MOSAIC CONCEPT

In the thirty years since the mosaic concept was proposed, it has received only grudging and limited acceptance. It is based on the Phase Rule principle of Willard Gibbs, which provides the intellectual framework to understand and ultimately predict the results of equilibrated forces. The mosaic concept was formulated at a time when knowledge of hypertension started to grow rapidly and theories of the pathogenesis, especially of essential and renovascular hypertension, soon followed. It was a period of growing confusion and confrontation.

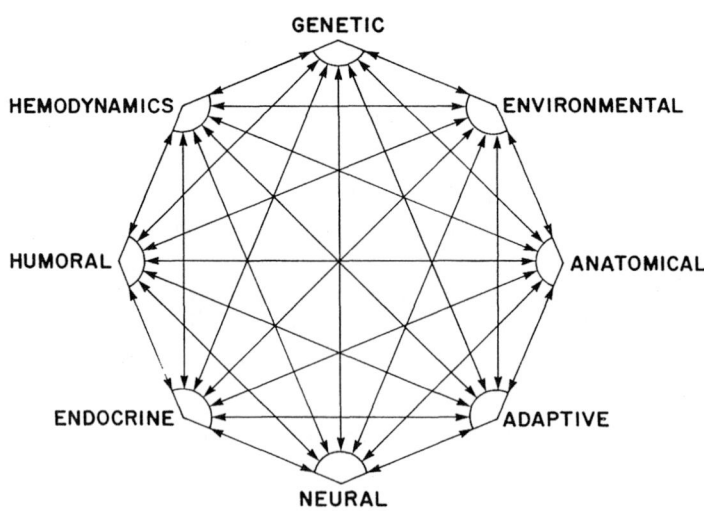

The mosaic concept aims only to provide a construct that will encompass the many mechanisms modulating blood pressure and tissue perfusion and allow predictions from quantitation of each component. It tacitly accepts a multiplicity of regulators and aims to define and measure their participation. Hypertension, then, becomes a 'disease of regulation,' in which many regulators participate in determining arterial pressure and tissue perfusion. Its current interpretation is illustrated in Table 1. It accepts the obvious, that all bodily functions ultimately are gene-directed. The eight concepts I have so cursorily described are all included, which makes no one but me happy – but I would warn there are several other concepts waiting in the wings ready to receive attention, which will also be eventually included in the mosaic!

It is understandable why 'hard' scientists find the concept either useless or suffering from swamp miasmosis. But in some ways, miasmogenesis is better than Procrustean restrictions or stretchings. Useless it is not, if the outline provided by it is remembered when examining a patient or incorporating new knowledge.

Table 1. A diagram illustrating current interpretations of the mosaic

Genetic configuration	SHR Salt-sensitive Essential hypertension Aldosterone plasma protein binding capacity
CNS	Reactivity – receptor responses Water-electrolytes-behavior Vasomotor actions
Kidney	Reactivity, receptor responses Water-electrolytes Antihypertensive actions
Heart	Cardiac output Inotropic response
Blood vessels	Reactivity Membrane potential Ion flux (sodium-potassium pump) Receptor affinity and number
Adrenal	Water-electrolytes Catecholamines Modulators
Pituitary	Water metabolism
Structural profile	Myocardial responses Vascular adaptations
Biochemical profile	Molecular configuration – receptor size and number Molecular affinities Biosynthesis and mass action
Biophysical profile	Mechanical Electrical

The mosaic is intended to include all valid knowledge concerned with regulators, so as to keep it integrated and equilibrated within the whole. It does not seek to add ephemera, for it recognizes that pouring oil on troubled waters may cause the trouble.

After thirty years, I have been unable either to explain the mosaic theory clearly or to convince most investigators of its usefulness. When it can be written, as it was recently, by one authority (Mendlowitz, 1979) that the mosaic 'does not account for such things as hereditary predisposition and the interrelationships and dynamics of hypertensive disease', and 'it also leaves about 85% of patients with hypertension still in the "essential" or "of unknown origin" category', I can only conclude that words mean different things to different people. It is exactly the interrelationships, on a genetic basis, that constitute the mosaic.

But then Mendlowitz concludes that essential hypertension is not one disease and that one hypertensive is unlike others, which is what the mosaic is supposed to say.

REACTIONS OF OTHER AUTHORS

From J.J. Brown et al. (1977): 'The central and possibly novel element in our proposal is the stepwise interaction of two pressor mechanisms (sympathetic overactivity or possibly ACTH and the kidneys'ability to sustain hypertension of non-renal cause), neither capable by itself of producing severe hypertension.'

From J. Genest (1977): 'Because of the complexity of the problem and the many facts of the "mosaic", it is quite probable that the solution of the pathogenesis of essential hypertension and the elucidation of the genetic factor will not be known before a second (or more?) edition of this textbook appears.'

From W.S. Peart (1977): 'I do not find too much satisfaction in mosaics, however, and think we still need more intensive study of well-defined circulatory states with the very best techniques we can bring to bear.'

From G.W. Pickering (1977): 'The raised pressure in essential hypertension is due to genetic and environmental factors.'

From A.C. Guyton: '. . . Figure 7 shows our form of the mosaic theory. And it was not meant to be significantly different from what Dr Page first expressed. The only real difference is that actual quantitated values are given for each of these lines and for each of the blocks.'

From S. Julius (1977): 'The part of the theory that has not been proven is that tissue perfusion takes precedence and that hypertension develops in response to tissue needs to keep perfusion at a normal level. The concept is useful insofar as it puts me on guard.'

But then, Franz Gross wrote: '. . . the mosaic theory is not a mosaic and is not a theory. The term mosaic theory should not be pursued any longer, instead we should analyse the various systems. The term reminds me of a slogan used by drug companies. The mosaic theory is past history, it is outdated.'

Perhaps, but so are most of us!

CONCLUSIONS

After 55 years of association with the slowly developing field of hypertension, I have cast my lot with two concepts: 1) most hypertensions are multifaceted, or multifactorial, diseases of regulation; and 2) angiotensin and salt are at the core of these mechanisms. Many agents modulate these mechanisms, such as aldosterone, and possibly kinins and prostaglandins, all acting on a genetically conditioned organism. These mechanisms cannot be dissociated from those controlling tissue perfusion.

In my opinion, there have been four major trends which support these generalities: 1) development of a variety of experimental models of hypertension, 2) isolation and synthesis of angiotensin, 3) synthesis of angiotensin antagonists and angiotensin converting-enzyme inhibitors, and 4) recognition that all hypertensive patients differ.

REFERENCES

Genest J, Kuchel O, Hamel P, Cantin M: Hypertension, Physiopathology and Treatment, 2nd Ed., McGraw-Hill, New York 1983
Page IH, McCubbin JW (Eds): Renal Hypertension. Yearbook, Chicago (1968)
Pickering G: High Blood Pressure, 2nd Ed., Grune and Stratton, New York (1968)

DISCUSSION

Commentary

The following discussion on the mosaic theory has taken place at a conference. The editor has considered this exchange of thought as a very valuable addition to Dr. Page's text and it is therefore included in this chapter.

Dr. A.F. Lever: I wonder whether Franz Gross and Arthur Guyton are both correct: perhaps the mosaic theory isn't a theory of the pathogenesis of hypertension, but a map explaining how the various control mechanisms might react in the event of something causing hypertension. In other words, I don't think the mosaic theory identifies the cause of hypertension or the area in which the blood pressure might be caused to rise, if you see what I mean – but it could explain very nicely how the control mechanisms would react once the blood pressure was raised by some process. So, in the sense that Gross says, it is not a theory of pathogenesis, I would agree, but in Guyton's sense, that it does explain, just as his theory does, how the system would react, I would also agree. So, perhaps there may be reconciliation there.

Dr D.F. Bohr: The mosaic theory describes, as Tony just pointed out, things wrong in various places and the interdependence of these regulating systems: if something goes haywire in the neurogenic control, it is apt to upset the endocrine, and that may upset the kidneys, and it's hard to decide which is the prime mover. It just might be that there is a prime mover in all these areas, the neurogenic, renal, endocrine, and particularly the salt problem – the salt problem, as Blaustine pointed out and you recognize, which may or may not be active. Something is happening in all these systems, something that exists in the systems themselves. If there were a primary fault in the cell membrane, this could reflect itself in all the systems. This has been emphasized recently by the abnormalities that have been seen in systems that probably don't have any role at all in blood pressure regulation, such as Yamori and others finding of the abnormal red blood cell membrane. I wonder whether looking at systems not involved in pressure regulation for a primary fault that could be also present in the various regulatory systems wouldn't be an important route to go.

Dr F.O. Simpson: I have, of course, for many years, heard Sir Horace Smirk talk about his multifactorial theory of hypertension, which I think really has many aspects in common with the mosaic theory. It seems to me that the question really at issue isn't – as Tony Lever says – that these are simply methods by which the blood pressure is kept up, but whether by this mechanism, little steps can produce little abnormalities, sort of piling up, which eventually lead to a high blood pressure. Would it not be the case, then, Dr Page, that within the mosaic theory there is the possibility that a tiny abnormality in each step could eventually lead to a fairly major abnormality, as it were. Is that not the crux of the message?

Dr I.H. Page: That is what I believe. I think it is the multiplicity of the regulatory facets which finally initiates and maintains hypertension. With so many regulatory echanisms available, all interacting with one another, it is understandable why a single cause is hard to identify. That is why I think there is value in talking about diseases of regulation. I can see the philosophical concept that Dr Lever is talking about, but it reminds me of the dilemma that the physicists got themselves into by always looking for one single cause and then finding they encountered the uncertainty principle. So, when you ask them what's the cause, they say, 'It is only probable. What occurs will be the statistical result of many things that happen.' The mosaic is a plan by which you can integrate and equilibrate a vast body of knowledge concerned with regulation.

Dr R. Tarazi: I always thought discussions about the mosaic theory should differentiate between three levels of application: the first deals in events responsible for the pathogenesis of hypertension, the second concerns the mechanisms regulating blood pressure after an initial stimulus has initiated a pressor course, and the third is that of the complications and subsequent evolution of hypertension. Acceptance of the mosaic theory differs according to the level to which it is applied. For instance, a statement about the third level – that many factors participate in the evolution of hypertensive disease once it is started, would not, I think, produce any controversy. To state that many factors are activated to regulate arterial pressure at a new value following an initial disturbing stimulus (second level) also would not lead to any controversy. The most lively controversy is at the first level; whether one postulates that all hypertensions are essentially (in the scholastic meaning of the term) of multiple causation, or whether there are some types of hypertension that are due to a single cause activating secondarily a multifactorial disturbance. An example could be an aldosterone-producing tumor triggering one disturbance to which the body reacts by multiple mechanisms. I understand the mosaic theory to mean, however, that hypertension is from the very first, in its very nature, the result of multiple factors, at least one of which would be a genetic predisposition. The differentiation of the level at which one is discussing the mosaic theory might help make the discussion more precise.

Dr. I.H. Page: I think that expresses it very well. Is there further discussion?

Dr J.D. Swales: I wonder if I could follow-up what Tony Lever said because I think it is quite an important point. There used to be a pundit on BBC radio in England colled Joad. He always began every answer to a question by saying it all depends on what you mean by. I think this applies to the mosaic theory – it all depends on what you mean by a theory. I think there is an acid test for a theory, and I would like to shorten the debate by throwing that ball back to you, Dr Page. The test of a theory should be: can you state clearly a prediction that can then be validated or invalidated experimentally? If you can't do that, then it becomes a concept or descriptive framework, or what have you. I don't think that's at all disreputable. This is, as most people no doubt recognize, the Popperion philosophy of science (Popper KR. The Logic of Scientific Discovery. Hutchinson, London, 1959). Popper does not regard Darwinian natural selection as a theory, for instance, so you are in very good company if you decide that this should be a concept rather than a theory. But can you imagine a situation where the mosaic theory would actually make a prediction that could be either validated or invalidated experimentally?

Dr I. Page: I think the answer is, yes, you can predict from the mosaic theory. Arthur Guyton does it on a quantitative basis. I think that when we get all the regulatory factors together, and we understand how each one is interrelated with the others, then we will be able to make clear predictions, I hope ultimately, not only as to how to treat patients, but as to what's going to happen to them. Something that is evident, I think, to anybody who has had broad experience in the treatment of hypertension, is that each individual 'essential' hypertensive patient seems to be different from the others. Some of them respond beautifully, for instance, to rigid low-salt diets, and others do not. We have tried that repeatedly under critical metabolic conditions. You are all aware of the variety of our therapeutic agents, some of which work very well in some people and very badly in others. You can argue that we are treating only different phases of the disease, which is perfectly possible. Structural changes appear, and then the question is, how fast and how severe. For instance, if we had some way of knowing biochemically what changes cause hypertrophy or the changes in the media of the vascular wall, this would immeasurably help us clinically to find out what is going to happen to a patient. Is there going to be a very rapid thickening of the vessels and production of target organ ischemia?

I've never known how to handle the wide variety of definitions of concepts and theories. According to some definitions in the dictionary, they often may be used interchangeably. The variety of philosophical interpretations baffles me.

Dr M.P. Sambhi: I would like to follow-up on what has been said about the patients with essential hypertension; let's exclude the secondary hypertensive for now. Do essential hypertensives fall into such clear, different categories where multiple initiating causes can be identified? Are there some patients whose hypertension is really initiated by the nervous system; are there some patients whose essential hypertension is really initiated by a steroid abnormality; are there really hypertensive states initiated at the kidney? Dr Guyton, if I quote him correctly, would tell us that abnormalities in other systems can be regulated in such a way that the blood pressure would return to normal, except when the abnormality is in a single place like the kidney.

This, then, essentially comes back to a single initiating cause. Dr Guyton who has been keeping quiet till now will have to speak up. I think that it is the distinction we have to make: is it a single initiating cause that can start and then sustain hypertension, or are all these multiple abnormalities capable of initiating and maintaining essential hypertension?

Dr A.C. Guyton: One thing I have learned in the past few years is the lack of understanding of language, just as Dr Page has emphasized today. I don't think I have ever said that there is one necessary cause of hypertension, and I am sure I never said that it had to originate in the kidney, and yet I've been quoted many times as having said that. What I have said is that it is impossible to have hypertension unless in some way the kidney is prevented from going into the pressure natriuresis phenomena. There are many ways in which this can happen: one is to have constriction of the blood vessels to the kidney, another to have aldosterone stimulation of the kidney, a third to have nervous stimulation of the kidney. In other words, the kidney is a key point, capable of preventing hypertension caused by anything else, unless the kidney itself is incapable of preventing pressure natriuresis. Now, getting back to the mosaic theory – all that was in the mosaic theory. The point that we have made was that we examined quantitatively many of the different steps in the mosaic theory, and reached the conclusion that this is one particular peculiar step that has a great potency that some of the others don't have and therefore it must be satisfied. But I think that everyone has to start with the mosaic type of theory, separate its pieces, and work on each one of those pieces to see how they all fit together; I believe that is the essence of what Dr. Page stated from the very beginning. Now this can be very, very useful, because it doesn't just say how the circulation reacts once you have hypertension. It says, if you have an abnormality anywhere in your body, will it cause hypertension; or, if you have many different abnormalities in the body, can they cumulatively cause hypertension. And I believe that is the essence of what you meant by the mosiac theory – is it, Dr Page?

Dr I.H. Page: From now on, I am going to turn the explanation of the mosaic theory over to you, Dr Guyton.

Dr A.G. Doyle: I am really not at all clear about some of the finer points of the mosaic theory. Let me perhaps sharpen it up and ask whether you could explain it to me in terms of three models. The first is pheochromocytoma, and illness in which there is almost always high blood pressure, which is relieved instantly by the removal of the tumor; that is to say, a situation in which, as you know, patients with pheochromocytoma may be seen by doctors for some time and appear to have essential hypertension – and yet, when the cause is removed, the circulation apparently returns to normal very rapidly. The second problem is not dissimilar, and is the situation of an animal with a single kidney which is clipped. Again, when that clip is removed, the blood pressure comes back to normal within hours; so, if there are other factors within the mosaic theory, they then appear, in those two situations at least, not to be essential for the maintenance of hypertension once the initiating cause is removed.

The third model is the Conn syndrome situation, primary aldosteronism due to a tumor. Here we have a situation in which the tumor is present, and yet we know that when the tumor is removed the blood pressure doesn't always return to normal. The question I think we have to ask about that is, are there patients with aldosterone-secreting tumors who do not become hypertensive, and are there patients whose tumors are removed yet do not return to normotension? Those examples seem to me in need of an answer in terms of the mosaic theory. If you could answer, it might help me at least to understand exactly what is meant by this theory.

Dr I.H. Page: What we are talking about is that there is a wide variety of methods that can produce hypertension. The interplay of the various regulatory mechanisms is what really is pointed out. My thinking began with the Phase Rule of Willard Gibs. The quantitative application of the mosaic theory is what I believe Dr Guyton is proposing. I realize that having been educated in the school of a single cause for a single disease, it is difficult to accept a dynamic multifactorial concept. All I can say, Dr Doyle – to try to make it clear – is that there are many, many regulatory mechanisms that ultimately can affect the arterial pressure, and that's what makes hypertension such an interesting disease and provides tenure for us.

Dr A. Zanchetti: I think that the mosaic theory, as I've always understood it, has been in some way the physiological or the physiopathological counterpart of Pickering's observation of the continuous distribution of blood pressure values. If the blood pressure is continually distributed, and the control of blood pressure is multifactorial, then it is likely that the activity of all the single mechanisms controlling blood pressure is continually distributed, and so it is likely that in different individuals higher blood pressure can result from a different setting of one or the other mechanism.

Dr I.H. Page: Are you assuming that, when blood pressure rises, there is nothing abnormal about it? This is the problem with the question of a dividing line between normotension and hypertension. We can only say the dividing line is useful because if you are on one side of it you do not develop signs of vascular disease, yet on the other side, you do.

Dr. Zanchetti: But, of course, you develop signs for intermediate values as well; it depends on the number or the severity of the signs that are developing – this is the concept, you know. There is not health nor disease, in a given sense. If there is a progressive setting up of one or the other factors regulating blood pressure and a progressive increase in blood pressure, there will be a progressive incidence of vascular signs. I think the value of the mosaic theory is to suggest that there is no real dividing line between normal and abnormal for any of the factors regulating blood pressure. If there is a continuous distribution of values of all factors, there is no normal nor abnormal sympathetic tone, no normal renin nor high renin, etc. I think the Glasgow group (Malliani A, Pagani M, Bergamaschi M: Positive feedback, sympathetic reflexes and hypertension. Am J Cardiol 44: 860–865, 1979.) produced some evidence that plasma renin values are continuously distributed, and the same can be true for norepinephrine. Other factors cannot be so easily measured, so you cannot be sure there is a continuous distribution.

Dr I.H. Page: I cannot disagree what that.

Dr S. Julius: Dr Page, I was always interested to know, and I was wondering whether there is a central thesis to the theory in that there is a purpose for blood pressure to maintain perfusion. Now, is there, in your own mind, a priority of hierarchy on whether tissue perfusion is the purpose for the maintenance of blood pressure? I know what Dr Guyton would say, but there are some situations in which, at least on the short haul, it looks as if the body were doing everything it can to maintain the blood pressure, regardless of the underlying hemodynamics. For example, during static exercise blood pressure will go up so there is an increase in cardiac output. If a beta blocking agent is given, there will be the same increase in blood pressure, now through increased vascular resistance. Another example: patients with borderline hypertension, that is, with only a 10 mm increase in blood pressure. With propranolol, they can first be converted from high-output hypertension to high-resistance hypertension; then an alpha blocking agent can remove the vascular resistance, yet they still remain hypertensive. It is only a 10 mm increase in blood pressure, but they jealously keep those 10 mm no matter what is done.

Dr I.H. Page: I don't quite get the point.

Dr Julius: Is there a primacy of flow or pressure regulation?

Dr I.H. Page: I would say that, under ordinary circumstances, the real purpose of blood pressure is to provide the *vis a tergo* for tissue perfusion, to get the right amount of blood to the right place.

Dr Julius: What I had in mind – is it possible that hypertension is a state of confusion in which the body, indeed, wants to keep the blood pressure up?

18

Dr I.H. Page: I think the body, in ordinary circumstances, is a little bit smarter than we are – strangely enough. The remarkable thing to me is that if you injure, for instance, the nervous system, through either total sympathectomy or cord section at C-6, the blood distribution is almost normal within a few days, which shows that even without the vagi the organism still distributes blood adequately. Quadraplegic patients also adjust very well. The only difference is that they are inclined to develop hypertension.

Dr J.C. Fasciolo: Dr Page you mentioned that in some cases, for instance in hyperaldosteronism, you may remove the tumor and the pressure still stays elevated. I wonder whether that may be due to changes in the arteriolar bed, as sometimes there is an increase of the muscular layer or a reduction of the lumen because of the arterial tissue increase, so that the pressure will be elevated as a consequence of hypertension and not because of other factors that may be involved. I should like to know your opinion.

Dr I.H. Page: We were all brought up on the notion that in hypertension a structural change always occurs which results in an irreversible stage. The thing that struck me was the fact that when we learned how, we could lower pressure, no matter how 'irreversible' it had been: it can still be lowered, and very quickly. For instance, I have never seen a patient in whom the pressure will not drop precipitously with sodium nitroprusside. And the interesting thing about it is that when it drops (except when it gets excessively low) the tissue perfusion, particularly the cerebral tissue perfusion, does not suffer. If structural change produces total irreversibility, how can the blood pressire fall?

Dr Fasciolo: I was thinking not only of the anatomical changes, but also of the increase in the muscular layer of the arterioles, which will increase their reactivity to the vasoconstrictor substances.

Dr R. Bevan: The phrase 'structural change' should not be equated with fibrosis because it also includes a change in smooth muscle content, and muscle has tone, thus nitroprusside or any drug affecting tone can reduce blood pressure.

Dr. I.H. Page: I would agree, insofar as structural change involves fibrosis, among other changes.

2. SIR GEORGE PICKERING'S VIEWS ON HYPERTENSION

Thomas G. Pickering

Allbutt [1] defined his hyperpiesis, which we now term essential hypertension, as 'a malady in which at or towards middle life blood pressure rises excessively' – a definition that has never been improved. The cause of this excessive rise is the outstanding problem concerning the malady. Two main possibilities exist: the cause may be genetic or environmental. On the basis of the evidence presently available, the contribution of these two factors is probably equal. Population studies [2] have shown that there is no natural dividing line between normal blood pressure and hypertension, the distribution curve of blood pressure at any particular age being continuous and unimodal. Thus any dividing line is artifactual and arbitrary. Evidence for a genetic influence on the rise of blood pressure with age comes from a study of the blood pressure of family members, which showed that first degree relatives tend to resemble each other in graded or quantitative form, as exhibited in polygenic inheritance. Miall and Oldham [3] calculated that the genetic contribution to blood pressure was around 33%, but more recently Cayalli-Sforza and Bodner [4] estimated that this figure might be as high as 84%. Arterial pressure tends to rise with age (at any rate in Western societies), but it rises more in some subjects than in others. In 1973, Harlan et al. [5] showed that 'tracking' of blood pressure tends to occur in a population: those subjects who rank in the top ten in one examination tend to remain in that position subsequently. Zinner et al. [6] demonstrated that this tracking is likely to show familial aggregation and it thus probably inherited. Such a quantitative pattern of inheritance makes it most unlikely that hypertension is inherited through a single Mendelian dominant gene, as suggested by Platt [7], or that it is manifested by a single biochemical fault.

Of the environmental factors that might significantly alter blood pressure, obesity is the only one so far convincingly identified in Western societies. Persons whose blood pressure rises fastest in middle age are also those who tend to put on weight, and conversely, weight reduction in the obese usually leads to a fall or arterial pressure [8].

By far the most popular environmental factor to be indicted in hypertension is excessive intake of sodium chloride. Four lines of evidence are cited in support of this hypothesis: the study of primitive peoples, the study of salt intake in Western societies, the effect of gross salt restriction on blood pressure, and the effect of

Sambhi, M.P. (ed.) Fundamental fault in hypertension
© *1984, Martinus Nijhoff Publishers. Boston/The Hague/Dordrecht/Lancaster.*
ISBN 978-94-010-9006-3

ingestion of excessive amounts of salt. There is no doubt that arterial pressure tends to be low in many races living in 'primitive conditions' in tribal societies and that in such people arterial pressure does not rise in middle age, although it does rise when they adopt the life style of Western societies. However, change in salt intake is only one aspect of the differences between the two life styles, and there are many others, such as the social organization of the societies, which could be equally good explanations. In Western societies, despite the contentions of Dahl and Love to the contrary [9], there is no good evidence that salt intake and blood pressure are correlated. Well-controlled studies in the USA [10], England [11], and New Zealand [12] all found that individuals with the highest pressures in a population eat and excrete no more salt than those with the lowest pressures.

The answers to the two other questions, namely will restriction of salt intake lower arterial pressure, and will excessive salt intake raise it?, are both yes, but the changes have to be extreme. Kempner's rice diet was the first really successful salt-restrictive regimen for the treatment of hypertension, and had a daily sodium intake of around 150 mg per day [13]. While this was often (but by no means always) able to lower arterial pressure, Watkin et al. [14] found that there was a prompt return of arterial pressure to its previously elevated level with as little as 1 g per day. Experiments in which normal volunteers varied their salt intake over a wide range have led to similar conclusions, because only extremely high levels (e.g., 800 mEq/day) produced a significant change of pressure [15].

What these results demonstrate is the remarkable ability of the normal human body to regulate the sodium content of its plasma despite enormous changes in sodium intake. The data also allow the conclusion that manipulating the dietary salt intake within the range of 2–10 g/day or recommending that Americans reduce their salt intake from 10 to 6 g/day is utterly meaningless.

Another approach to the problem of essential hypertension is to examine the circulation from a physiological point of view and to ask what is the basic fault or faults in the circulation, of which the raised arterial pressure is the outward sign? It is clear that in the vast majority of cases the pressure is high because of an increased peripheral resistance, with the cardiac output being normal. Reports of 'high cardiac output hypertension' probably reflect nothing more than an exaggerated orienting or defense reflex occurring in response to the circumstances in which the hemodynamic measurements are made.

The increased resistance is generalized in the systemic, but not the pulmonary, circulation: it affects all tissues more or less equally except that the kidney has a little more and muscle a little less than other areas; it remains during exercise so that distribution of blood changes in the same way as in normal subjects, and it seems to remain during reactive hyperemia. Thus, in uncomplicated essential hypertension the circulation seems to be conducted in the same general way as in normal subjects, except that the level of arterial pressure and peripheral resistance are higher; the responses to exercise and sleep are normal [16].

The increase of peripheral resistance in hypertension could be caused by three kinds of change; overaction of the sympathetic nerves, humoral agents, or changes originating in the vessels themselves. Evidence for sympathetic overactivity is indirect and unconvincing; no humoral agent has so far been identified whose activity is consistently altered in essential hypertension. Transfusion of fresh whole blood from subjects with hypertension produces no greater rise of pressure in anemic recipients than does normal blood [17], and the concentrations of renin and angiotensin, still the most likely humoral mediators, may be high, normal, or low.

It is tempting to bring all these fragmentary pieces of knowledge together and ask whether, if the arterial pressure is raised repeatedly and for long periods by those environmental circumstances (e.g., states of mind), as might be a cause of essential hypertension, or by more specific chemical mechanisms, as in secondary hypertension, there could develop a generalized change in the peripheral vessels which would fit all these characteristics. Such a change could be constituted by altered physical properties of the arterial vessel wall. Evidence to support such structural changes came from an experiment by Folkow, Grimby, and Thulesius, who showed that during reactive hyperemia, when vasodilatation is maximal, the pressure–flow relationship indicates a persistently increased resistance in hypertensive patients, which was attributed to hypertrophy of the walls of the resistance vessels [18]. Animal experiments are also consistent with this view. In rabbits made hypertensive by constriction of the abdominal aorta there is an initial phase of hypertrophy of vascular smooth muscle and a later phase of increased numbers of smooth muscle cells [19]. And in spontaneously hypertensive rats a decrease in the number of arterioles per unit volume of tissue has been demonstrated; such an abnormality could contribute to the increased peripheral resistance without invoking any hypertrophy of the vessel wall [20]. Certain individuals might have a genetic predisposition to developing such vascular hypertrophy, which might lead to a progressive structural change in the circulation enabling it to maintain its hemodynamic equilibrium at a higher level of pressure and resistance. Such a change would also account for the persistence of hypertension that is sometimes seen when the original cause is removed, as in coarctation.

The traditional view of the causation of the disease is that it is characterized by a unique and specific fault of a qualitative nature. Those with the disease have the fault, those without do not. So it is supposed that there is a fundamental distinction between normotension and hypertension. When, however, we come to the realization that there is no natural dividing line between normotension and hypertension, and that the inheritance is polygenic, it becomes clear that there can be no single fault, of 'Holy Grail' of hypertension. Arterial pressure, like body height or temperature, is a quantity, and as such is the end product of a variety of different processes, both genetic and environmental. It may become raised in a number of diseases in which a specific physical or chemical fault is probable or proven, such as coarctation, Conn's syndrome and pheochromocytoma. But in all these conditions, and in essential hypertension, where no single fault can be identified, the end result is the same. If the pressure reaches a high enough level, the disease enters the malignant phase, characterized by a destruction of the arteriolar wall, with seepage of plasma and red cells into the wall leading to fibrinoid necrosis. Such lesions can occur at any age, and in both primary and secondary hypertension provided only that it is severe [21]. If the pressure is lowered, by whatever means, these tragic consequences are reversible. The explanation for these relationships is of course, that arterial pressure is a quantity, and its adverse effects are related numerically to it [22]. The 'disease' essential hypertension, representing the consequences of raised pressure without evident cause, is thus a type of disease not hitherto recognized in medicine, in which the defect if one of degree not of kind, quantitative not qualitative.

These considerations may be summarized as follows. The raised pressure in essential hypertension is due to genetic and environmental factors. The genetic factor tends to determine arterial pressure at any age. What is inherited may be a structural or biochemical peculiarity of the vessels which may influence their response to stimuli. As life proceeds, episodes occur which tend to raise or lower blood pressure. These episodes, if prolonged, tend to leave an imprint on the vessels, probably by increasing the size of the media when the pressure is high and diminishing it when it is low.

REFERENCES

1. Allbutt TC: Diseases of the arteries, including angina pectoris. MacMillan, London, 1915
2. Hamilton M, Pickering GW, Roberts JAF et al.: The aetiology of essential hypertension, I. The arterial pressure in the general population. Clin Sci 13: 11, 1954
3. Miall WE, Oldham PD: The hereditary factor in arterial blood-pressure. Br Med J 1: 75, 1963
4. Cavalli-Sforza LL, Bodner WF: Genetics, Evolution, and Man. Freeman, San Francisco, 1976, p 472
5. Harlan WR, Oberman A, Mitchell RE et al.: A thirty year study of blood pressure in a white male cohort. In: Onetsi G, Kim KE, Moyer JH (eds), Hypertension: Mechanisms and Management. Grune & Stratton, New York, 1973
6. Zinner SH, Levy PS, Kass EH: Familial aggregation of blood pressure in childhood. N Engl J Med 284: 402, 1971
7. Platt R: Heredity and hypertension. Lancet 1: 899, 1963
8. Reisin E, Abel R, Modan et al.: The effect of weight loss without salt restriction on the reduction of blood pressure in overweight hypertensive patients. N Engl J Med 298: 1, 1978
9. Dahl LK, Love RM: Evidence for relationship between sodium (chloride) intake and human hypertension. Arch Int Med 94: 525, 1954
10. Dawber TR, Kannel WB, Kagan A et al.: Environmental factors in hypertension. In: Stamler J, Stamler R, Pullman TN (eds), Epidemiology of hypertension. Grume & Stratton, New York, 1967

11. Thomas GW, Ledingham JGG, Beilin LJ et al.: Reduced renin in hypertension. Kidney Int 13: 513, 1978
12. Simpson FO, Waal- Manning HJ, Bolli P et al.: Relationship of blood pressure to sodium excretion in a population survey. Clin Sci Mol Med 55: 373, 1978
13. Kempner W: Treatment of hypertensive vascular disease with rice diet. Am J Med 4: 545, 1948
14. Watkin DM, Froeb JF, Hatch FT et al.: Effects of diet in essential hypertension. Am J Med 26: 428, 1959
15. Murray RH, Luft FC, Block R, Weyman AE: Blood pressure responses to extremes of sodium intake in normal man. Proc Soc Exp Biol Med 159: 432, 1978
16. Pickering GW: High Blood Pressure. Churchill London, 1968
17. Pickering GW: The effect of introducing blood from patients with essential hypertension into other human subjects. Clin Sci 2: 185, 1936
18. Folkow B, Grimby G, Thulesius O: Adaptive structural changes of the vascular walls in hypertension and their relation to the control of peripheral resistance. Acta Physiol Scand 44: 255, 1958
19. Bevan RD, Eggena P, Hume WR, VanMarthens E, Bevan JA: Transient and persistent changes in rabbit blood vessels associated with main rained elevations in arterial pressure. Hypertension 2: 63, 1980
20. Chen IIH, Prewitt RL, Dowell RF: Microvascular rarefaction in spontaneously hypertensive rat cremaster muscle. Am J Physiol 241: H306, 1981
21. Pickering GW: The relationship of benign and malignant hypertension. J Mt Sinai Hospital 8: 916, 1942
22. Pickering GW: Normotension and hypertension: the mysterious viability of the false. Am J Med 65: 561, 1978

3. FACTS, INTERPRETATIONS AND EXTRAPOLATIONS ON THE MECHANISMS THAT CAUSE ARTERIAL HYPERTENSION

JUAN CARLOS FASCIOLO

When one presents a discussion on the 'fundamental fault in hypertension', one must decide which of the ten or more models of experimental hypertension represents human hypertension. In my opinion, all models are applicable. Hypertension must be the consequence of the failure of one of the several mechanisms related to the control of the circulation and the blood pressure.

The numerous vasoactive substances seem to belong to systems that regulate different vascular parameters through changes in the tonus of the smooth muscle of the resistance vessels. The increase of this tonus may result in arterial hypertension.

Most likely, there will be general agreement on the *facts* presented in this paper. Also the orthodox *interpretations* of these facts will probably receive general approval. However, opinions may differ concerning the *extrapolations* made by the author and concerning his personal interpretations which are still without substantial experimental support.

The pressure within the arterial tree is caused by the distension of its elastic walls by the volume of blood contained within the arteries. This volume is replaced several times every minute; its constancy depends upon the equality between the blood entering the arteries (cardiac output) and the blood leaving the arteries for the capillaries and veins during the same period (arterial output).

The arterial pressure in a given subject depends on the volume of blood contained in the arterial tree. Changes in arterial pressure are the result of the transference of blood from the venous-capillary compartment to the arteries when the blood pressure rises, and from the arteries to the capillaries and veins when it falls. Since the volumes of blood transferred in both directions are very small in relation to the blood volume, the change of pressures produced in the venous-capillary compartment is negligible.

The regulation of the blood pressure is achieved by regulating the volume of blood contained within the arterial tree, mainly by controlling the arterial output. The arterial output is a function of the arterial pressure and of the resistance that the small arteries and arterioles oppose to

Sambhi, M.P. (ed.) Fundamental fault in hypertension
© *1984, Martinus Nijhoff Publishers. Boston/The Hague/Dordrecht/Lancaster.*
ISBN 978-94-010-9006-3

the progression of the blood from the arteries to the capillaries. When this resistance is increased, the resulting arterial hypertension may be looked upon as a compensation to allow the arterial output to increase as to reach the level of the cardiac output. Changes in the arterial output are also produced when the caliber of the resistance vessels is altered. These changes are brought about mainly by increasing or reducing the tonus of the smooth muscle of these vessels, setting the blood pressure at a level where the arterial output equals the cardiac output.

The tonus of the smooth muscle is controlled by various vasoactive agonists, some carried out by the blood, some released at the nervous terminals or formed in the walls of the arteries or in their proximity. These agonists may be grouped into 3 systems that seem to have different physiological significance (Fig. 1). The *nervous regulation* is concerned with the blood pressure level and its adaptation to the various physiological requirements. The vascular agonists involved are the catecholamines, serotonin and acetylcholine. These agonists are released at the nerve terminals in the smooth muscle of the vessels.

The *humoral regulation* is involved in the regulation of the blood volume and in the adaptations of the vascular system to its changes, in order to maintain a normal arterial pressure. The agonists, angiotensins, kinins and vasopressin are carried out by the blood stream.

The *idiovascular regulation* seems to be involved in the control of the blood flow through the tissues. Their vascular agonists are formed in the arterial walls or their proximity, and reach the smooth muscle cells by simple diffusion. Among these agonists there are vasoconstrictors such as the isorenins and within the vasodilators, prostacyclins and isokallikreins.

The ten or more vascular agonists mentioned influence the tonus of the vascular smooth muscle and the arterial pressure. They are released in response to different physiological requirements not always related to the regulation of the arterial pressure. The final tonus of the smooth muscle of the resistance vessels and the arterial pressure will result from the complex interaction of these agonists and from the reactivity of the effector muscle cells. The analysis of the influence of one or several agonists on the vascular effect of the others has not yet been completed.

All mechanisms, including the biological ones, are fallible and what may fail will eventually do so. Disturbances of the mechanisms that control the vascular tone may lead to its increase and to the development of arterial hypertension. I will consider now very briefly the 3 systems already mentioned and some of their disorders that may produce hypertension.

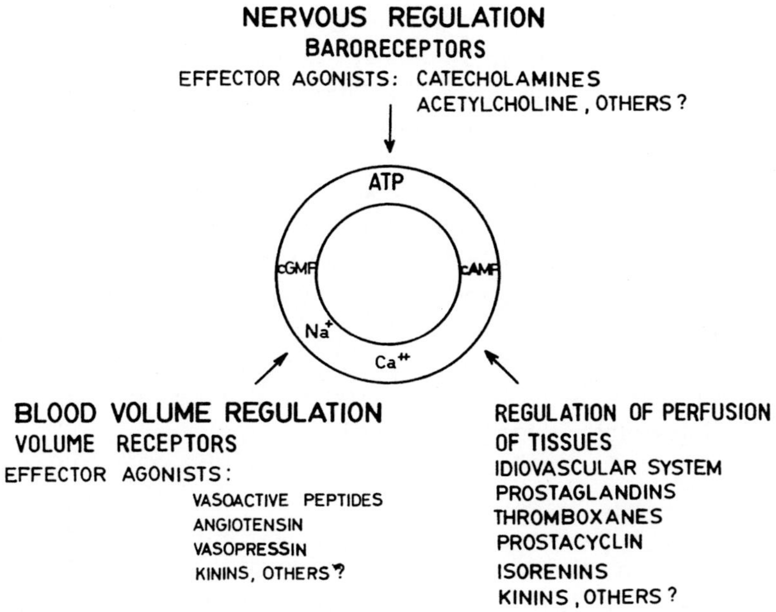

NERVOUS REGULATION
BARORECEPTORS
EFFECTOR AGONISTS: CATECHOLAMINES
ACETYLCHOLINE , OTHERS ?

BLOOD VOLUME REGULATION	REGULATION OF PERFUSION
VOLUME RECEPTORS	OF TISSUES
EFFECTOR AGONISTS:	IDIOVASCULAR SYSTEM
VASOACTIVE PEPTIDES	PROSTAGLANDINS
ANGIOTENSIN	THROMBOXANES
VASOPRESSIN	PROSTACYCLIN
KININS, OTHERS ?	ISORENINS
	KININS , OTHERS ?

Figure 1. Vasoactive agonists of the body may be grouped in three main regulatory systems: the nervous regulation of blood pressure, the humoral regulation of blood volume, and the idiovascular regulation of blood flow. The three systems are not completely independent, but show many interrelations. All these agonists may be involved in hypertension. Another possibility is a change in the contractile mechanism that would increase either vascular sensitivity to vasoconstrictor agonists or myogenic tonus.

NERVOUS REGULATION OF THE BLOOD PRESSURE

The nervous regulation in concerned primarily with maintaining an adequate level of the blood pressure. This adequate level does not necessarily mean a constant one, since it may change according to physiological requirements.

The central part of the nervous organization are the vasomotor centers of the medulla. These centers have an intrinsic or idioneurogenic tone and maintain the tonus of the smoth muscle of the resistance vessels, especially those in the splanchnic area that are involved in blood pressure regulation. The neurogenic tone of the vasomotor centers is modulated by *nervous, humoral* and *metabolic* factors. These modulators give the vasomotor centers more versatility to meet physiological requirements.

The arterial baroreceptors modulate the tonus of the vasomotorcenters through inhibitory impulses. When the blood pressure rises, the firing of the inhibitories impulses increases thus reducing the tonus of the vasomotor centers; as a consequence the release of catecholamines at the end of the sympathetic nerves diminishes and this results in vasodilatation. The opposite happens when the blood pressure falls. When other agonists produce vasoconstriction, the efficiency of the baroreceptor regulation is severely impaired because most of its control on the vasocular tonus is lost. This may explain why in arterial hypertension the baroreceptors are unable to normalize the peripheral vascular resistance.

The nervous modulation of the vasomotor tonus has been shown to be very complex and is under intensive study at present. The medullary vasomotor centers receive suprasegmentary projections which may enhance or depress their tonus. The ablation or the stimulation of some areas of the central nervous system may produce a rise in blood pressure or may inhibit experimentally induced hypertension.

The best known humoral modulator of the vasomotor center is angiotensin. Angiotensin is not only a direct vasoconstrictor substance, but acting upon the vasomotor centers at medullary and diencephalic levels, it raises the blood pressure by increasing the vasomotor tone. Part of the pressor effect of angiotensin seems to be due to its central effect; this must be taken into consideration when discussing the role played by angiotensin in hypertension.

The vasomotor tonus is also influenced by metabolic factors: Low PO_2 and high PCO_2 stimulate the vasomotor neurons producing a rise in blood pressure. Chronic ischemia of the vasomotor centers has been re-

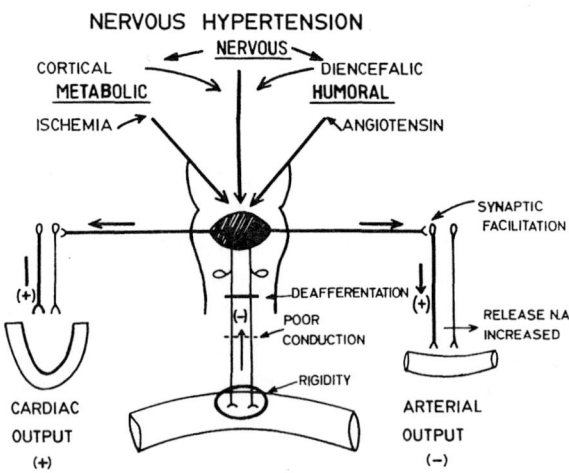

Figure 2. Nervous hypertension results from an increased vasomotor tonus. Since the tonus of the vasomotor centers is modulated by arterial baroreceptors and by nervous, humoral and metabolic factors, the hypertony may arise from alterations in one or various of these modulators.

ported to produce hypertension, probably through a decrease of PO₂ and an increase of PCO₂ at the capillaries of the vasomotor center.

Nervous hypertension will result from an increase of the tonus of the vasomotor centers either primary or secondary to the activity of the various modulators. (Fig. 2). The idea that hypertony of the vasomotor centers may cause arterial hypertension is not new. In 1920 von Monakow postulated that arterial hypertension had a neurogenic origen, a theory backed by the baroreceptor deafferentation experiments of Koch and Mies in 1929.

Reduction of the signal traffic in the baroreceptor nerves will lead to hypertony of the vasomotor centers and arterial hypertension. Several circumstances may lead to a reduction of the afferent inhibitory impulses reaching the vasomotor centers. Rigidity of the arterial wall, where the baroreceptor terminals are located, will hinder their elongation thus reducing the frequency of the inhibitory signals. Modals of experimental neurogenic hypertension by peripheral or central deafferentation of the baroreceptors or by preventing the elongation of the receptors have been described.

It has been found that in hypertension the baroreceptors adapt to the new pressure levels, so instead of lowering the pressure, they tend to maintain it, a phenomenon described as 'ressetting' of the baroreceptors. This failure of the baroreceptors to cope with increased blood pressure may be due to an increase of the tonus of the vasomotor centers. The

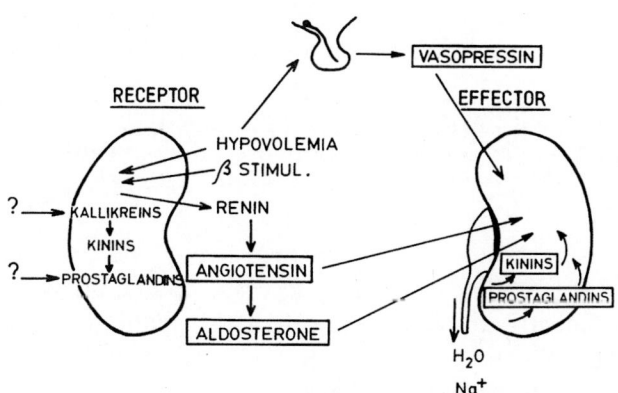

KIDNEY IN BLOOD VOLUME REGULATION

Figure 3. The kidney plays a central role in the regulation of plasma volume. Acting as a volume receptor it releases renin when the intra-renal arterial pressure is reduced. It is also the target organ for aldosterone and vasopressin. Renal prostaglandins and kallikrein may also control sodium and water excretion by the kidney.

firing of an inhibitory stimulus that will bring the pressure back to normal when the tonus of the vasomotor center is normal, will be unable to do so if the tonus is increased.

HUMORAL REGULATION OF THE BLOOD PRESSURE

The role of angiotensin, vasopressin and bradykinin in the regulation of blood pressure is controversial. These vasoactive polypeptides are clearly related to the regulation of blood volume and, all three are very potent vasomotor substances.

Plasma angiotensin is released by renal renin. Renin secretion by the kidney is increased when the sensor mechanisms signal a reduction in blood volume. Angiotensin not only produces vasoconstriction by direct and neural mechanisms but also increases the secretion of aldosterone which in turn increases sodium reabsorption by the kidney. So the kidney plays a dual role, first as a volume receptor that signals hypovolemia and releases renin, secondly as the target organ not only for aldosterone but for vasopressin and most probably for bradykinin and other kinins (Fig. 3).

Two forms of renal hypertension may be distinguished, namely renovascular and renoparenchymal. The former is a disorder of the kidney as a volume receptor. Dispite the normovolemia and because of its reduced blood perfusion, the kidney signals hypovolemia. The release of substances such as renin that help to maintain the arterial pressure when the blood volume is reduced will produce hypertension when the blood volume is normal.

In renoparenquimal hypertension there is a drastic reduction of the nephron population, and the excretion of sodium, water and other substances is impaired and may be responsible for the increase in blood pressure.

Vasopressin is released from the neural hypophysis not only when the plasma osmolarity is increased but also by a reduction in blood volume. Its strong vasoconstrictor action may help to adapt the vascular bed to the reduced blood volume and to maintain in normal pressure.

Bradykinin and related kinins are strong vasodilator substances but their participation in the regulatory mechanisms of blood pressure is only conjectural. There is, however, some evidence that the kinins may increase water excretion by the kidney thus having probably a role in blood volume regulation.

Some researchers believe that the kidney kallikrein-kinin system is involved in hypertension. According to their views, arterial hypertension may result from a reduction in the release of kinins by the kidney. Kinins are believed to mediate the antihypertensive action of the kidney.

The adrenal cortex is involved in the regulation of blood volume through the secretion of aldosterone and its effect on renal sodium excretion. The hypertension of aldosteronism is sodium dependent. High doses of aldosterone or D.C.A. will not induce hypertension in the absence of sodium in the diet, and the administration of extrasodium potentiates the hypertensive effect of these steroids.

There is no general agreement on the role played by the substances mentioned in arterial hypertension. Angiotensin and aldosterone are considered to be responsible for some types of experimental or clinical hypertension. The role of vasopressin or the kinins is still unsettled.

IDIOVASCULAR REGULATION OF BLOOD FLOW

Most tissues are able to regulate their blood flow according to their metabolic needs. This local regulation would produce changes in blood pressure if the baroreceptors would not make up for the changes in peripheral resistance by constricting or dilating other vascular areas.

The mechanism of auto-regulation of blood flow is poorly understood. Vasoconstrictor and vasodilator agonists are synthesized in the arterial wall or its proximity. This system of vasoactive substances (the intrinsic or idiovascular system) is believed to produce the vasomotor changes responsible for the auto-regulation of blood flow. The evidence for that, however, is still poor.

Among the vasoconstrictor substances of the idiovascular system are the so-called isorenins. They may release 'in situ', from a tissue or a plasma substrate, small amounts of angiotensin that can increase the tonus of vascular muscle. The thromboxans which belong to the group of prostaglandins that are synthesized in the arterial wall are also very strong vasoconstrictor substances.

Among the vasodilators, prostacyclin and prostaglandins of the E type have been found. Arteries and other tissues also have small amounts of a kallikrein-like enzyme which after prolonged incubation with a plasmic substrate releases small amount of kinins with strong vasodilating action.

The physiological role of the idiovascular vasomotor system, and of course its participation in the mechanisms of arterial hypertension, is only hypothetical at present. We may substitute speculations for experimental data, with the well known risks of that approach and postulate that increased release of vasoconstrictor agonists (or a reduced release of vasodilator ones) in the wall of the resistance vessels may enhance the smooth muscle tone, thus increasing peripheral resistance and leading to hypertension when this increase is widespread. This hypothesis is being tested nowadays in various laboratories, especially concerning the role of the prostaglandins in hypertension.

THE VASCULAR SMOOTH MUSCLE

Any of the vasoconstrictor agonists of the three different systems described may be able to increase the vascular tone and produce hypertension. The fault however may be within the smooth muscle cells giving rise to an increased reactivity towards vasoconstrictor agonists (or a reduced reactivity toward vasodilators), or to an increase in the myogenic tonus.

The sensitivity of arterial vessels to vasoconstrictors in various models of experimental hypertension has been extensively investigated, but the results have been far from uniform. This was to be expected since there are great variations in vascular sensitivity according to the agonist and the vascular bed considered. In the case of angiotensin tested on isolated smooth muscle preparations, the development of tachyphylaxis and of the potentiation of the vascular response complicate the interpretation of the findings.

A modern approach is to study the changes that occur in the vascular smooth muscle during the development of hypertension. It is known that the vasoconstrictor agonists attach to specific receptors and through secondary messengers, release calcium ions attached to the endoplasmic reticulum and other cellular organelles. The concentration of citosolic calcium rises and, by activating calmodulin and a myosin phosphorilase, brings about the contraction of the myofibrils. The vasodilators revert the process.

The miogenic tonus of the vascular smooth muscle is increased when the concentration of the sarcoplasmic Ca^{++} rises above 10^{-8} M. Since the concentration of the extracellular Ca^{++} is many thousand times higher than the intracellular one, Ca^{++} must be extruded from the cell to maintain its low concentration. It is believed that the energy necessary to extrude the Ca^{++} against a large electrochemical gradient is derived from the entrance of Na^+ to the cell. When the intracellular Na^+ concentration rises the extrusion of Ca^{++} is impaired and its sarcoplasmic concentration and the tonus of the smooth muscle increase. Changes in the Na^+ permeability of the cells and in the activity of the Na-K pump have been found in human and experimental hypertension and have been considered responsible for the disease.

Several biochemical changes of the arterial vessels have been described in hypertension. However, the question arises as to whether these changes are the cause or the consequence of hypertension.

CONCLUSIONS

The train of thought of this essay is that the various mechanisms that control the vascular tone may fail and their failure may lead eventually to an increase of this tonus and to arterial hypertension. So arterial hypertension may be caused by many different mechanisms.

These mechanisms are interrelated and the target organ, the vascular smooth muscle, is common to them all. One fault in one of the vascular smooth muscles will alter the balance and produce changes in the others. In other words, an increase of humoral agonists may impair the regulation of the vascular tone by the baroreceptors; an increase in the angiotensin content of the blood will raise the tonus of the vasomotor centers; an increase in the sympathetic nervous tone will increase the renin release by the kidneys, and so on.

Most cases of arterial hypertension are classified as essential hypertension, that is to say, of unknown origin. I believe that under the label of essential hypertension, patients with different hypertensive diseases are grouped. It may be argued that patients with essential hypertension form a rather homogeneous group with similar clinical and hemodynamic characteristics and therefore it is unlikely that the disease could be caused by so many different mechanisms. The vascular and cardiac consequences of hypertension, however, depend mainly on the level of the blood pressure rise and on its duration. Therefore, we would expect any long lasting hypertension, if high enough, to have the well known deleterious effects on the heart and the arterial tree regardless of its underlying mechanism. On the other hand, since a given mechanism may be more prone to fail than others, a large group of essential hypertensives may have a common mechanism.

Coming back to the title of this book, I think that after all, in spite of the numerous mechanisms that may raise the arterial pressure, there might be a 'fundamental fault' in hypertension. In arterial hypertension the tonus of the vascular smooth muscle and the peripheral resistance are above normal values. When hypertension results from an increased cardiac output, the peripheral resistance may be normal but it should be reduced to allow the arterial output to increase and to make up for the higher cardiac output.

The fundamental fault of arterial hypertension seems to be the increased tonus of the smooth muscle of the resistance vessels produced, either by the interplay of the numerous vascular agonists, or by disturbances of the contractile mechanism. This increase is mediated by a rise in the concentration of the sarcoplasmic Ca^{++}. One is tempted to consider the increase of the sarcoplasmic Ca^{++} of the vascular smooth muscle as the 'Fundamental Fault of Arterial Hypertension'.

4. THE INFINITE GAIN PRINCIPLE FOR ARTERIAL PRESSURE CONTROL BY THE KIDNEY-VOLUME-PRESSURE SYSTEM

ARTHUR C. GUYTON, THOMAS E. LOHMEIER, JOHN E. HALL, MANIS J. SMITH, PHILIP R. KASTNER

About ten years ago, one of the authors (ACG) coined the term 'infinite gain principle' for pressure control that applies to the kidney-volume-pressure control mechanism. The purpose of the present chapter is to elaborate on this principle and to explain it in more detail, especially because it has been misunderstood by many if not most workers in hypertension research. There have always been special qualifiers to this principle that in the main have been overlooked by others in their application of it. But, even more important, only a few have understood the universal applicability of the principle for the control of arterial pressure under all long-term stabilized pressure conditions. Please bear with us in the hope that we will be able to explain this principle so that it will be meaningful and useful.

Basically, the infinite gain principle states that, for a given intake of salt and a given functional state of the kidneys, there is only one single arterial pressure that will provide a balance between intake and output of salt, and because of this the arterial pressure, in the long run, will always attempt to return exactly to this pressure level. Please note the two qualifiers: (1) for a given level of salt intake, and (2) for a given functional state of the kidneys. If either of these two factors should change, then the exact pressure level to which the arterial pressure will be controlled would change accordingly. Therefore, this principle does not state that the arterial pressure will always return exactly to the same level, and it does not even state how the pressure will reach that level. It simply states that in the long run the pressure will get to that level, or else the person will continue to retain fluid forever until dying of edema, or will continue to lose fluid until dying of dehydration.

Thus far, the principle is very simple. It is simply a restatement of the fact that, over the long term, a person must remain in fluid balance and that arterial pressure control is one of the factors that helps to establish a balance between input and output of salt and water.

There is a much more far-reaching consequence of the infinite gain principle, however. This is the fact that it gives the kidney-volume-pressure control system the almost magical power to override the other pressure control systems in determining the final long-term level at which the arterial pressure is controlled. That is, if the intake of salt remains constant but the capability of the kidney to

Sambhi, M.P. (ed.) Fundamental fault in hypertension
© *1984, Martinus Nijhoff Publishers. Boston/The Hague/Dordrecht/Lancaster.*
ISBN 978-94-010-9006-3

36

excrete salt becomes diminished, then the consequence is an automatic increase in the arterial pressure over a period of days, up to that level at which intake and output become exactly in balance. The other pressure control systems can affect this final pressure level only by either changing the rate of intake of salt or changing the kidney's capability for excreting salt. Thus, the infinite gain principle of the kidney-volume-pressure control system places an extreme limitation on the ways in which the final pressure level can be controlled – this can be achieved only by altering one of two factors: (1) the level of salt intake, or (2) the capability of the kidneys to excrete salt. We shall see later in this chapter that all of the mechanisms for control of long-term pressure do indeed alter one or both of these two factors, most frequently the capability of the kidneys to excrete salt.

In the next few pages, we will review the basic hemodynamics of arterial pressure control and then develop from these basic hemodynamics the physiological basis of the infinite gain principle.

ARTERIAL PRESSURE CONTROL IN THE BASIC CIRCULATION WHEN THERE IS NO RENAL FUNCTION

The basic hemodynamic circuit of the circulation is illustrated in Figure 1, which shows the heart and the flow of blood through the arteries, capillaries, and viens. The figure also lists the different quantitative factors that must be considered in analyzing (a) flow of blood through the circuit, (b) control of cardiac output, and (c) control of pressures in all the different segments of the circulation, including

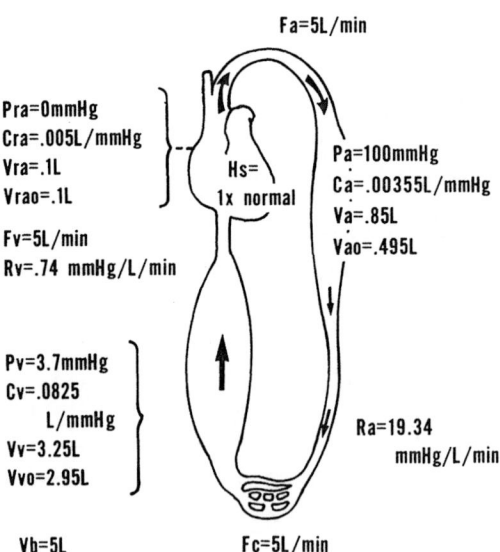

Figure 1. A simple hemodynamic circuit of the circulation without functioning kidneys. (Reprinted from Guyton [9].)

the arterial pressure. These basic factors include the pumping strength of the heart, the resistance to blood flow in each segment of the circulation, the capacitance of each capacitative area of the circulation, and blood volume. Using these quantitative values and also the standard hemodynamic equations available in all circulatory physiology texts, it is possible to program the function of this basic circulatory schema on the computer. The computer can then be used to calculate the effect on the dependent variables of the circuit when any one of the basic parameters of function is changed. For instance, what is the effect on arterial pressure of changing the heart strength? Or, what is the effect on the arterial pressure of changing the arterial resistance, and so forth? Now let us see what the computer predicts when we do change some of the important parameters of function.

Effect of increasing the pumping capability of the heart

There is a common belief that increasing the pumping capability of the heart will increase both the cardiac output and the arterial pressure. Figure 2 shows the computer solution to this problem, utilizing the simple equations from the schema in Figure 1. The X point on this figure represents the normal mean arterial pressure, in this instance 100 mm Hg. The figure shows that, as the heart strength decreases below normal, so also does the arterial pressure decrease, not so much at first, but very considerably with greater decreases in heart strength – as would be expected. On the other hand, when the heart strength is increased above normal, indeed up to three times normal, as illustrated in the figure, there is hardly any increase in arterial pressure. The reason is an inability of the heart to

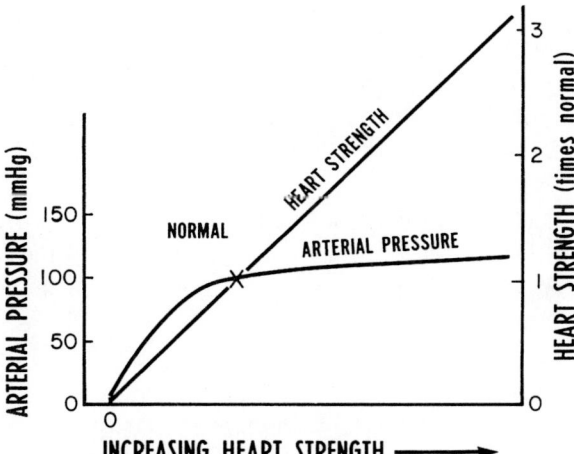

Figure 2. Effect on arterial pressure caused by progressive increase of heart pumping capability from zero to three times normal. (Reprinted from Guyton [9].)

pump any more blood than will flow from the veins into the right atrium. It is well known that the veins leading to the heart are very easily collapsible, and any time that the heart pumps with excess strength, the veins leading into the chest do indeed begin to collapse, which prevents still additional blood flow into the central venous reservoir. Consequently, the amount of blood that can be pumped by the heart is automatically limited. Even normally the pumping capability of the heart is considerably greater than the rate of flow of blood into the heart, demonstrated by the fact that an instant transfusion into the right atrium can increase the cardiac output about $2^1/_2$-fold. But normally, despite this great excess pumping capability of the heart, the cardiac output is limited by the venous return. Therefore, it also follows that, if increasing the pumping capability of the heart cannot increase the cardiac output, neither can it increase the arterial pressure. Thus, Figure 2 shows that even an increase in the cardiac pumping capability to three times normal will increase the arterial pressure by only a few percentage points.

Effect of vascular capacitance changes on the arterial pressure

The capacitance of a blood vessel (or of a whole segment of the circulation) is defined as the change in volume for a given change in pressure, or $\triangle V / \triangle P$. The normal capacitance of the entire circulatory system in the human being is approximately 100 ml of blood per mm Hg change in the so-called 'mean circulatory filling pressure', which is the pressure in the circulation when the heart is stopped and all pressures are brought to equilibrium [22]. A decrease in the capacitance of the system causes the pressure to rise all through the circulation because there is then less of a capacitative reservoir for storage of the blood. The increase in pressures in the peripheral vessels also increases flow of blood into the veins and thence into the right atrium, thus increasing the venous return. Consequently, the cardiac output and arterial pressure also increase. Figure 3 illustrates this effect, a marked increase in both cardiac output and arterial pressure when the vascular capacitance decreases. Conversely, both of these decrease when the vascular capacitance increases.

Note in Figure 3 the upper limit to which both the cardiac output and arterial pressure may rise. This is determined by a limit in the pumping capability of the heart, i.e., it is the greatest amount of cardiac output that the heart can pump before it fails to respond to still additional venous return. This is also the point at which blood begins to dam up in the right atrium, so that the venous pressures begin to rise significantly.

We can conclude that, in the basic hemodynamic circuit, it is possible to cause very marked changes in arterial pressure as a result of changes in vascular capacitance.

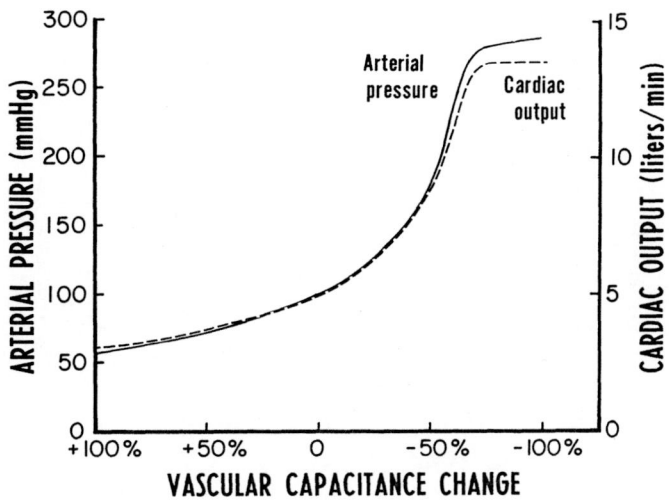

Figure 3. Effect on cardiac output and arterial pressure caused by changes in vascular capacitance between the limits of 100% below normal to 100% above normal. (Reprinted from Guyton [9].)

Effect on arterial pressure of changes in total peripheral resistance

We have all been taught that increasing the total peripheral resistance always has a profound effect in increasing the arterial pressure. Yet, careful study of Figure 4 shows that this basic principle is *not* always true. Indeed, it is not always true even of the basic hemodynamic circuit itself, much less of the actual circulatory system with all its special controls.

Note in the lower panel of Figure 4 two separate curves that relate total peripheral resistance to arterial pressure. One of these curves is the effect on arterial pressure when the total peripheral resistance is increased as a result of increased arterial resistance. Note from this curve that the arterial pressure does indeed increase very markedly when that is the cause of the increased total peripheral resistance. The other curve is equally as important, however, showing the effect on arterial pressure of increased total peripheral resistance when this results from increased venous resistance. In this instance, instead of a rise there is an obvious and very profound decrease in arterial pressure. The obvious reason is that increased venous resistance causes much more decrease in cardiac output (because of decreasing venous return) than it increases the total peripheral resistance. Therefore, the product of these two effects is a greatly diminished arterial pressure.

These differential effects on arterial pressure caused by changes in arterial resistance versus changes in venous resistance have been confirmed many times in basic experimental studies, one of which was a quantitative analysis of the phenomenon dating from over 10 years ago [1].

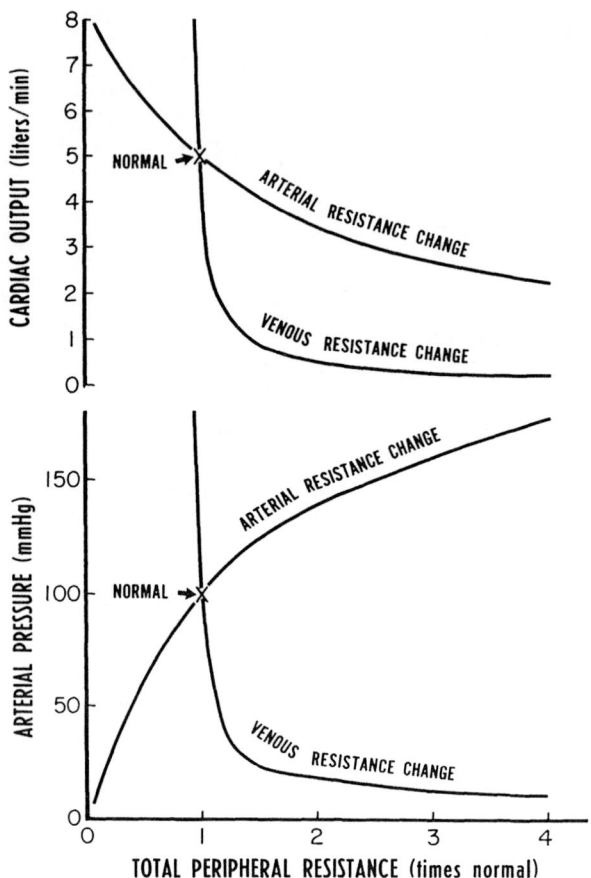

Figure 4. Effect on cardiac output and arterial pressure caused by progressively increasing the total peripheral resistance in two different ways, by increasing the arterial resistance and by increasing the venous resistance. (Reprinted from Guyton [9].)

Thus it can be readily seen that it would be most incorrect to assume that an increase in total peripheral resistance will necessarily increase the arterial pressure. Indeed, there are many instances in the function of the circulation in which this is not true. To give a simple illustration (that will be addressed more fully later), when an arteriovenous fistula is closed in a human being who had the fistula for many months or even years, the total peripheral resistance often increases as much as 100 to 200%. However, the arterial pressure hardly changes. And even if it were to change a small amount acutely, another hemodynamic phenomenon (to be discussed later) would still bring the pressure exactly back to the normal level over the next few days.

Before leaving this subject, it is appropriate to suggest that our understanding of arterial pressure control might be greatly enhanced if we would train ourselves to think in terms of arterial pressure being related mainly to the *ratio of arterial resistance to venous resistance,* and not by either of these alone.

HEMODYNAMICS OF ARTERIAL PRESSURE CONTROL WHEN THERE IS A
FUNCTIONING KIDNEY IN THE CIRCUIT

In this section we would like to explain the profound difference in pressure
control that occurs when the circulatory system is endowed with a functioning
kidney, in contrast to arterial pressure control when there is no mechanism for
control of body fluid balance, as was the case in the basic hemodynamic circuit
discussed thus far. We shall see that the kidney exerts a profound long-term
stabilizing influence on pressure. Let us see how this works.

Figure 5 illustrates the same basic hemodynamic circuit shown in Figure 1, with
the addition of several factors: (1) a functioning kidney, (2) a continuous intake of
salt (and a proportionate amount of water to go along with the salt), and (3) a
tissue space reservoir in continuous dynamic fluid equilibrium with the circulatory system. This third factor, the tissue space reservoir, plays no role in long-
term pressure regulation, even though it does determine in almost all instances
the speed at which the pressure will aproach any new pressure level. Therefore,
for the purpose of the present discussion, which is concerned with long-term
pressure regulation, we shall deal only with the first two of the above factors, the
renal excretion of salt and water and the intake of salt and water.

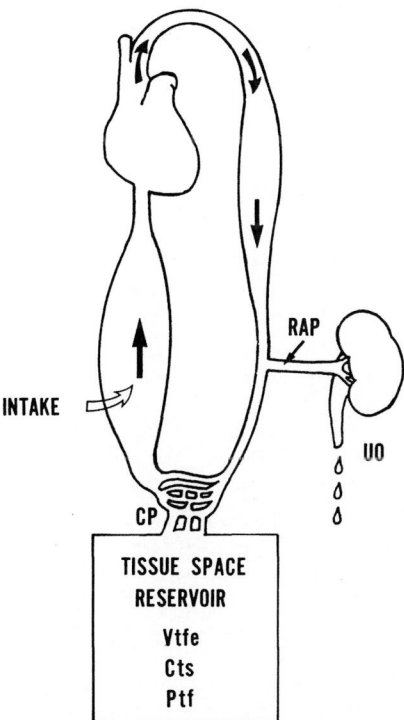

Figure 5. Circulatory schema with a functioning kidney and a tissue space fluid reservoir. (Reprinted
from Guyton [9].)

When the kidney is added to the hemodynamic circuit, it is essential to assign to it appropriate quantitative functional characteristics for excretion of salt. In Figure 6 the curve labeled 'renal output' designates the relationship between renal arterial pressure and renal output of salt and water, as measured by a great many different investigators, including Selkurt [23], Thompson and Pitts [25], Shipley and Study [24], and several different investigators in our laboratory.

Figure 6 also shows the net intake level of salt and water; the point at which the two curves in the figure cross is called the 'equilibrium point'. This equilibrium point will become a major factor of dicussion in the next few sections of this paper, and it will be a basic part of our quantitative explanation of the infinite gain principle; please note it carefully. In the next two sections we will demonstrate the role of the kidney-volume-pressure system in the long-term stabilization of the arterial pressure and, at the same time, hopefully explain in more depth the significance of the infinite gain principle.

Stabilization of the long-term arterial pressure by the kidney-volume-pressure control system

Note in Figure 6 that an increase in arterial pressure has a profound effect to increase the renal output of both salt and water. This is the phenomenon called

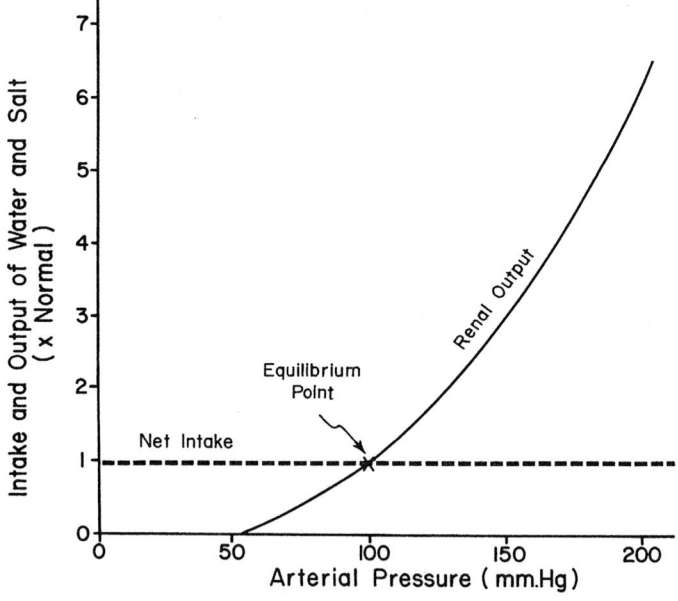

Figure 6. A 'pressure-analysis diagram' showing a line that depicts the intake of salt and water and a curve that shows the normal effect of pressure on renal output of salt and water by the isolated kidney. The point at which these curves cross, the 'equilibrium point', represents the 'set-point' at which the kidney-volume-pressure control system maintains the long-term arterial pressure level. (Reprinted from Guyton [9].)

pressure natriuresis and diuresis. It is this basic mechanism that allows the kidneys to return the arterial pressure back toward normal whenever the pressure rises too much.

Figure 7 illustrates this stabilizing effect of the kidney-volume-pressure control system. This figure is a computer record of the predicted changes (as computed from the mathematical equations describing the circulatory system in Figure 5) in arterial pressure, cardiac output, blood volume, and urinary output when (a) the total peripheral resistance was altered, (b) the vascular capacitance was altered, or (c) the heart strength was altered. The following is an explanation of the important details in the figure.

Note at the top of the figure the successive time periods when resistance, capacitance, or heart pumping capability (heart strength) was altered. The sequential stages are:

(1) *Effect of opening and then closing an A–V fistula.* Note the changes in arterial pressure when the fistula was opened and then closed. This fistula was large enough to decrease the total peripheral resistance exactly 50% when the fistula was opened, and then to increase the total peripheral resistance exactly 100% when the fistula was closed. The immediate effect of opening the fistula was

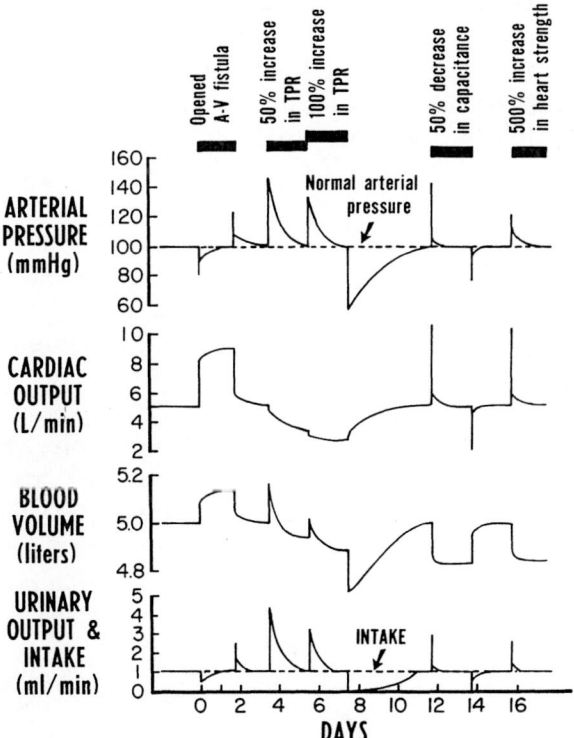

Figure 7. Computer simulation of the effect of changes in total peripheral resistance (TPR), vascular capacitance, and heart strength on arterial pressure, cardiac output, blood volume, and urinary output. (Reprinted from Guyton [9].)

a marked increase in cardiac output and a very slight fall in arterial pressure. Thus, the tremendous change in total peripheral resistance had only a slight effect on arterial pressure. Then, during the next day or so the arterial pressure returned entirely and exactly to the normal level. The bottom curve gives the explanation: the return of the pressure to normal resulted from a slight amount of fluid volume retention by the kidneys. Once the pressure had returned to its normal level, the kidneys stopped retaining additional fluid. Then, when the fistula was closed, exactly the reverse sequence took place – an immediate rise in pressure that was mainly compensated within a few minutes but was fully compensated during the next day as a result of salt and water loss through the kidneys. Thus, the arterial pressure once again became absolutely and completely stabilized back to its original level despite the 100% increase in total peripheral resistance that oc-curred when the fistula was closed.

(2) *Effect of increasing the total peripheral resistance as a result of increased arterial resistance.* Note at the top of Figure 7 the two time periods in which the peripheral resistance was increased first to 50% and then to 100% above normal. At each stage the arterial pressure rose markedly when the resistance was first increased. After each elevation of pressure, however, there was an immediate and marked increase in urinary output of water and salt, as illustrated by the lowermost curve in the figure. This caused loss of blood volume and thereby decreased the cardiac output. As a result, the arterial pressure returned exactly and completely back to the original control level within a day or so after each increase in resistance. Finally, when the resistance was returned to normal, the arterial pressure fell dramatically at first, but diminished urinary output caused salt and water to collect in the body during the next few days, and once again the pressure returned exactly and completely back to its normal level.

(3) *Effect of decreased capacitance of the circulation.* Now, note the time period when the capacitance of the circulatory system was drastically decreased. The instantaneous effect was a dramatic increase in arterial pressure. Most of this increase in pressure was compensated within the next few minutes as a result of fluid loss out of the blood into the interstitium through the capillary membranes. There was still a very slight elevation of pressure, however, corrected by a small amount of fluid loss through the kidneys during the next day or so. When the capacitance was returned to normal, exactly reverse events ensued.

(4) *Effect of a tremendous increase in heart strength.* Finally, the heart strength was increased to five times normal, and once again the arterial pressure rose a slight amount acutely. This pressure was also corrected during the next few hours to days because of loss of fluid through the kidneys, with decrease in blood volume. The final result was an exact and complete return of the arterial pressure to the normal value.

It is clear, therefore, that the kidney-volume-pressure mechanism has a pro-found stabilizing effect on the arterial pressure – in fact, such a profound effect that over the long run the arterial pressure will return to exactly the same value if the functional status of this system is not altered. Therefore, to change the pressure to some new long-term level, it becomes necessary to make some alteration in this pressure control system. This can occur in many different ways, but the possible ways are quite different from the usual concepts of simply changing the total peripheral resistance, heart strength, or vascular capacitance.

An experimental demonstration of the infinite gain principle of the kidney-volume-pressure system

Though Figure 7 was derived entirely from the computer output of a mathematical model of the circulation, the principles of that mathematical analysis have been demonstrated experimentally in many different ways. One very dramatic demonstration of the principle is illustrated in Figure 8, which shows the profound effect on the arterial pressure of an initial increase in blood volume; it also shows the subsequent course of the arterial pressure for the next hour as the kidney-volume-pressure system functioned to return the pressure back to normal [4]. This experiment was performed in a series of dogs whose nervous systems had

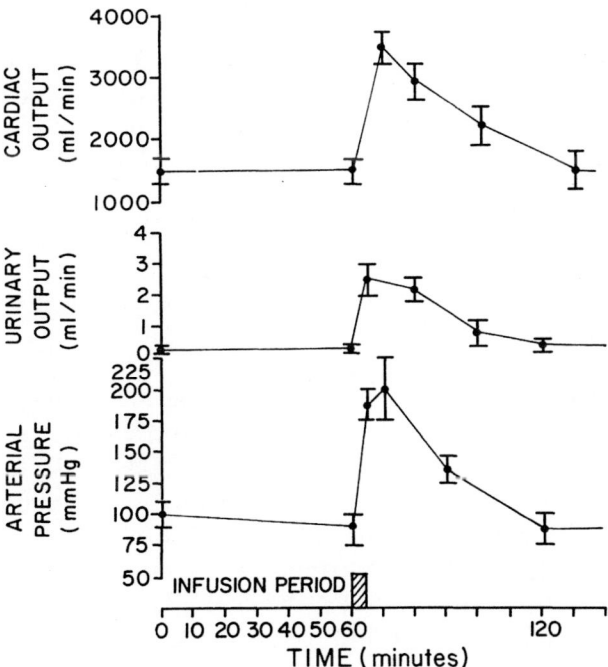

Figure 8. An experiment illustrating the applicability of the infinite gain principle for control of arterial pressure by the kidney-volume-pressure servocontrol system. Note the increase in arterial pressure when the blood volume is increased, and its return precisely to normal an hour after the infusion period. Note also the high rate of urine output as long as the pressure is above normal and its return also to normal as the pressure reapproaches the normal value. (Drawn from Data in Dobbs [4].)

been destroyed by removing the head and injecting alcohol into the spinal canal to destroy all spinal cord function. After a one-hour control period, 400 ml of blood were transfused into each animal over a period of 4 minutes; this represented approximately a 40% increase in blood volume. Note the instantaneous rise in arterial pressure, a rise to 135% above the control level. There was approximately an equal amount of increase in cardiac output, which was the cause of the greatly elevated pressure. But, especially important, please note the tremendous increase in urinary output as well. As soon as the pressure rose to this very high level, the urinary output increased 12-fold, and remained above normal all during the following hour, until the arterial pressure returned exactly and precisely back to its original control level.

In the normal animal with a normal nervous system it is difficult to demonstrate the function of this kidney-volume-pressure control system when the volume is greatly expanded because the nervous system provides an extreme pressure-buffering mechanism that literally hides the arterial pressure control function of this basic fluid volume system. However, the fluid volume system is always present, despite the buffering function of the nervous system. Furthermore, all the long-term studies thus far made on reflex pressure control by the nervous system have shown that this mechanism adapts over a period of one to three days [14, 15, 19, 20], so that after that time it can no longer buffer the long-term changes in arterial pressure. Thus, it is essential to use some other pressure control system besides the nervous system beyond the first few days. Yet, the kidney-volume-pressure mechanism does not adapt. Therefore, when the nervous system has run its course in controlling the pressure, the kidney-volume-pressure mechanism is still functioning to provide long-term stabilization of the arterial pressure.

Stabilization of the long-term arterial pressure level in clinical conditions that change the total peripheral resistance

Since the kidney-volume-pressure control mechanism is a long-term pressure controller, it is important to examine its function for stabilizing the arterial pressure in long continued clinical abnormalities of the circulation. Figure 9 illustrates an examination of the role of this system in stabilizing the arterial pressure in a series of conditions that are known to cause primary changes in total peripheral resistance: (1) beriberi, (2) arteriovenous fistula, (3) thyrotoxicosis, (4) anemia, (5) pulmonary disease, (6) Paget's disease, (7) loss of all four limbs, and (8) hypothyroidism. The first five decrease the total peripheral resistance, while the last two increase the total peripheral resistance.

The two curves in Figures 9 show the relationship of the total peripheral resistance in all the different conditions to the cardiac output, and the relationship of changes in total peripheral resistance to the arterial pressure. Although it is very difficult to find in the literature any special studies on the arterial pressure in

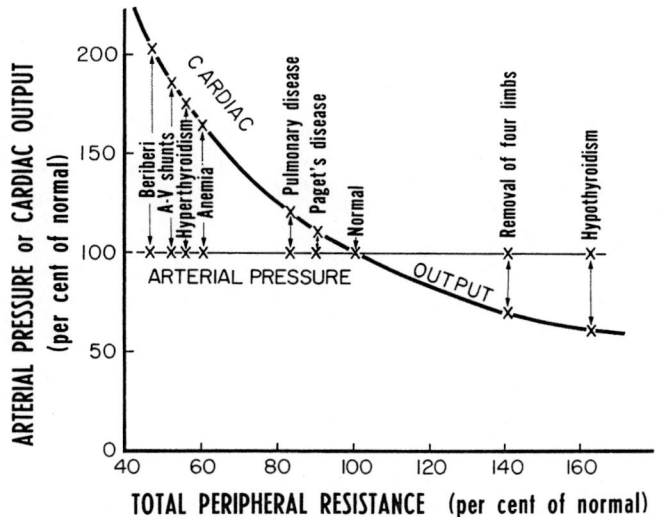

Figure 9. Applicability of the infinite gain principle for control of arterial pressure in various clinical conditions that alter the total peripheral resistance. Note that in all of these the long-term arterial pressure level is exactly normal, while the cardiac output is inversely related to the abnormality of the total peripheral resistance. (Reprinted from Guyton [9].)

all of the different conditions listed above because none of them are known to change the mean pressure significantly from normal), in the few instances in which definitive studies have been made the arterial pressure is indeed exactly normal. For instance, Warren and his colleagues [26] studied a large series of patients with long-term A–V fistulas, measuring their arterial pressures before and after surgical closure of the fistula. They were unable to find a statistically significant change in pressure.

On the other hand, in each of the separate listed conditions, the cardiac output is exactly inversely related to the change in total peripheral resistance.

It is clear that some active mechanism is controlling the arterial pressure to a very exact level, but this is not true for the control of cardiac output. If we return to our previous discussion of the stabilizing influence of the kidney-volume-pressure control system, and especially if we study Figure 7 once again, we can readily understand why the pressure is controlled exactly to normal in all of the conditions listed: the kidney-volume-pressure mechanism causes retention or loss of fluid until the pressure returns exactly to the control level as set by the kidney-volume-pressure mechanism itself. Thus, the cardiac output is altered up or down as a result of fluid volume changes until it becomes exactly inversely proportional to the change in total peripheral resistance. Furthermore, these changes in volume and cardiac output do not stop until the arterial pressure in each instance is stabilized at the normal control level.

A further explanation of the infinite gain principle

Now that we have demonstrated both in a computer model and in a number of practical examples the extreme stabilizing influence of the kidney-volume-pressure control system on the long-term level of arterial pressure, we can provide still further insight into the infinite gain principle. Please refer once again to Figure 6, which shows the intake level of salt and water as well as the rate of renal output of salt and water at each respective pressure level. Note once again the equilibrium point between the intake line and the output curve; it is only at this point that a person can remain indefinitely in salt and water balance. What is the effect of increasing the arterial pressure to a level greater than that represented by the equilibrium point? Or, what is the effect of decreasing the pressure to a level lower than the equilibrium point?

If the pressure is increased to a value greater than normal, one can immediately see that the renal output will rise to a level far greater than the intake. This obviously cannot continue forever because it would eventually remove all the salt and water present in the body. Therefore, it is clear that, as the salt and water content of the body falls, there eventually comes a time when the pressure will reapproach exactly and precisely the equilibrium point.

Conversely, if the pressure falls below normal, then the intake becomes greater than the output. This also is a condition incompatible with life should it continue forever, because so long as it does persist there will be progressive retention of salt and water. Either the body responds with an increase in pressure up to the equilibrium point level or, conversely, the person will die of congestive heart failure. Indeed, a very good functional definition of decompensated heart failure is failure of the pressure to rise to a level high enough to achieve balance between fluid output and intake.

Therefore, it is clear that the long-term arterial pressure level must inexorably approach the equilibrium point, and that the arterial pressure must remain very near to this equilibrium point as long as the functional capability of the kidney to excrete salt and water remains unchanged and as long as the intake remains unchanged. *This is the infinite gain principle.*

SERVOCONTROL OF ARTERIAL PRESSURE – FUNCTION OF THE KIDNEY-
VOLUME-PRESSURE CONTROLLER AS A SERVOCONTROLLER

If the kidney-volume-pressure control system has such an infinite capability for controlling the arterial pressure, how is it possible for the long-term arterial pressure level ever to change from the normal value? The answer is a very simple one: it can be achieved by changing the status of the kidney-volume-pressure mechanism itself. For those familiar with the principles of servocontrol, it is immediately apparent that the kidney-volume-pressure mechanism is a servo

NON-TUBULAR FACTORS AFFECTING PRESSURE

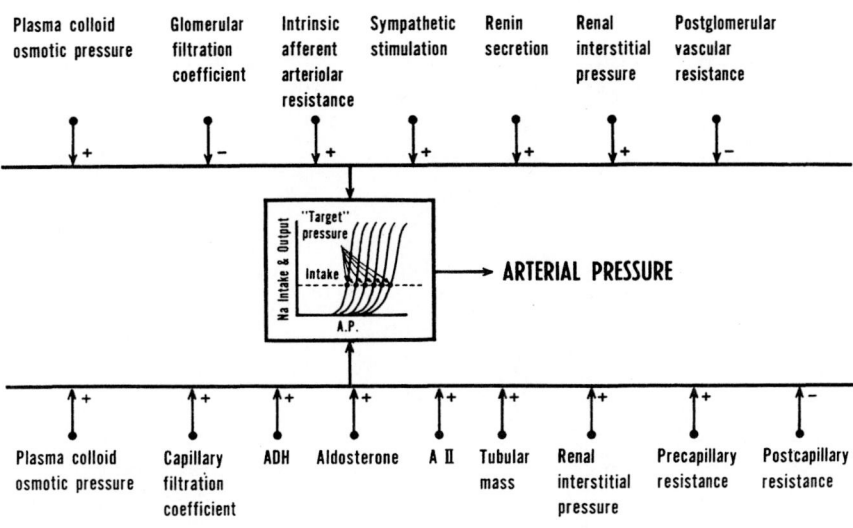

Figure 10. Diagram illustrating the servocontrol function of the kidney-volume-pressure mechanism for determining the long-term arterial pressure level. See text. (Reprinted from Guyton [9].)

system that stabilizes the arterial pressure to an exact level. Any factor that alters the function of this servo system itself can change the pressure to a new level. For instance, sympathetic stimulation of the kidneys depresses their functional capability to excrete salt, and this shifts the 'set-point' of the kidney-volume-pressure servocontroller to a higher pressure level. Therefore, as long as the sympathetic stimulation continues, the kidney-volume-pressure servocontroller will attempt to adjust the arterial pressure to the new elevated set-point level.

In addition to sympathetic stimulation, the kidney-volume-pressure servo-controller can be regulated by still many other factors. Figure 10 illustrates some of these. But, first, an explanation of the figure itself. At the center is a graph showing an intake level of salt and water and several renal function curves. At the top, most of the different factors known to change the rate of glomerular filtration, either positively or negatively (as indicated by the plus or minus signs) are listed. At the bottom, most of the known factors that can change tubular reabsorption, again either positiviely or negatively, are also listed. A change either in the capability of the kidneys to filter into the tubules or in reabsorption may change the slope and/or shift of the renal function curve along the pressure axis. Therefore, any one of the factors listed in the figure may not only change the renal function curve but may also shift the pressure level of the point at which it crosses the intake line. Thus, the equilibrium point for control of arterial pressure can be shifted either to a higher or to a lower pressure level in many different ways. Expressing this in terms of servocontrol principles, the pressure set-point of the servocontroller can be adjusted upward or downward by any one or all of these separate factors.

Note especially the following among the different factors that can change the set-point of the kidney-volume-pressure servocontroller:
1. Sympathetic stimulation of the kidneys
2. Aldosterone stimulation of the kidneys
3. Angiotensin stimulation of the kidneys
4. ADH stimulation of the kidneys
5. Effect of electrolytes on kidney function

These five factors help to control kidney function; therefore, they also play important and continuing roles in the long-term control of arterial pressure.

Note also the pathological factors listed in the figure, such as:
1. Decreased glomerular filtration coefficient
2. Increased vascular resistances
3. Excess reabsorption of electrolytes and fluid by the kidney tubules

Thus, pathological abnormalities of kidney function can also alter the level to which the arterial pressure adjusts over a long period of time.

Interaction of other pressure control systems with the long-term kidney-volume-pressure servocontroller

At this point we need to issue a caution and a reservation. All that we have discussed thus far has been the long-term pressure control function of the kidney-volume-pressure control mechanism. Nothing should be construed in anything that has been said to imply there are no other pressure control mechanisms functioning at the same time. Indeed, under acute conditions the nervous controls of pressure play an extremely important role in buffering the arterial pressure and in controlling it for short periods of time, as needed by the body. Similarly, the renin-angiotensin system has profound influences on the control of arterial pressure both acutely and for long periods of time. While its acute function is exerted mainly through changes in peripheral resistance, its long-term effect is exerted by shifting the renal function curve and thus increasing the set-point of the kidney-volume-pressure servocontroller. We will say more about this in a subsequent section.

Thus, the kidney-volume-pressure servocontroller does not operate by itself in a vacuum, but as part of a major complex of pressure control systems. Nevertheless, its infinite gain capability puts it in a fundamental and unique position for the long-term control of pressure. However profoundly the other pressure control systems affect the arterial pressure for short-term periods, the only way in which they can affect the pressure long-term is to control the servocontroller itself, as explained above. Thus, the long-term effect of sympathetic stimulation for the control of arterial pressure is exerted not by the vasoconstrictor effect of sympathetic stimulation on the non-renal blood vessels, but rather by elevation of the set-point of the kidney-volume-pressure servocontroller. Likewise, the short-term effect of the angiotensin system functions almost entirely by vasoconstriction, but its long-term effect works by altering the set-point of the servocontroller. The same can be said for aldosterone and the effects of various electrolytes on the long-term pressure level, and also for the different pathological conditions that alter arterial pressure.

THE INFINITE GAIN PRINCIPLE IN LOW VOLUME AND LOW CARDIAC OUTPUT
HYPERTENSION

Probably the most disastrous interpretation of the infinite gain principle has been that it requires an increase in blood volume in all types of hypertension. This is the farthest from the truth. The infinite gain principle makes no statement about the final volume; it makes no statement about the final cardiac output; it makes no statement about how the arterial pressure reaches the new set-point level of the kidney-volume-pressure servocontroller. It simply states that the set-point of the kidney-volume-pressure servocontroller is the final determinant of the long-term pressure level. If the pressure arrives at this level as a result of some vasoconstrictor factor acting on the peripheral circulation, so much the better; under such conditions, the kidney-volume-pressure mechanism need not operate at all. However, if the vasoconstrictor mechanism fails to bring the arterial pressure exactly to the set-point level, then, and only then, will the kidney-volume-pressure servocontroller function.

If the pressure caused by the vasoconstrictor is too high, then the kidney-volume-pressure servocontroller will function negatively by excreting excess amounts of salt and water and decreasing blood volume and cardiac output until the pressure falls to the set-point level.

If the vasoconstrictor mechanism fails to bring the arterial pressure to a level as high as the set-point level, then the kidney-volume-pressure servocontroller will function positively, causing accumulation of salt and water and an increase in both blood volume and cardiac output until the pressure rises to the set-point level.

It is clear that the final levels of volume and of cardiac output may be either above or below normal. In types of hypertension that have a strong vasoconstrictor component, one would expect both the volume and the cardiac output to be less than normal. On the other hand, in types of hypertension where the vasoconstrictor component is weak, one would expect the volume and cardiac output to be elevated slightly above normal.

All who truly wish to understand the infinite gain principle of pressure control by the kidney-volume-pressure servocontroller must be especially careful not to fall into the naive trap of assuming that the infinite gain principle requires increased volume and cardiac output.

Other factors can also decrease volume or cardiac output to below normal in hypertension. One is a pathological decrease in the volume-holding capacity of the vascular system; this will decrease the blood volume. Another is pathological constriction of the arteries or arterioles, a condition actually observed in spontaneously hypertensive rats; this can decrease both cardiac output and blood volume below normal.

Finally, when volume or cardiac output is elevated or depressed in the different types of hypertension, the elevation or depression is rarely large, usually no more than 5 to 10%, except in very unusual circumstances. Careful study of the autoregulation mechanism which has been explained in detail in many publications [6, 11, 12] will show why. For instance, in volume-loading hypertension, which generally tends to increase volume and cardiac output to above normal, the autoregulation mechanism automatically returns the cardiac output back toward normal while increasing the total peripheral resistance; at the same time, this mechanism also reduces the volume back toward normal. In a subsequent section we shall show that, after a few weeks of volume-loading, one can hardly measure an increase either in blood volume or cardiac output.

Conversely, in the types of hypertension in which there is a strong vasoconstrictor component, the primary effect of the autoregulation mechanism is drastic reduction of blood volume and cardiac output. A full understanding of the autoregulation principle will show, however, that autoregulation in this instance operates in a negative direction, preventing the disastrous vasoconstriction that might occur and thereby preventing the cardiac output from falling much below normal. Even in types of hypertension in which there is extreme vasoconstriction, as occurs in patients with pheochromocytomata, the blood volume has been reported to be only slightly below normal in some patients and almost exactly normal in others [17]. And the same is also true for cardiac output.

Therefore, we once again express the hope that the reader will study the principle of infinite gain of the kidney-volume-pressure control system in enough detail to understand the applicability of this principle even in low-volume–low-cardiac output types of hypertension.

SOME EXAMPLES OF FACTORS THAT INCREASE THE SET-POINT OF THE KIDNEY-VOLUME-PRESSURE SERVOCONTROLLER

It is important not to go further without full understanding of the principle illustrated in Figure 10 – that any shift of the renal function curve in the high pressure direction will increase the pressure leven of the servocontroller set-point. On this basis, we can proceed to explain how different pressure controlling factors can cause long-term sustained elevations of arterial pressure.

Effect of angiotensin infusion

Figure 11 illustrates three separate renal function curves measured in dogs. The almost vertical solid curve shows normal renal function [3]; the reason for the shape of the normal curve will be discussed subsequently. To the right is the renal function curve in dogs infused with a very low level of angiotensin, enough to increase circulating angiotensin about three-fold [3]; this infusion was continued for approximately a month, while the different levels of the curve were measured on subsequent days, after prolonged equilibration before each measurement. To the left is a similar renal function curve, measured when the renin-angiotensin system was blocked by continuous infusion of the converting enzyme inhibitor, SQ-14225 [10]. Note the shift of the function curve toward a higher pressure level during continuous angiotensin infusion, and the shift toward lower pressure when the natural formation of angiotensin II had been blocked.

Thus, it is clear that an increase in the circulating level of angiotensin will shift the set-point of the kidney-volume-pressure servocontroller to a higher than normal pressure level. Consequently, it is to be expected that continuous infusion of angiotensin should cause chronic hypertension. Furthermore, it is this ability of angiotensin to shift the renal function curve that causes the hypertension, not its capacity to cause vascular vasoconstriction in the non-renal parts of the circulation. If the reader has difficulty in understanding this, it would be good to return to the full discussion of the infinite gain principle.

It is also clear that blocking the renin-angiotensin system will shift the renal function curve to the left, which tends to decrease the arterial pressure. This will occur only at low salt intake levels, however.

Now, let us explain why the normal renal function curve is almost vertical. The quantitative values written on the curves are the approximate levels of angioten-

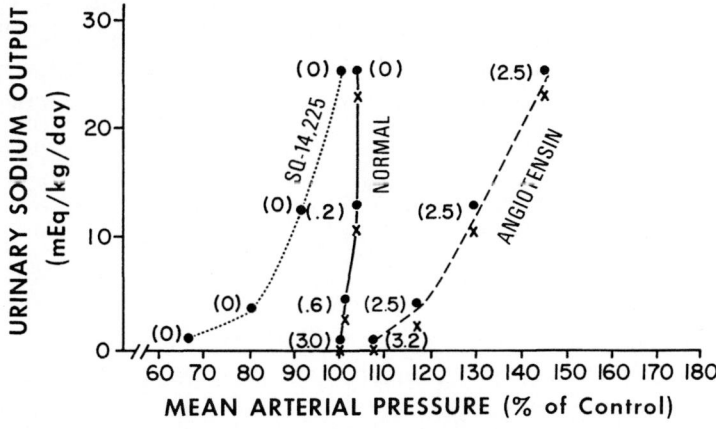

Figure 11. Renal function curves in three different states: normal (center), during continuous infusion of angiotensin at a very low rate (right), and during continuous infusion of a blocker of the renin-angiotensin system, SQ-14225 (left). (Reprinted from Guyton [9].)

54

sin activity in the circulating blood under the different conditions. When angiotensin is infused, the circulating angiotensin remains high all the time, and the changes in endogenous angiotensin have little effect. On the other hand, when the converting enzyme inhibitor is infused, the level of circulating angiotensin remains essentially zero all of the time. In the normal animal, the level of circulating angiotensin changes markedly depending on the conditions. For instance, when salt intake is low, and therefore salt output is also low, the rate of angiotensin formation in the body increases markedly. Consequently, at the bottom end of the normal function curve in Figure 11, which represents low salt intake and low salt output, the person is actually functioning on the angiotensin infusion curve. Yet, at the upper end of the normal curve, which represents the high salt intake–high salt output state, the amount of circulating angiotensin in the normal person falls essentially to zero; therefore, the person is then operating on the zero angiotensin curve. Thus, careful study of the diagram and consideration of its implications will show that the renin-angiotensin system is a very potent mechanism for keeping the arterial pressure very near a constant level despite vast changes in salt intake. When the salt intake is low, the renal function curve is shifted to the right, which mainly nullifies the effect of low salt intake on pressure. Conversely, when salt intake is very high, the renal function curve shifts to the left, which mainly nullifies the effect of high salt intake to increase the pressure. Therefore, the so-called 'normal' renal function curve in Figure 11 is not the 'acute' renal function curve, but rather the 'chronic' renal function curve. And it should also be remembered that this chronic curve includes the effects of not only the pressure-diuresis mechanism but also of the active control systems such as the renin-angiotensin system, the aldosterone system, and others that function in association with the pressure diuresis mechanism to defend the normal arterial pressure level. Even though we will not have time in the present chapter to explain it, this still does not invalidate the infinite gain principle. Instead, the interaction of these other control systems and the steepening effect they have on the 'chronic' renal function curve serves a very useful role in sharpening the precision with which the kidney-volume-pressure control mechanism maintains the long-term arterial pressure level near normal.

Effect of aldosterone on the renal function curve and on the set-point of the servocontroller

Figure 12 shows a series of function curves, beginning on the left with the normal 'chronic' renal function curve as determined in dogs. To the right, there are four different renal function curves, measured or calculated for aldosterone infusion in different dog experiments. The crossmarks on the curves represent specific data points measured in multiple dog series.

Note that the renal function curve during aldosterone stimulation does not shift

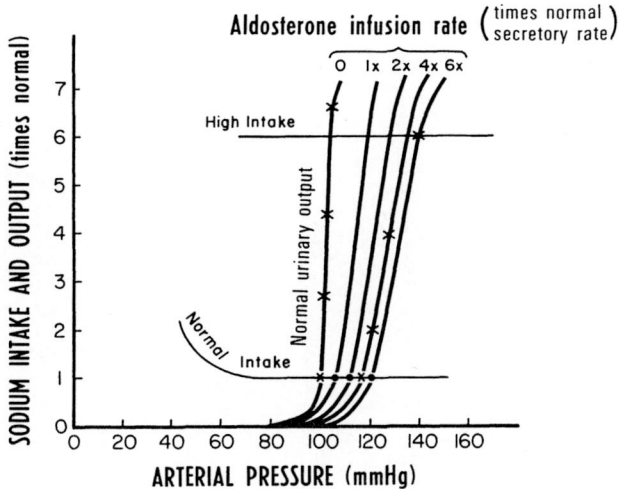

Figure 12. Renal function curves at different rates of continuous infusion of aldosterone, showing only a mild shift of the renal function curve toward higher pressure levels. (Reprinted from Guyton [9].)

as far to the right as it does during angiotensin infusion, even though the curve shown farthest to the right in Figure 12 represents approximately the maximum amount of aldosterone infusion the dog could tolerate, and even though the angiotensin infusion curve of Figure 11 represents only a minimal level of angiotensin infusion. Therefore, infusion of aldosterone in maximal amounts can shift the set-point of the servocontroller only 15–20 mm Hg when the salt intake is normal (in the dog). It is easy to understand why it is very difficult to cause large increases in arterial pressure in the dog by aldosterone infusion.

Shift of the renal function curve, and of the pressure set-point, in the spontaneously hypertensive rat

Figure 13 illustrates renal function curves as measured in the normal rat (WKY) and in Okamoto spontaneously hypertensive rats (SHR) [21]. Note that there is approximately a 40 mm Hg shift in the function curve toward higher pressure; one can understand readily why the set-point for arterial pressure control is very high in the SHR. Thus, it appears that the basic cause of the hypertension in these rats is this abnormal shift of the renal function curve. The cause of the shift itself is not yet known; it might be a pathological condition of the kidneys themselves, which is very likely; or, less likely, it might be some factor from outside the kidney – some investigators believe that it might be increased sympathetic stimulation.

56

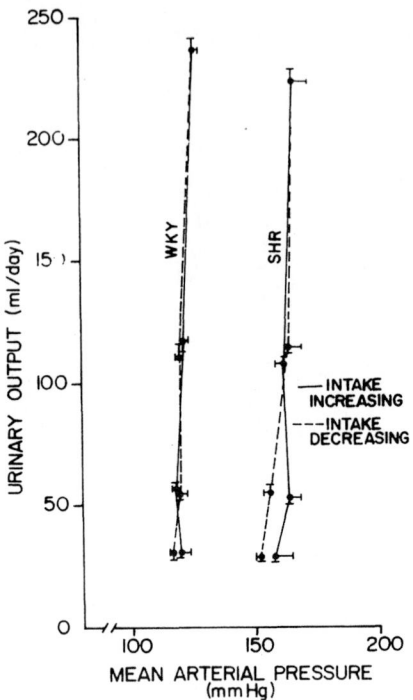

Figure 13. Renal function curves as determined in a series of normal rats (WKY) and in another series of spontaneously hypertensive rats (SHR). (Reprinted from Norman et al., [21].)

Shift of the renal function curve in essential hypertension – elevated pressure set-point

Figure 14 illustrates the normal renal function curve and also a postulated renal function curve for the essential hypertensive drawn by one of the authors a number of years ago on the basis of data in the literature [8]. More recently, Bartter and his associates measured portions of the renal function curve in essential hypertension patients, and found curves shifted far to the right, similar to the curve in Figure 14; some of their curves had slightly steeper slopes than the one illustrate in this figure, and some had slightly less steep slopes [13]. Those that are less steep are said to be salt-sensitive, those that are very steep are said to be salt-insensitive. That is, the less steep the curve, the greater the change in arterial pressure when the patient ingests excessive amounts of salt.

At any rate, it is clear that the renal function curve in essential hypertension is shifted far to the right, and therefore the set-point of the kidney-volume-pressure servocontroller is also raised to a continuously elevated pressure level. Again, it is not known why the curve is shifted far to the right. Many different reasons have recently come to the fore suggesting intrinsic kidney pathology as the cause of the shift. This intrinsic pathology might have resulted from events in the history of the

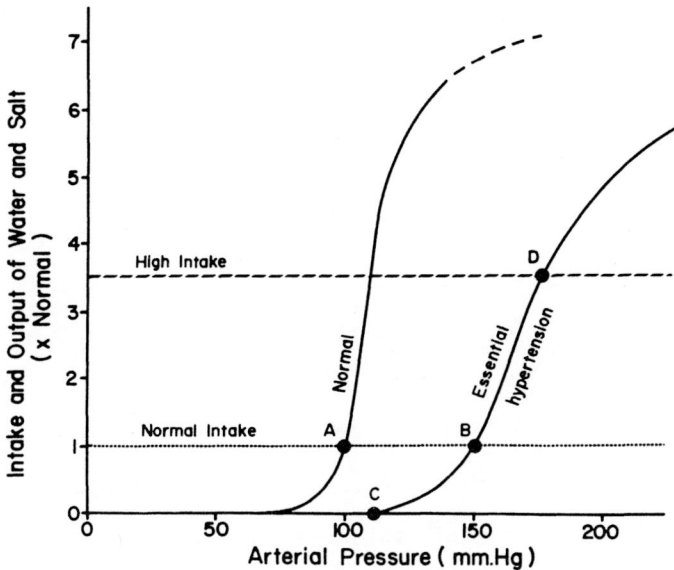

Figure 14. Shift of the renal function curve from the normal (left) to approximately that which occurs in essential hypertension (right). (Reprinted from Guyton et al. [9].)

kidney – for instance, episodes of excess sympathetic stimulation, episodes of excess aldosterone, episodes of disease, genetic deterioration of the kidney, etc. Anyhow, as the function curve is shifted far to the right, and as removal of any or all the different factors normally believed to control kidney function still does not return the arterial pressure to normal in most patients with essential hypertension, it can be assumed that the hypertension is maintained not by factors extrinsic to the kidney but by the fact that the renal function curve has indeed been shifted far to the right because of some intrinsic renal factor. This almost certainly results from permanent changes in the kidneys themselves.

Increase in the servocontroller set-point and the development of hypertension in low kidney mass dogs that are volume-loaded

Figure 15 shows renal function curves for the normal dog and for dogs in which 70% of the kidney mass has been removed (removal of one kidney and the two poles of the opposite kidney). The figure also shows two levels of salt intake. At the lower level of salt intake, reduction of the kidney mass shifts the servo-controller set-point only about 6 mm Hg – from point A to point B on the diagram. Therefore, removal of the kidney mass by itself causes almost no elevation of arterial pressure as long as the animal remains on a normal salt intake.

On the other hand, if the salt intake is suddenly increased in the animal with

58

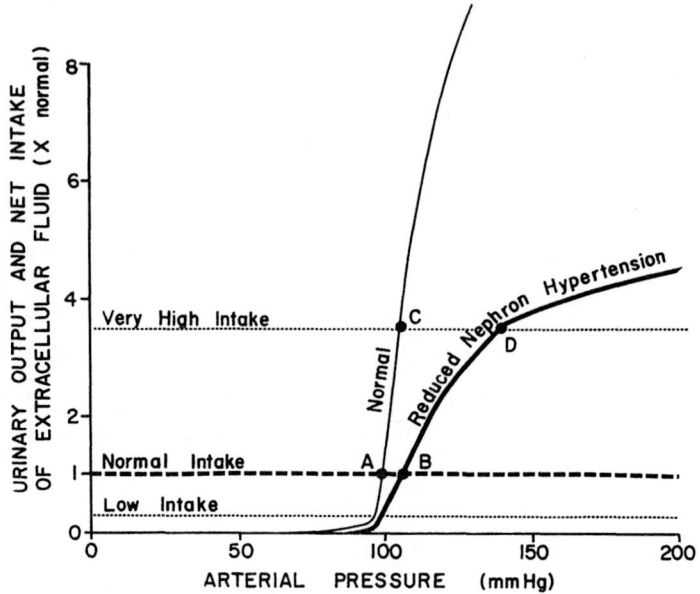

Figure 15. Change of the renal function curve from the normal as a result of reducing the renal mass to 30% of normal. This creates a highly salt-sensitive state, causing severe hypertension during large intakes of salt, and normotension without the high salt intake.

low kidney mass, the set-point of the servocontroller becomes point D on the diagram – the point where the high salt intake level crosses the reduced kidney mass function curve. We have performed this type of experiment many times in our laboratory to study the hemodynamics and pathogenesis of volume-loading hypertension. Figure 16 illustrates the approximate summated results of our experiments, beginning in 1961 up to the present [1, 2, 5, 16, 18]. After an appropriate control period, the set-point of the servocontroller was suddenly raised approximately 45 mm Hg by placing the dogs with low renal mass on a salt intake five to seven times normal. Note at the bottom of the figure that the instant these dogs were placed on such a salt intake their set-point rose 45% above the control level. However, the pressure itself did not rise immediately. Instead, the kidney-volume-pressure servocontroller required several days to bring the pressure up to the set-point level; then it rose slightly above this level for a few days, and finally settled back at exactly the level dictated by the set-point.

But, how did the pressure reach this elevated level? The upper curves in the figure illustrate the mechanism. Immediately after the high level of salt intake began, the extracellular fluid volume, blood volume, cardiac output, mean circulatory filling pressure, and pressure gradient for venous return, all increased far above normal. It was during these first few days that the arterial pressure rose up to the set-point level. Thus, the cause of the elevated pressure was increased volume and increased cardiac output.

It is equally as instructive to look at the next-to-the-bottom curve, depicting the changes in total peripheral resistance, which decreased during the first few days of salt loading, which was also the time when the arterial pressure rose up to the set-point level. Then, the total peripheral resistance increased progressively during the next two weeks while the volume and cardiac output returned toward normal. The most likely explanation for this effect is that the excess cardiac output caused progressive arteriolar vasoconstriction throughout the body. This is the *blood flow autoregulation mechanism.* As a consequence, the cardiac output returned back toward normal while the total peripheral resistance increased. Yet the arterial pressure still remained at the elevated set-point level. Thus, the autoregulation mechanism provides a means for converting high cardiac output hypertension into high resistance hypertension. Furthermore, as the increase in total peripheral resistance results almost entirely from increased arteriolar resistance, this tends to reduce both the capillary pressure and the

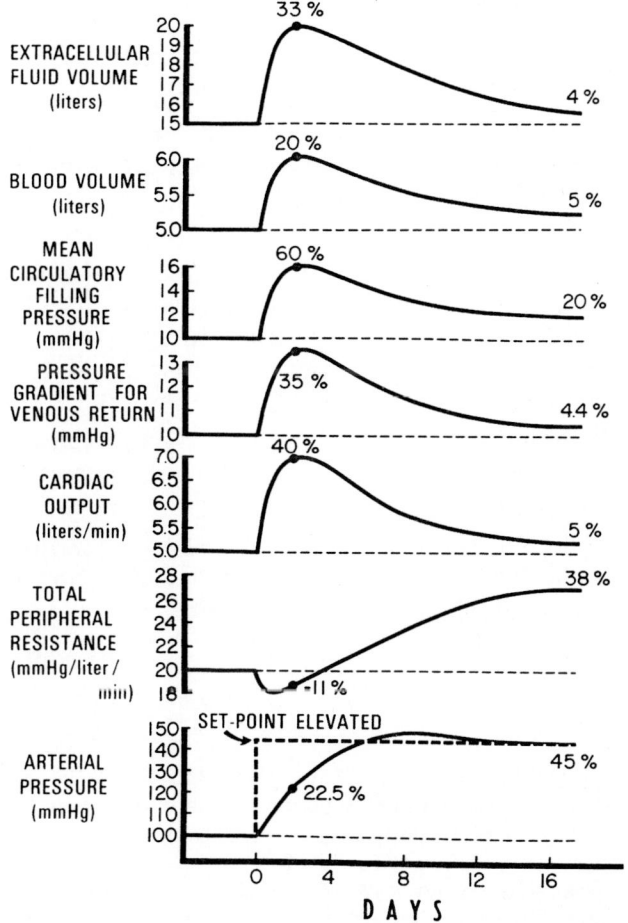

Figure 16. Salt-loading hypertension in dogs with low renal mass and high salt intake. The sequential changes shown in this figure for the different circulatory variables have been observed in several series of experiments in our laboratory since 1961. (Reprinted from Guyton [9].)

venous pressure back toward normal. Therefore, both the extracellular fluid volume and the blood volume also returned back toward normal. Thus, at the end of several weeks, despite the fact that the hypertension had been caused by volume loading, it was almost impossible to show either an elevated cardiac output or an elevated blood volume. This is an exceedingly important observation, as it indicates that even pure volume-loading hypertension in the chronic state is not manifest by increases in blood volume and cardiac output that can be measured reliably by the usual techniques. All of these phenomena are described in far greater detail elsewhere [9] and deserve thorough study and understanding, as so many workers in the hypertension field still believe that a high total peripheral resistance always means that there is a circulating vasoconstrictor substance in the blood. This is almost certainly nonsense.

SUMMARY

The purpose of this paper has been to explain in detail the infinite gain principle for blood pressure control by the kidney-volume-pressure servocontrol system. It has especially been emphasized that this principle does not require that hypertensive patients have increased blood volume or increased cardiac output. Indeed, in most types of hypertension, both of these are either normal or even subnormal, but this does not invalidate the infinite gain principle. In fact, in types of hypertension associated with a very strong vasoconstrictor factor, the kidney-volume-pressure servocontrol mechanism itself often decreases the blood volume and cardiac output to below normal.

The essence of the infinite gain principle is that it is impossible ever to have hypertension unless the set-point level of the kidney-volume-pressure servocontrol mechanism is raised to an elevated pressure level. The reverse of this is also true: if ever the set-point of this controller is elevated to a high pressure level, then hypertension either will ensue, or the person will eventually die of congestive heart failure while trying to reach that pressure level.

REFERENCES

1. Coleman TG, Guyton AC: Hypertension caused by salt loading in the dog. III. Onset transients of cardiac output and other circulatory variables. Circ Res 25: 152, 1969
2. Cowley AW, Jr, Guyton AC: Baroreceptor reflex contribution in angiotensin II induced hypertension. Circulation 50: 61, 1974
3. DeClue JW, Guyton AC, Cowley AW, Jr, Coleman TG, Norman RA, Jr, McCaa RE: Subpressor angiotensin infusion, renal sodium handling, and salt-induced hypertension in the dog. Circ Res 43: 503, 1978
4. Dobbs WA, Jr: Relative importance of nervous and intrinsic mechanical factors in cardiovascular control systems. PhD Thesis, University of Mississippi School of Medicine, Jackson, Mississippi, 1970

5. Douglas BH, Guyton AC, Langston JB, Bishop VS: Hypertension caused by salt loading. II: Fluid volume and tissue pressure changes. Am J Physiol 207: 669, 1964

6 Folkow B, Gurevich M, Hallback M, Lundgren Y, Weiss L: The hemodynamic consequences of regional hypertension in spontaneously hypertensive and normotensive rats. Acta Physiol Scand 83: 532, 1971

7. Guyton AC, Abernathy JB, Langston JB, Kaufman BN, Fairchild HM: Relative importance of venous and arterial resistances in controlling venous return and cardiac output. Am J Physiol 196: 1008, 1959

8. Guyton AC, Coleman TG, Cowley AW, Jr, Scheel KW, Manning RD, Jr, Norman RA, Jr: Arterial pressure regulation: overriding dominance of the kidney in long-term regulation and in hypertension. Am J Med 52: 584, 1972

9. Guyton AC: Arterial pressure and hypertension. WB Saunders Company, Philadelphia, 1980

10. Hall JE, Guyton AC, Smith MJ, Jr, Coleman TG: Blood pressure and renal function during chronic changes in sodium intake: role of angiotensin (in preparation)

11. Johnson PC (ed): Autoregulation of Blood Flow. Proceedings of an International Symposium. Am Heart Assoc, New York, 1964

12. Jones RD, Berne RM: Intrinsic regulation of skeletal muscle blood flow. Circ Rec 14: 126, 1964

13. Kawasaki T, Kelea CS, Bartter FC, Smith H: The effect of high-sodium and low-sodium intakes on blood pressure and other related variables in human subjects with idiopathic hypertension. Am J Med 64: 193, 1978

14. Kezdi P, Wennemark J: Baroreceptor and sympathetic activity in experimental renal hypertension. Circulation 17: 785, 1958

15. Krieger EM: Time course of baroreceptor resetting in acute hypertension. Am J Physiol 218: 486, 1970

16. Langston JB, Guyton AC, Douglas BH, Dorsett PE: Effect of changes in salt intake on arterial pressure and renal function in nephrectomized dogs. Circ Res 12: 508, 1963

17. Manger WM, Gifford RW, Jr: Pheochromocytoma. Springer-Verlag, New York, 1977

18. Manning RD, Jr, Coleman TG, Guyton AC, Normal RA, Jr, McCaa RW: Essential role of mean circulatory filling pressure in salt-induced hypertension. Am J Physiol 236: R40, 1979

19. McCubbin JW, Green JH, Page IH: Baroreceptor function in chronic renal hypertension. Circ Res 4: 205, 1956

20. McCubbin JW: Carotid sinus participation in experimental renal hypertension. Circulation 17: 791, 1958

21. Norman RA, Jr, Enobakhare JA, DeClue JW, Douglas BH, Guyton AC: Renal function curves in normotensive and spontaneously hypertensive rats. Am J Physiol 234: R98, 1978

22. Richardson TQ, Stallings JO, Guyton AC: Pressure-volume curves in live, intact dogs. Am J Physiol 201: 471, 1961

23. Selkurt EE, Hall PW, Spencer MP: Influence of graded arterial pressure decrement on renal clearance of creatinine, ϱ-amino hippurate and sodium. Am J Physiol 159: 369, 1949

24. Shipley RE, Study RS: Changes in renal blood flow, extraction of insulin, glomerular filtration rate, tissue pressure, and urine flow with acute alterations of renal artery blood pressure. Am J Physiol 167: 676, 1951

25. Thompson DD, Pitts RF: Effects of alterations of renal arterial pressure on sodium and water excretion. Am J Physiol 168: 490, 1952

26. Warren JV, Nickerson JL, Elkin DC: The cardiac output in patients with arteriovenous fistulas. J Clin Invest 30: 210, 1951

5. HYPERTENSION RESEARCH: A VIEWPOINT

W.H. BIRKENHÄGER, P.W. DE LEEUW

The search for the fundamental fault in (essential) hypertension remains one of the main challenges to biological and clinical science. The only concensus at present concerns the rather vague concept that essential hypertension is probably the result of an interaction between genetic and environmental factors.

When one takes it from there, the fundamental disorder is likely to be camouflaged by changes that occur as a consequence of the hypertensive process itself. It may be argued, therefore, that the search for the prime mover should be based on the investigation of the earliest recognizable stage of hypertension, and perhaps even of the prehypertensive state. Figure 1 may be of help in framing our thoughts while we try to arrange some of the points raised in this Volume.

It is obvious that the primary problem is hemodynamically oriented: should the increase in blood pressure be explained in terms of a cardiac or rather of a vascular mechanism? In young subjects with mild hypertension cardiac output is not infrequently found to be elevated, in comparison with age- and sex-matched controls. Dr Julius supposed that this subjects with borderline hypertension were hyper-responsive to the stress of the procedure, adding that anxiety may be all that is needed to develop hypertension. We feel that part of all this is an artifact, as informed hypertensives tend to have pronounced feelings where investigations of their condition are concerned. This sense of personal involvement is of course absent in those who have been explicitly selected for control studies. In *unsuspecting* early hypertensives we failed to find an elevation of cardiac output. The possibility that a raised cardiac output in the resting state is an emotional artifact is also suggested by the observation that the difference between the average cardiac output of hypertensives and normotensives disappears when they are exercised, resulting in a consistent difference in total peripheral vascular resistance [1].

Follow-up studies also tend to diminish the importance of a raised cardiac output. Lund-Johansen [4], for instance, found a decline in cardiac output after 10 years of observation in subjects aged 20–30 years and 30–40 years respectively. In the first study 30–40-year old subjects had a considerably higher cardiac index than those who had arrived in that age range by the time of the second study. Recently, the Göteborg group completed a follow-up study in hyperkinetic and normokinetic subjects with mild blood pressure elevation. After 5 years the

Sambhi, M.P. (ed.) Fundamental fault in hypertension
© *1984, Martinus Nijhoff Publishers. Boston/The Hague/Dordrecht/Lancaster.*
ISBN 978-94-010-9006-3

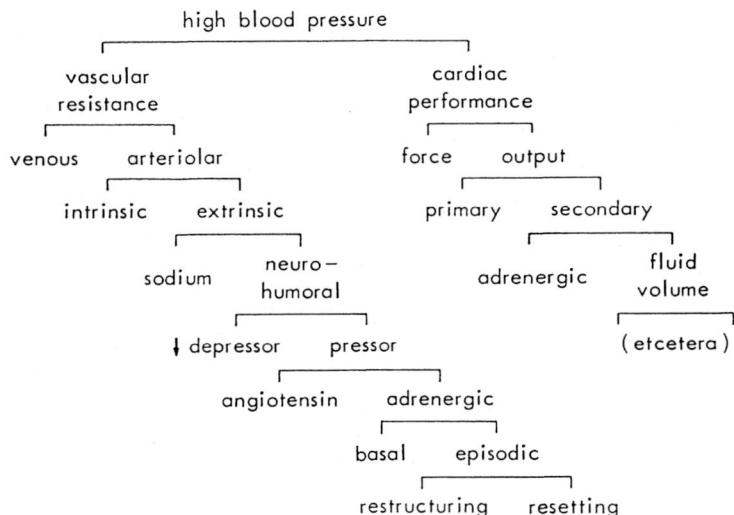

Figure 1. One way of balancing the priorities in looking for a prime mover in essential hypertension.

hyperkinetic group had normalized their cardiac output but without any change in blood pressure and without any evidence for the development of vascular abnormalities (Andersson et al.).

Even though an increase in vascular resistance already is the main hemodynamic feature in early hypertension, a contributory role for the heart (in terms of rate of pressure rise and generation of positive vascular reflexes, as proposed by Dr Tarazi) cannot be denied.

The increase in vascular resistance can be viewed from many angles.

Some of us have difficulties in visualizing hypertension as an intrinsic membrane disorder. To those, a lack of depressor control or an excess of pressor activity are more plausible mechanisms. Although Drs Carretero and Scicli and Dr Muirhead have presented a lot of convincing material illustrating the potential of depressor systems the relevance to essential hypertension remains to be proven.

The main pressor systems, the renin – angiotensin – and the adrenergic system can indeed induce structural alterations in the arteriolar wall.

The systemic aspects of the renin angiotensin system have been extensively discussed in this volume. On the basis of earlier findings [1] we felt that the activity of the system in uncomplicated essential hypertension tends to be fed back to subnormal levels rather than being stimulated. The contributions of Dr Lever, Dr Sambhi and Dr Haddy and his colleagues indeed focus on low renin hypertension. Dr Swales admirably exposed the weaknesses in the arguments of those who try to salvage a role for renin. Whether or not hypertensive subjects respond to angiotensin analogues or angiotensin conversion blockers (Dr Lijnen and his colleagues) is probably beside the point in identifying the prime mover. We found it difficult to come to grips with renin substrate as a pathogenetic factor, as it tends to adapt to changes in renin. Angiotensin II concentrations reflect the tendency of renin to be suppressed.

By contrast, the adrenergic system remains a (seasoned) candidate. Dr Doyle has highlighted some of his vast experience and rather convincingly stated that the development of hypertension automatically involves the autonomic nervous system. Dr Zanchetti contrasted the well-preserved integrity of short-term blood pressure regulation with the loss of baseline control. The main target organ, the arteriolar wall, appears to be hyper-reactive (Dr Bevan) or supersensitive (Dr Doyle) by virtue of its increased smooth muscle mass (both seem to agree on that), but this is no specific expression of adrenergic activity. Do circulating catecholamines truly reflect adrenergic activity? It is generally recognized that there is a vast latitude for misinterpretation. The early claim that catecholamines are raised in a considerable proportion of early hypertensives, could not be maintained under better controlled conditions.

In our laboratory similar levels were found in a group of mild to moderate hypertensives and an appropriate control group consisting of normotensive patients with unrelated ailments; both were studied under basal metabolic ward conditions with a fixed sodium intake [3]. This lack of a difference in basal norepinephrine levels, however, does not preclude a role for the adrenergic system. This has been amply demonstrated by Philipp et al. [5] who found an inverse (hyperbolic) relationship between plasma levels of endogenous norepinephrine and vascular reactivity to infused norepinephrine. Compared to normotensives this relationship was shifted to the right in hypertensives. Therefore, what has in fact been demonstrated is that norepinephrine levels – in contrast to renin or angiotensin levels – fail to become *suppressed* in the face of an increased arterial pressure and presumed hyper-reactivity of the arteriolar wall. With some reservations – and defying Dr Swales – one could propose, that the adrenergic system operates at an inappropriately normal level.

Such an interpretation extends to the intrarenal part of the adrenergic system. As Dr Doyle rightly put it, reflecting Dr Guyton's view, the adrenergic system by virtue of its effect on the renal arterioles prevents the pressure diuresis and natriuresis which would otherwise offset the rise in arterial pressure. Incidentally, this could be one area where the vascular effects of adrenergic activity could be tied in with ambient sodium concentration, such as demonstrated by dr Doyle. The predominant problem with salt seems to be, that the impact of salt on blood pressure remains undefined in volumetric or hemodynamic terms. One possibility is that sodium exerts its pressor effect through an intracellular mechanism in vascular smooth muscle cells [2]. On the other hand, it is conceivable that the inner brain will turn out to be the main site of interaction. The role of the central catecholaminergic neurons has been discussed by Drs De Jong, Lovenberg and Brody, and the latter associated one particular area (AV3V) with salt metabolism.

In the clinical setting the inner brain is a rather remote area, and one therefore has to make do with indirect indices. The theme raised by Dr L.B. Page in his presentation may be relevant to the present one. It has been repeatedly demonstrated that body weight is a consistent correlate of blood pressure. In our hands it was already demonstrable in a small population sample, when we compared young adults with low grade hypertension with normotensive matched for age, sex and height. The hypertensives were on the average 5 kg overweight. Although weight and blood pressure appear to be to some extent causally related, the weight losses needed to bring the blood pressure down are in excess of the order of magnitude we are now discussing. We therefore like to propose, that the association between overweight and high blood pressure may run in parallel rather in series, indicating a common pathogenesis originating from adjoining or overlapping hypothalamic areas that regulate appetite and baseline blood pressure.

REFERENCES

1. Birkenhäger WH, De Leeuw PW, Schalekamp MADH: Control mechanisms in essential hypertension. Elsevier Biomed. Publishing Company, Amsterdam, 1982
2. Blaustein MP: Sodium ions, calcium ions, blood pressure regulation and hypertension: a reassessment and a hypothesis. Am J Physiol 232: C165, 1977
3. De Leeuw PW, Wester A, Punt R, Falke HE, Birkenhäger WH: Noradrenaline levels in essential hypertensives and normotensive controls. Neth J Med 22: 145, 1979
4. Lund-Johansen P: Spontaneous changes in central hemodynamics in essential hypertension – a 10 year follow-up study. In: Onesti G, Klimt ChR (eds), Hypertension: Determinants, Complications and Intervention. Grune & Stratton, New York, 1977, pp 201–209
5. Philipp T, Distler A, Cordes U: Sympathetic nervous system and blood pressure control in essential hypertension. Lancet ii: 959, 1978

II. HOW IMPORTANT IS THE SALT INTAKE?

6. DETERINANTS OF BLOOD PRESSURE IN POPULATIONS

LOT B. PAGE

The origins of primary hypertension are controversial. Nevertheless, there is general agreement on the determinants of adult blood pressure beginning to operate very early in life. The great importance of heredity as one major determinant is universally accepted. The relative importance of other determinants is in dispute, but most will agree that body mass, dietary electrolyte intake, and psycho-social stress factors are among the principal contenders.

Major difficulties arise in translating the determinants of blood pressure identified in population studies into disturbances of blood pressure control understandable by known physiologic principles. I should like to defend the value of population studies, and at the same time to point out the inherent limitations of this type of research. If these strengths and weaknesses are understood, strategies may be devised for testing hypotheses derived from population studies in controlled experiments.

Population studies in many parts of the world have usually shown blood pressure rising progressively with age, although varying in level and slope from one population to another. An increase in blood pressure with age may be considered a prerequisite to primary hypertension; it results in a cumulative increase in hypertension prevalence in successive decades, the magnitude of which depends on the chosen cutting point.

Contrary to the general trend, more than twenty different populations have been described in various parts of the world that show little or no tendency for blood pressure to rise with age. In the Epstein. Eckoff [13] classification (Figure 1), these populations have blood pressures at levels a or b and slopes of 0 to 1.

Populations that show no tendency for blood pressure to rise with age are called 'low blood pressure populations.' All are traditional, unacculturated groups living in isolation from Western cultural influences [21]. When they migrate or become acculturated through exposure to Western cultural influences, an age-related upward trend in blood pressure appears [8, 9, 17, 20]. Three examples of this change are shown in Figure 2. This trend is common to all races and groups; it begins to appear quite early in the acculturation process.

Before discussing specific blood pressure determinants, it is appropriate to consider broadly the biologic consequences that ensue when a primitive population becomes acculturated or modernized. Several interdisciplinary projects,

Sambhi, M.P. (ed.) Fundamental fault in hypertension
© *1984, Martinus Nijhoff Publishers. Boston/The Hague/Dordrecht/Lancaster.*
ISBN 978-94-010-9006-3

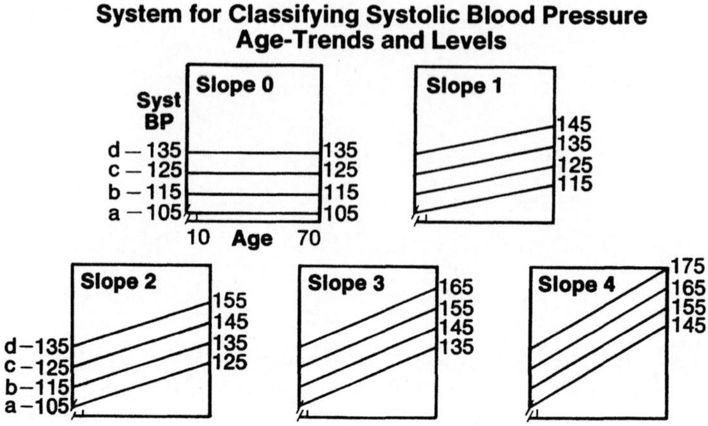

System for Classifying Systolic Blood Pressure
Age-Trends and Levels

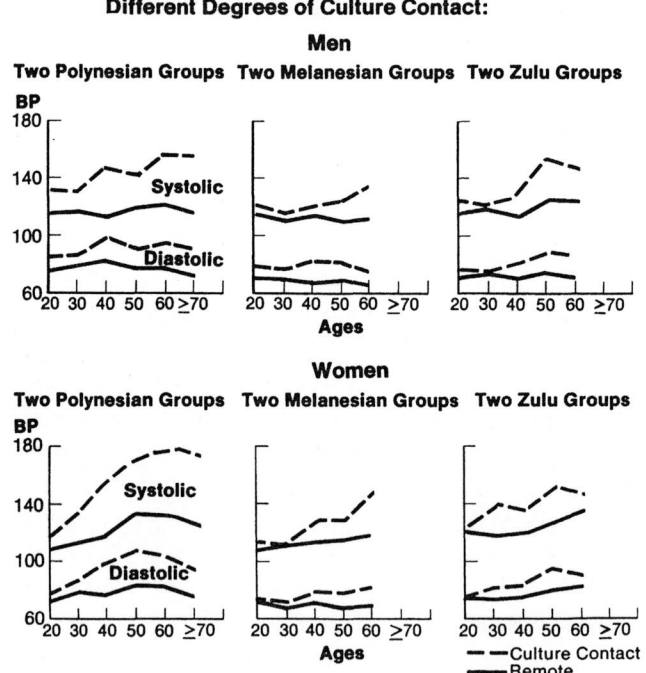

Figure 1. System for classifying age-related trends of systolic blood pressure in populations by level and slope. Modified from Epstein and Eckoff [13].

Figure 2. Effects of culture contact on age-related blood pressure trends. Modified from Cassel [5].

including the Tokelau Island Migrant Study [27], the Samoan Population Study [2] and the Harvard Solomon Islands Project [22] are engaged in examining interrelations between culture change, disease, and human biology.

The emerging science of human biology is concerned with the impact of environment on population structure and biologic fitness.

An example of the analytic approach of human biology is shown in Figure 3 [2]. The influence of modernization on various structural indicators of biologic fitness in the population has measurable consequences. Some examples will help to illustrate this. With modernization, certain genetic diseases such as sickle cell anemia will decline as malaria is eradicated; others, such as hemophilia, may increase because of prolonged life span of afflicted persons. With access to medical care, infant mortality is reduced and a population explosion in the youngest ages develops, gaining impetus as fecundity increases, the age of menarche declines, and the age of menopause recedes. Infectious desease declines and life expectancy increases. From these interwoven influences, demographic structure and population size are irreversibly changed.

Further biologic changes also ensue: growth rate in children accelerates and a secular trend in adult height usually appears. Sons and daughters progressively grow taller than their parents. Diet, work, and activity patterns change; body weight and fatness increase. Maximal oxygen consumption and other measures of physical fitness decline. All these changes and many others have been docu-

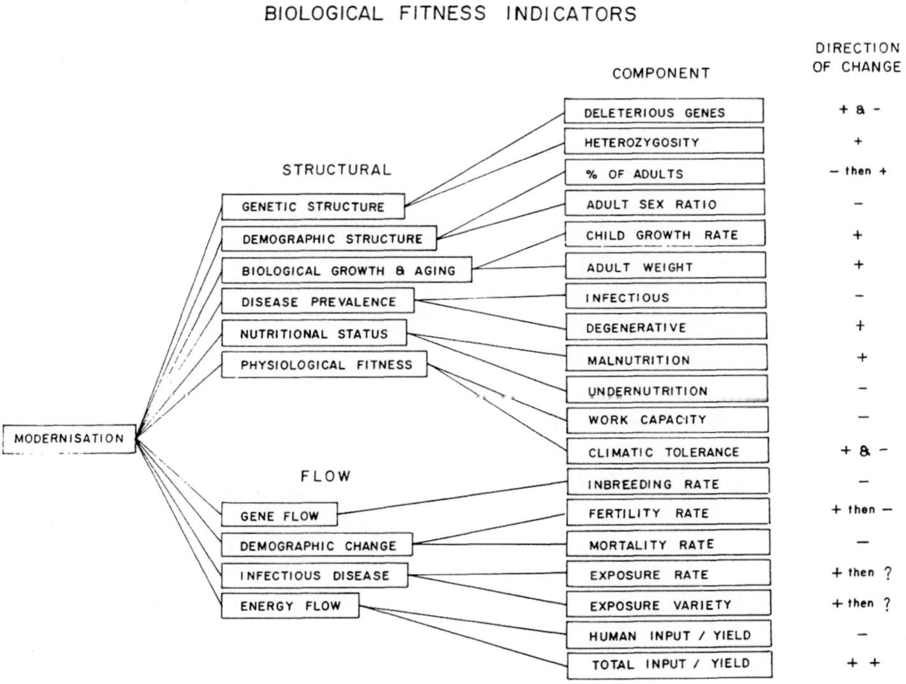

BIOLOGICAL FITNESS INDICATORS

STRUCTURAL	COMPONENT	DIRECTION OF CHANGE
	DELETERIOUS GENES	+ & −
	HETEROZYGOSITY	+
GENETIC STRUCTURE	% OF ADULTS	− then +
DEMOGRAPHIC STRUCTURE	ADULT SEX RATIO	−
BIOLOGICAL GROWTH & AGING	CHILD GROWTH RATE	+
DISEASE PREVALENCE	ADULT WEIGHT	+
NUTRITIONAL STATUS	INFECTIOUS	−
PHYSIOLOGICAL FITNESS	DEGENERATIVE	+
	MALNUTRITION	+
	UNDERNUTRITION	−
	WORK CAPACITY	−
MODERNISATION	CLIMATIC TOLERANCE	+ & −
FLOW	INBREEDING RATE	−
GENE FLOW	FERTILITY RATE	+ then −
DEMOGRAPHIC CHANGE	MORTALITY RATE	−
INFECTIOUS DISEASE	EXPOSURE RATE	+ then ?
ENERGY FLOW	EXPOSURE VARIETY	+ then ?
	HUMAN INPUT / YIELD	−
	TOTAL INPUT / YIELD	+ +

Figure 3. Effects of modernization on biologic fitness. After Baker [1].

72

mented repeatedly in emerging populations. Behind and associated with the biologic trends are a vast array of cultural and psycho-social changes. the overall result is paradoxical. Mortality declines and life expectancy increases, but biologic fitness deteriorates. Risk factors for cardiovascular disease appear, and middle-age mortality emerges.

Against such a kaleidoscopic background, any single hypothesis about the relationship of environment and biologic change becomes unprovable. Even when the data show the expected relationship, the interaction of other variables prevents any final statement of cause and effect. This, then, is the central limitation on studies of free living human societies. Some strategies for reducing the uncertainties of confounding variables have been devised. These include *1.* the study of relatively static populations, *2.* the accumulation of large data bases in interdisciplinary projects, *3.* data analysis based on a multivariate mathemetical models, and *4.* studies of migrants in relation to non-migrants. The special needs of studying genetic/environmental interaction also require studies of extended kindreds (rather than random population samples) in contrasting environments. Final conclusions are obtained, if ever, only from carefully controlled experiments based on hypotheses generated by population studies.

Turning to blood pressure determinants in populations, many investigators have been attracted by the psycho-social hypothesis that relates rising blood pressure to the direct emotional stress of acculturation. The results of several multidisciplinary studies of culture change and blood pressure have thus far suggested that physical and dietary factors are far more potent as determinants of blood pressure than are various indicators of sociocultural mobility and psycho-social stress, at least in the early stages of culture change [3, 16, 20]. Further study of social stress factors should, of course, be encouraged to continue, and to improve and refine methodologies.

Body mass and electrolyte intake remain the two environmental determinants of blood pressure for which the most impressive evidence has accrued. Low blood pressure populations are generally lean and active, with little or no tendency for weight to increase with age. In addition, all low blood pressure populations that have been well studied habitually use diets that tend to be low in sodium and high in potassium; there are no exceptions to this that have ever been well documented. This is an important part of the evidence supporting the importance of dietary electrolytes as determinants of blood pressure. With acculturation, westernized dietary items progressively supplant traditional foods. Consumption of sugar, flour, meat, and fat increase. Total caloric intake increases and physical activity diminishes, with a consequent increase in body weight and fatness. Salt use also increase. Often these changes occur simultaneously, making interpretation difficult. Fortunately, there are a few populations in which some of these changes occur independently or sequentially.

Both weight and other measures of body mass are highly correlated with blood pressure in all populations studied throughout the world [6, 24]. The relationship is not concerned only with obesity. Correlations of blood pressure with body mass are as strong in lean and normotensive populations as in the obese, and even hold true in the unacculturated 'low blood pressure populations.'

Figure 4 shows body weight in three sub-populations of Samoans. Western Samoans are unacculturated, those in American Samoa and in Hawaii are progressively more Westernized. Heights of the three groups are not significantly different, but weight differences are dramatic [2]. mean blood pressures at different ages in these same three groups (Figure 5) range from among the lowest

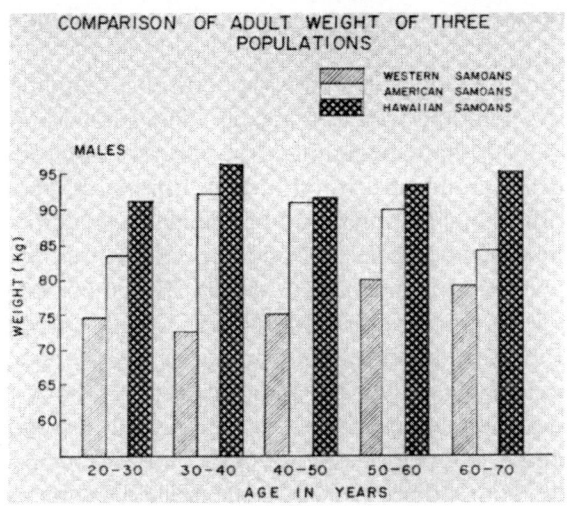

Figure 4. Adult weight in three populations of Samoan males. [2].

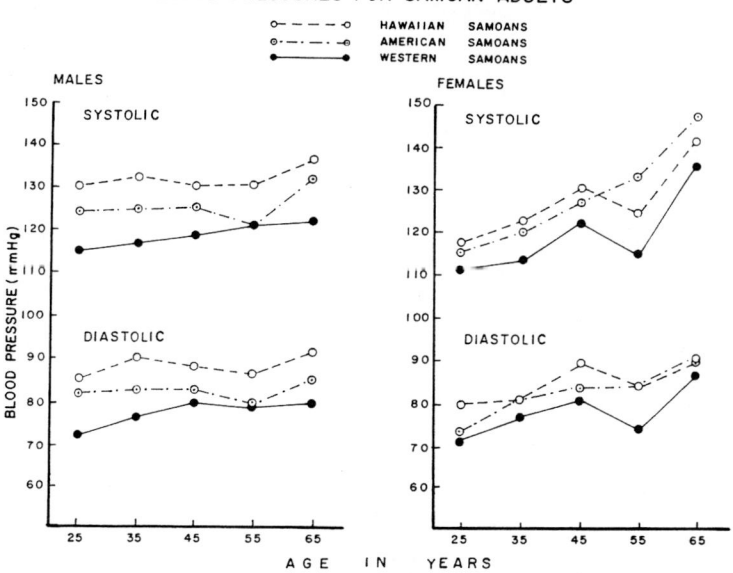

Figure 5. Mean blood pressure by deciles of age for three populations of adult Samoan males [2].

74

in the world in Western Samoa to among the highest in Hawaii. Polynesians seem
to be racially and/or culturally disposed toward obesity as an early result of
culture change.

Parenthetically, the available studies of maximum oxygen consumption in
unacculturated persons show very high values, denoting excellent fitness [2, 18].

Work capacity among a group of highly acculturated Samoans is strikingly
poor, as compared to other groups, including Americans, whose physical fitness
is usually considered to be poor (Figure 6). The interrelations of body mass, blood
pressure, and measures of physical fitness are only now beginning to be studied in
populations.

Colleagues and I are now analyzing follow-up data on Solomon Islands subjects
first studied between eight and twelve years ago. The Nagovisi of Bougainville,
when first studied in 1970, where beginning to acculturate, salt use had increased,
and they were showing an upward trend in blood pressure among the women
only. They were at that time lean, with no tendency for weight to increase with
age. By 1978, both males and females had shown a striking rise in blood pressure
associated with an average 4 kg increase in weight. Blood pressures of the same
Nagovisi men eight years apart are shown in Figure 7. Data such as these and the
strong intrapopulation correlations of body mass and blood pressure in all populations studies strongly suggest that the biologic effect of body mass on blood
pressure does not depend very much, if at all, on genetic susceptibility.

Because the primitive populations of the world are all changing so fast, it is
hard to find control populations that are not changing with time. However,

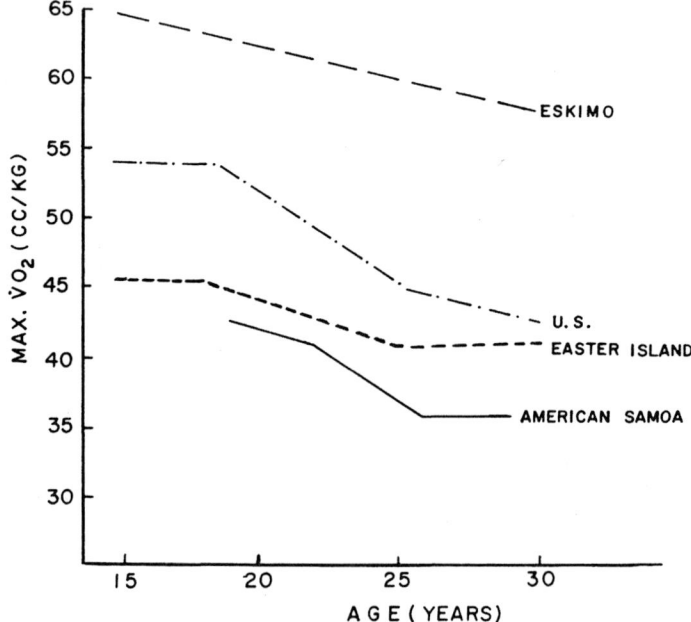

Figure 6. Maximal oxygen consumption in adult males from different population samples [2].

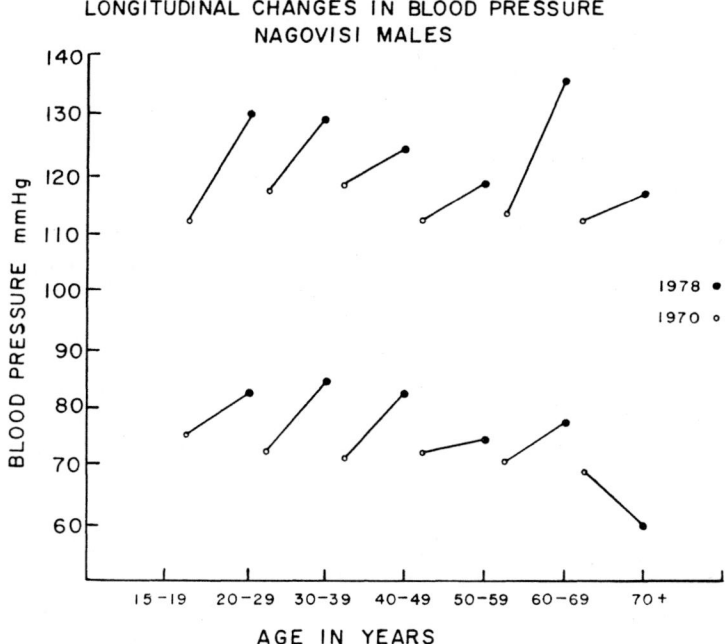

LONGITUDINAL CHANGES IN BLOOD PRESSURE
NAGOVISI MALES

Figure 7. Changes in blood pressure over eight years in Nagovisi men, Bougainville Island.

occasional examples remain. The Kwaio of the Solomon Islands were unacculturated primitives in 1966, and remained unchanged in culture in 1980, fourteen years later. They had not gained weight nor changed their diet. As shown in Figure 8, blood pressure in the same individuals twelve years apart remained virtually unchanged.

Data on the relationship of blood pressure and body mass in man are abundant and consistent. The physiologic mechanism nevertheless remains obscure, and good data on an animal model are lacking.

Data on the relationship between blood pressure and dietary sodium in humans have accumulated slowly and by fits and starts. Sodium excess regularly causes hypertension in several species of animals [10, 19]. In rats, wide variability in genetic susceptibility to sodium has been demonstrated [10]. In susceptible animals, sodium excess characteristically causes a slow inexorable rise in blood pressure which, once established, becomes irreversible. In the Dahl sensitive strain the young animal is more sensitive than the adult, and may go on to develop hypertension after even a brief exposure to excess sodium in infancy [11]. Yet the animal will remain normotensive throughout life if it is never exposed to excessive sodium. Large amounts of potassium seem to have some modifying effect on hypertension and its complications in this model [12].

The evidence now available from epidemiologic studies seems consistently to support the hypothesis that human populations resemble animals in their response to excessive sodium, with wide individual differences in genetic suscep-

76

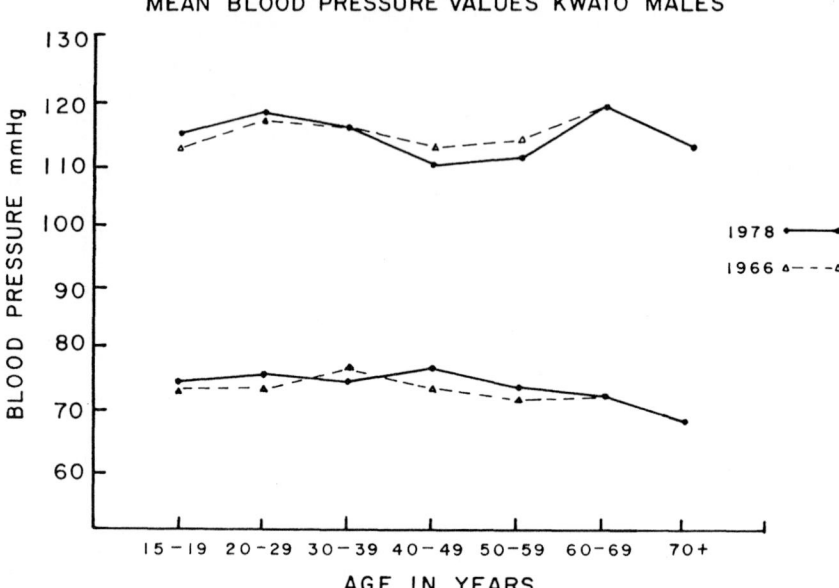

MEAN BLOOD PRESSURE VALUES KWAIO MALES

Figure 8. Comparison of blood pressure twelve years apart in Kwaio men of Malaita (Solomon Islands).

tibility. But more and better data are needed, using improved methodology and including potassium excretion, which has been little studied until recently.

Quantitative data on sodium intake or excretion in populations are still rather slim. Among truly 'low blood pressure populations', the most reliable data available are summarized in Table 1. Sodium excretion is below 70 mEq. per day in all except the Tarahumara Indians recently studied by Connor et al. [7], who average 85 mEq/day. The Tarahumara are exceptionally athletic and active people who live at an altitude of 8000 feet and often run as much as 200 miles in competitive games lasting several days.

Among the eight Solomon Island groups that we have studied, the five groups with low blood pressure had sodium intakes between 10 and 50 mEq/day, whereas in the three others blood pressure was rising somewhat with age at a median

Table 1. Hypertension and atherosclerosis in primitive and acculturating societies

Society	Sodium mEq/24 hrs
Yanomamo Indians, Brazil	± 1.5
Tukisenta, New Guinea	± 15
Kwaio, Baegu, Aita, Solomon Islands	10–15
Pukapuka, Cook Islands	± 65
Samburu, Uganda	± 50
Ontong Java, Solomon Islands	50
Tarahumara, Mexico	± 85

In 'Hypertension Updata', edited and published by Dialogues in Hypertension, Hunt, J.C. et al. 1980, p.6.

sodium intake of ±100 mEq/day in two, and rising more strongly at an intake of 150–230 mEq. in the third. Weight was falling with age in all eight Solomon groups. According to Shaper's study of Samburu warriors who entered the Army in Kenya, dietary sodium increased from 50 to 275 mEq/day [29]. Blood pressure in these young men (Figure 9) rose progressively from the second through the sixth year without associated weight change. We found rising blood pressure correlated with sodium excretion in the absence of weight gain in the Qash'qai Nomads of Iran [23]. Prior et al. [26] found independent effects of weight and sodium intake on blood pressure in Cook islanders. Extremely high prevalences of hypertension have been reported in Japanese [27] and Korean [15] populations in which sodium intake exceeds 300 mEq/day. There is, therefore, a considerable and consistent body of data supporting the role of sodium as an important blood pressure determinant, independent of the effects of body weight and accultura-tion. The several determinants may act independently at times, and may interact as well.

Many acculturating populations are increasing in weight and sodium intake simultaneously. Some, like the Solomon islanders, increase salt only at first and weight second. In the Tokelau islanders who have remained on the home island, the effect on blood pressure of weight gain alone is seen without excessive sodium intake [27]. As shown in Figure 10, the Tokelau women, in particular, are rather fat and gain weight progressively with age, yet sodium excretion remains in the range of 30 to 50 mEq/day. Blood pressure rises with age in Tokelau, especially in females. The main change is in systolic pressure, and the incidence of diastolic hypertension is very small.

High sodium intake in the absence of acculturation and weight gain is the

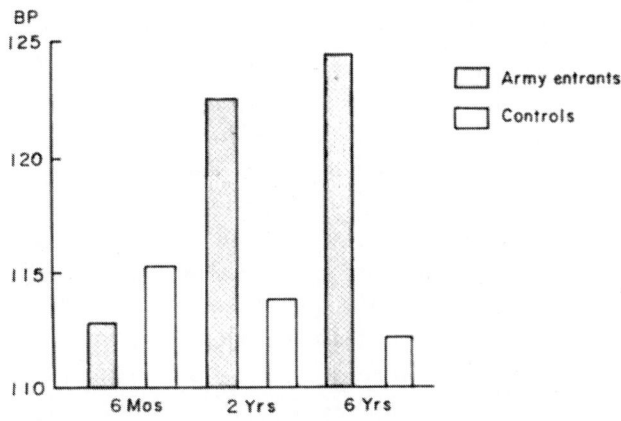

Figure 9. Changes in systolic blood pressure in Samburu men who entered the Kenyan Army, compared with age-matched controls. After Shaper et al. [29].

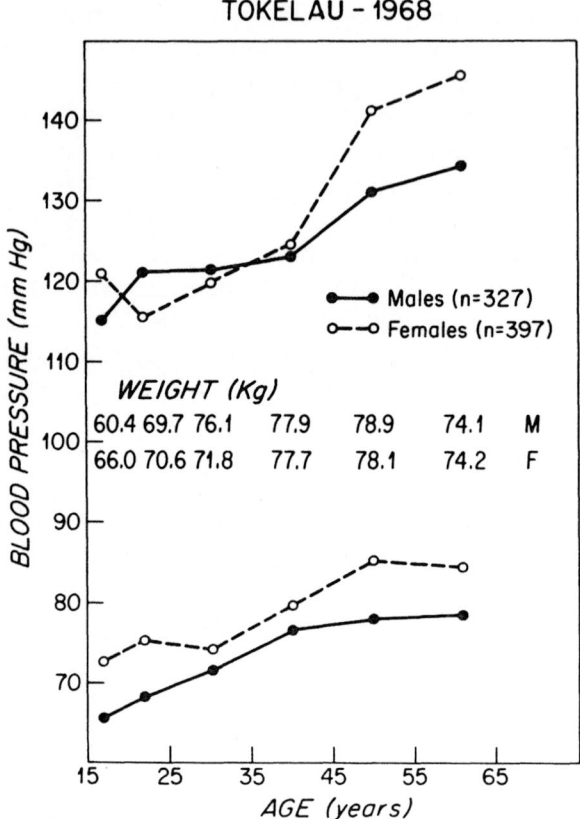

Figure 10. Mean systolic and diastolic blood pressure of Tokelau islanders by deciles of age. Prepared from data of Prior et al. [27].

obverse combination. This is seen in the Qash'gai nomads of Iran (Figure 11). The Qash'gai show no rise in weight with age, but sodium excretion is 150–190 mEq/ day. Blood pressure rises with age and correlates directly with sodium excretion. In comparison with the Tokelau, the level of diastolic pressure in the Qash'gai is higher, and prevalence of hypertension is greater.

The evidence relating sodium intake to blood pressure is based largely on comparisons between populations. Unlike the blood pressure/body mass relationship, intrapopulation studies have usually failed to show a correlation between sodium excretion and blood pressure of individuals. There may be methodologic reasons for this, and indeed blood pressure and sodium or Na/K ratio are correlated in several recent studies [4, 15, 23]. But if human subjects vary in their susceptibility to sodium as rats do, it is not surprising that this relationship is not seen consistently in random subjects all of whom are on a high sodium intake. It would clearly be of great value to know who is and who is not sensitive in the population.

Recently, Pietenen et al. [25] reported a study of normotensive adults whose

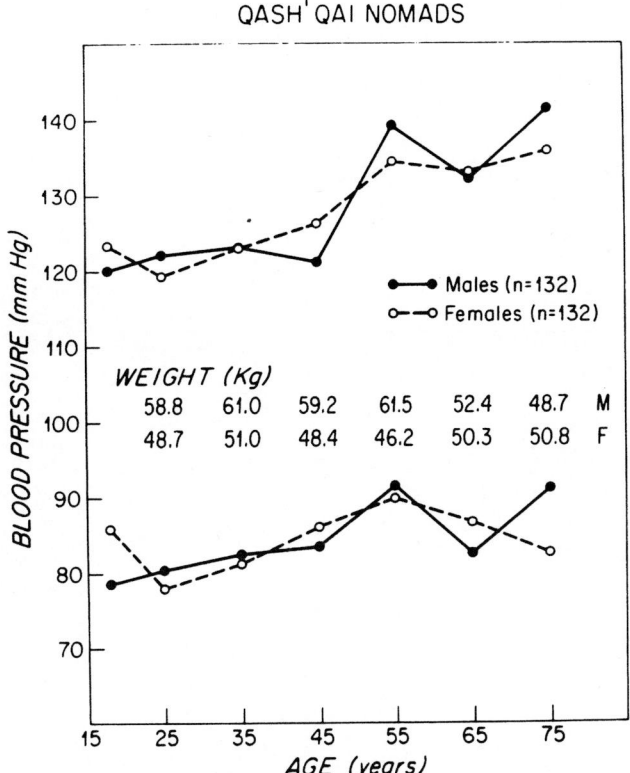

Figure 11. Mean systolic and diastolic blood pressure of Qash'gai nomads, southern Iran, by deciles of age.

first-degree relatives were hypertensive, and a similar normotensive group with no family history of hypertension. Twenty-four hour sodium excretion in the group with the positive family history correlated closely with blood pressure ($p<0.001$), whereas no correlation was found in the other group. (Figure 12) A similarly excellent correlation between blood pressure and Na/K ratio was found only in the group whose family history was positive for hypertension. In addition, there was high correlation between body weight and blood pressure, again confined to the group with the positive family history. It is noteworthy that a close relationship was found between weight and sodium excretion in both groups. Pietenen's study, if confirmed, seems to strike toward the heart of the problem, and suggests further experiments that may help to clarify these relationships.

One more topic remains to the considered. Does the human infant resemble the Dahl rat in having a greater susceptibility to the effects of sodium (and possibly weight gain) than the adult? Once upward tracking of blood pressure has become established in childhood, is it reversible, or is it inexorable? The answers to these questions is unknown at present, but should be taken into consideration in any study of the feasibility of primary prevention.

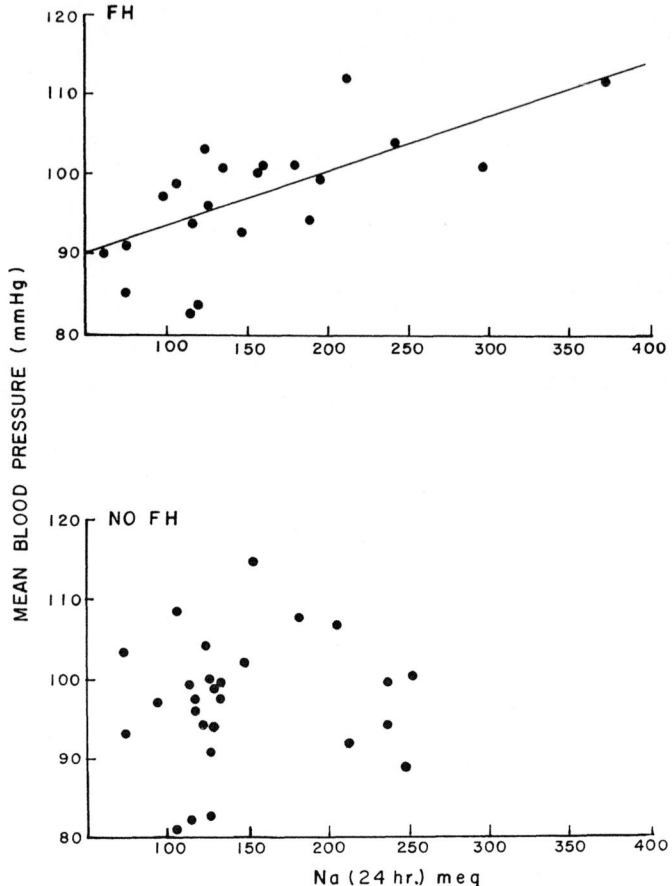

Figure 12. Relation of 24-hr sodium excretion to mean blood pressure. The upper panel shows data on normotensive subjects with a family history of hypertension. The lower panel shows data on similar subjects with no family history of hypertension. The equation of the linear relationship is $Y = 85.71 + 0.07X$. $r = 0.71$, $p < 0.001$. Modified from Pietenen et al. [25].

There are analogous situations, in which physiologic adaptations to environmental stress occur only during the developmental years. For example, in infants and children raised at high altitudes, respiratory and cardiovascular adaptations occur that enhance oxygen transport [14]. Persons who grow up at sea level cannot develop comparable adaptations even after living many years at high altitude. Other examples could also be adduced.

If a progressive 'hardening' of the blood pressure trend with age does occur in humans, preventive interventions such as reduction in dietary sodium and control of fatness will be progressively less effective as the population ages. Potentially, all susceptible persons may respond in the early years, but thereafter the response may be less, among fewer individuals. This is illustrated conceptually in Figure 13.

Sufficient evidence seems now to have accumulated to justify an attempt at

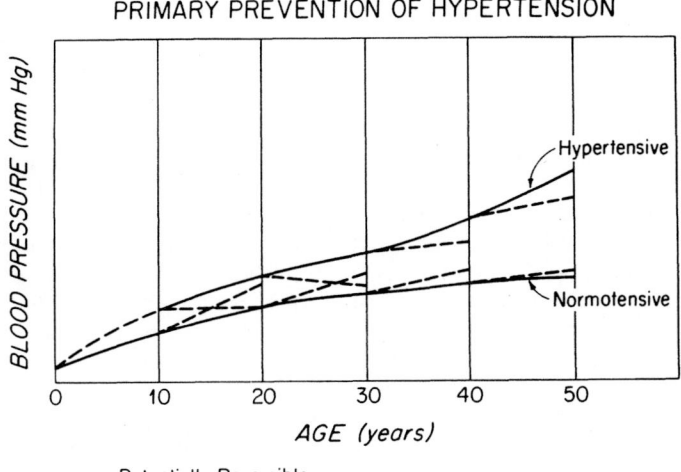

Figure 13. Conceptual representation of expected results of dietary intervention to prevent hypertension (see text for explanation).

primary prevention through dietary intervention. If such a study is truly well designed, it has the potential to answer many questions of fundamental physiologic importance, and if primary prevention is proved successful it has public health implications of truly great proportions.

REFERENCES

1. Baker PT: Migration and human adaptation. Proceedings of Seminar on Migration and Health, Wellington, N.Z (in press).
2. Baker PT, Hanna JM: Modernization and the biological fitness of Samoans. A progress report on a research program. In: Fleming C, Prior I (eds), Migration, Adaptation and Health in the Pacific. Wellington, N.Z, 1981.
3. Beaglehole R, Salmond CE, Hooper A, Huntsman J, Stanhope JM, Cassel JC, Prior IAM: Blood pressure and social interaction in Tokelauan migrants in New Zealand. J Chron Dis 30: 803, 1977.
4. Berenson GS, Voors A.W., Dalferes ER, Jr, Webber LS, Shulei SE. Creatinine clearance, electrolytes and plasma renin activity related to the blood pressure of white and black children – The Bogalusa Heart Study. J Lab Clin Med 93: 535, 1979.
5. Cassel JH: Studies of hypertension in migrants. In: Paul O (ed) Epidemiology and Control of Hypertension, pp 41. Stratton Intercontinental Medical Book Corp, New York, 1975.
6. Chiang BN, Perlman LV, Epstein FH: Overweight and hypertension – a review. Circulation 39: 403, 1969.
7. Connor WE, Argueira MT, Connor RW, Wallace RB, Molinow R, Casdorph HR: The plasma lipids, lipoproteins and diet of the Tarahumara Indians of Mexico. Am J Clin Nutr 31: 1131, 1978.
8. Cruz-Coke R, Etcheverry R, Nagel R: Influences of migration on blood pressure of Easter Islanders. Lancet 1: 697, 1964.

9. Cruz-Coke R, Donoso H, Berrera R: Genetic ecology of hypertension. Clin Sci Mol Med 45 (Suppl I): 55, 1973.
10. Dahl LK: Possible role of salt intake in the development of essential hypertension. Springer-Verlag, Berlin, 1960, p 53.
11. Dahl LK, Knudsen KD, Heine MA, Leith GJ: Effects of chronic excess salt ingestion, modification of experimental hypertension in the rat by variations in the diet. Circ Res 22: 11, 1968.
12. Dahl LK, Leith G, Heine M: Influence of dietary potassium and sodium/potassium molar ratio on the development of salt hypertension. J Exp Med 136: 318, 1972.
13. Epstein FH, Eckoff RD: The epidemiology of high blood pressure – geographic distributions and etiologic factors. In: Stamler J, Stamler R, Pullman TM (eds), Epidemiology of Hypertension. Grune & Stratton, New York, 1967.
14. Frisancho AP: Functional adaptation to high altitude hypoxia. Science 187: 313, 1975.
15. Kesteloot H, Song CS, Song JS, Park BC, Brems-Heyns E, Joosens JV: An epidemiologic survey of arterial plood pressure in Korea using home reading. In: Rorive G, Van Cauwenberge H (eds), The Arterial Hypertensive Disease. Mossen, Inc New York, 1976, p 141.
16. Labarthe D, Reed D, Brady J, Stallones R: Health effects of modernization in Palau. Am J Epidemiol 98: 61, 1973.
17. Maddocks I: Blood pressure in melanesians. Med J Austral 1: 1123, 1969.
18. Mann GV, Shaffer RD, Rich A: Physical fitness and immunity to heart disease in Masai. Lancet 2: 1308, 1965.
19. Meneely GR, Dahl LK: Electrolytes in hypertension: the effects of sodium chloride, the evidence from animal and human studies. Med Clin N Am 45: 271–283, 1961.
20. Page LB, Damon A, Moellering RC Jr: Antecedents of cardiovascular diseases in six Solomon Islands societies. Circulation 49: 1132, 1974.
21. Page LB: Epidemiologic evidence on the etiology of human hypertension and its possible prevention. Am Heart J 91: 527, 1976.
22. Page LB: Friedlaender J, Moellering RC Jr: Culture, human biology and disease in the Solomon Islands. In: Population structure and human variation, Cambridge University Press, Cambridge, 1977, p 143.
23. Page LB, Vandevert DE, Nader K, Lubin NK, Page JR: Blood pressure of Qash'gai Pastoral Nomads in Iran in relation to culture, diet, and body form. Am J Clin Nutr 34: 527, 1981.
24. Page LB: Dietary sodium and blood pressure: evidence from human studies. In: Lauer RM, Shekelle RB (eds), Childhood prevention of atherosclerosis and hypertension, Raven Press, New York, 1980, pp. 291–304.
25. Pietenen PE, Wong O, Altshul AM: Electrolyte output, blood pressure and family history of hypertension. Am J Clin Nutr 32: 997, 1979.
26. Prior IAM, Grimley-Evans J, Harvey HPB, Davidson F, Lindsey M: Sodium intake and blood pressure in two Polynesian populations. N Engl J Med 279: 515, 1968.
27. Prior IAM, Hooper A, Huntsman J, Stanhope JM, Salmond CE: The Tokelau Island migrant study. In: Harrison GA (ed), Population structure and human variation. Cambridge University Press, Cambridge, 1977, p 165.
28. Sasaki N: The relationship of salt intake to hypertension in the Japanese. Geriatrics 19: 735, 1964.
29. Shaper AG, Leonard PA, Jones KW, Jones M: Environmental effects on the body build, blood pressure, and blood chemistry of nomadic warriors serving in the Army in Kenya. E Afr Med J 46: 282, 1969.

III. THE CENTRAL ROLE OF THE KIDNEY

7. THE MECHANISM OF SODIUM-DEPENDENT LOW RENIN
    HYPERTENSION

F.J. HADDY, M.B. PAMNANI, D.L. CLOUGH

ROLE OF SALT IN HYPERTENSION

The influence of sodium chloride intake and excretion on blood pressure in
hypertensive subjects has been known for many years [17, 23, 24, 43, 60, 87].
Reduction in the dietary intake of salt or the administration of diuretics often
ameliorates hypertension, while increased salt intake or decreased excretion
often aggravates it. Certain studies suggest that salt also has a role in the genesis
of hypertension. Epidemiologic surveys reveal a higher incidence of hypertension
in acculturated societies, which ingest much salt, than in unacculturated societies,
which ingest little salt [23, 24, 71]. While a positive relationship between blood
pressure and the estimated level of sodium intake has been difficult to establish
within a society such as ours where intake is high, recent studies suggest that such
a relationship does in fact exist in normal subjects [29]. Furthermore, elevated
pressure can be induced in diabetic children [58] and normal adults [57, 64] by a
large increase in dietary salt intake over a short period of time. For example,
800 mEq/day for three days produces a significant rise in pressure in normal
adults [64]. There are no systematic studies on the effects on the blood pressure of
normotensive subjects of a more modest increase in salt intake over a prolonged
period of time, as occurs naturally. It may well be that only certain normotensive
subjects are susceptible to a high salt intake, just as only certain hypertensive
subjects respond to a low salt intake [18, 43].

Subtle abnormalities in the ability to excrete salt, perhaps genetic and age-
related, may determine individual susceptibility to a high salt intake. Black
subjects have a higher hypertensive morbidity and mortality and seem to be prone
to the low renin hypervolemic variety (see references in [54] and [12]). Normotensive black subjects excrete an acute intravenous sodium load over 24 hr less well
than normotensive white subjects [54, 55]. Blood pressure increases with age.
Normotensive subjects (mainly white) older than 40 years of age also excrete an
acute intravenous sodium load slowly when compared with normotensive subjects younger than 40 years [54].

This abnormality could result from functional or organic changes. For example, renal kallikrein (an enzyme that catalyzes the formation of kallidin, a
natriuretic, diuretic, and vasodilator peptide) is found by some investigators to be

Sambhi, M.P. (ed.) Fundamental fault in hypertension
© *1984, Martinus Nijhoff Publishers. Boston/The Hague/Dordrecht/Lancaster.*
ISBN 978-94-010-9006-3

excreted in lesser amount by normotensive black than by white normotensive subjects [52]. A decreased generation of kallidin for a given state of sodium balance might contribute to the blunted natriuretic response to sodium in normotensive black subjects. Nephrosclerosis increases with age [20, 42], and glomerular filtration rate decreases with age [80] in normotensive subjects. This too might contribute to the blunted natriuretic response. Regardless of the cause, blunted natriuresis for a given sodium load should result in increased sodium and water retention and hence higher blood pressure in black and aged subjects relative to white and young subjects. Normotensive black subjects do in fact respond to a large short-term increase in dietary salt intake with a greater blood pressure increase than normotensive white subjects [53]. Furthermore, following intravenous infusion of two liters of normal saline, blood pressure is significantly higher and plasma renin activity significantly lower in black subjects than in white subjects [54]. The higher prevalence of hypertension in the black population does not appear to be related to a greater dietary intake of sodium chloride as several groups have reported a similar intake of sodium in black compared to white subjects [28, 48, 54].

Excessive dietary sodium clearly raises pressure in animals, particularily when excretory function is impaired. Sapirstein et al. [81], Meneely et al. [59], Koletsky [45], and Dahl[17] were among the first to show that the common laboratory rat develops hypertension when fed excessive sodium chloride. In susceptible animals, blood pressure rises slowly over a period of months and is proportional to the amount of sodium chloride in the diet. A significant increase in pressure can occur with amounts comparable to those found in acculturated societies [17, 61]. The response is much more consistent and rapid if the ability to excrete salt is impaired by removal of both kidneys, removal of 70% of the renal mass, compression of the kidney, or administration of mineralocorticoids [46, 87]. Dahl [17, 18] puzzled over the inconsistency of the response in normal rats and then demonstrated a genetic substrate for sodium-dependent hypertension in this species. Through selective breeding, he developed two strains, one that regularly develops salt hypertension at an accelerated rate, and another that is insensitive to salt. Other studies suggest that the genetic defect in the susceptible animals is an inability to excrete salt normally [88], perhaps because of decreased papillary blood flow [26] subsequent to a deficiency in renal kallikrein [8]. The normal chicken, rabbit, dog, and monkey also slowly develop hypertension on a high salt intake [11, 25, 50, 91]. As in the rat, the dog and monkey can be made more sensitive to salt by reducing renal mass [11, 49]; blood pressure then rises more rapidly and to higher levels.

MECHANISM OF SALT EFFECT

The mechanism of the effect of sodium chloride on blood pressure is not clear.

The increased pressure does not seem to result from an immediate direct effect of the salt on blood vessels, as elevation of the sodium chloride concentration in the blood of isolated perfused vascular beds or in the bath surrounding isolated blood vessels causes relaxation rather than contraction (just as occurs when osmolality is raised with other agents, such as dextrose) (see references in Haddy [31]). Other studies suggest that the increased pressure is related to the increase in extracellular fluid volume rather than to the increase in salt. In the dog, alteration of extracellular salt while holding extracellular volume constant has little effect on pressure [36, 66]. On the other hand, in hypertensive man, a 1.5 liter expansion of extracellular fluid volume over a 60 to 90 min period with a 5% solution of glucose in water is associated with a 31% increase in mean arterial pressure [21].

The time-course of the changes in total peripheral resistance and arterial pressure following increase and decrease in volume suggests a slowly acting indirect mechanism [33]. The changes in resistance and pressure are too slow for classic overperfusion autoregulation, and too fast for vascular restructuring such as muscular hypertrophy [33]. They are in the wrong direction to implicate the renin-angiotensin-aldosteron [44, 64, 77] or the sympathico-adrenal systems [56, 79], i.e., plasma renin activity, aldosterone concentration, and catecholamine concentration all decrease as a function of dietary salt intake. There are, therefore, reasons to search for other mechanisms in the genesis of the increases in total peripheral resistance and arterial pressure that follow a high intake of dietary sodium or other procedures (administration of mineralocorticoids, reduction of renal mass, removal of one kidney and stenosis of the opposite artery, etc.) which produce low-renin, presumably volume-expanded hypertension.

UNKNOWN HUMORAL AGENT

Certain studies in the old and recent literature suggest the presence of an unknown slowly acting pressor agent in the blood. In 1940, Solandt et al. cross-circulated blood between two dogs, one with one-kidney, one-clip or one-kidney, one wrapped hypertension, and the other smaller and acutely nephrectomized but normotensive (Figure 1), and found that pressure rose in the small acutely nephrectomized animal (Figure 2). The pressor response was delayed in onset, taking about one hour to appear. In 1953, Gordon et al. circulated blood for 30 to 60 min between two rabbits, one with one-kidney, one-clip hypertension, and the other salt-loaded but normotensive, and found that pressure rose in the normotensive salt-loaded assay rabbit (Figure 3). Again, the response was delayed in onset and prolonged. The maximum rise in pressure was not reached for two to three hours after completion of the 30–60 min cross circulation. Gordon was unable to reproduce these results at a later date (personal communication).

In 1965, Hinke noted that plasma from rats with one-kidney, DOCA, salt hypertension increased the vasoconstrictor response of an isolated perfused rat

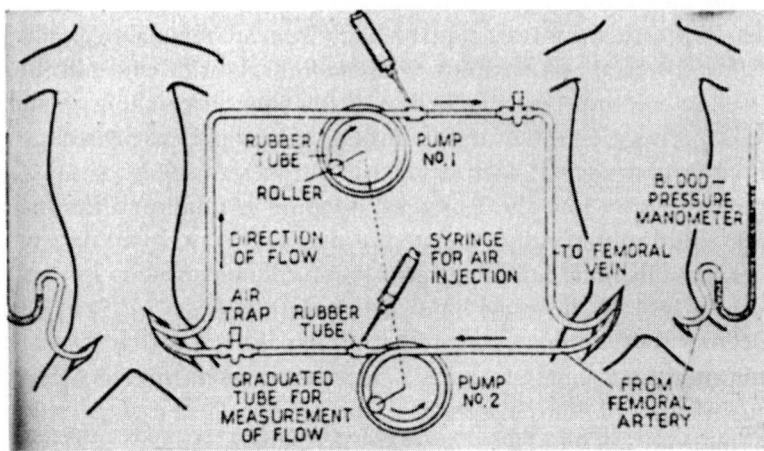

Figure 1. Cross-circulation method used by Solandt et al. [85] to search for a humoral pressor agent in one-kidney, one-clip hypertension in dogs. Hypertensive animal on the left, normotensive acutely nephrectomized small bioassay animal on the right.

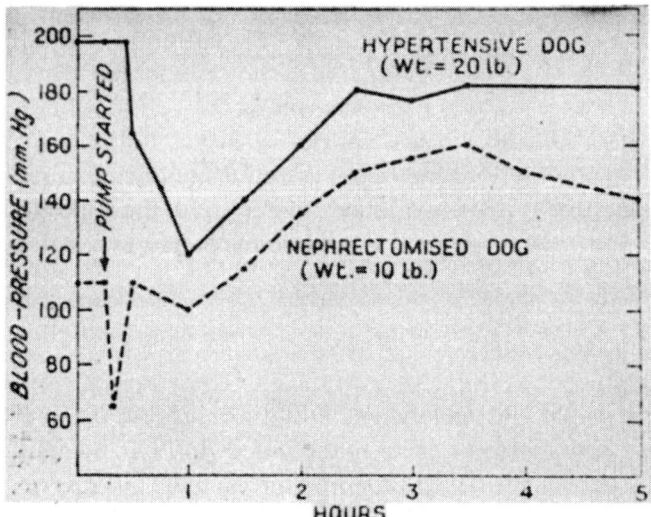

Figure 2. Findings of Solandt et al. [85] in one experiment. Note that the pressor response in the small nephrectomized bioassay animal appeared one hour after establishment of cross circulation.

tail artery to norepinephrine. Something in the plasma made the vessel more sensitive to norepinephrine. In 1969, Dahl et al. placed their salt-resistant rat in parabiosis with their salt-sensitive rat, and found that the resistant rat also developed hypertension when both animals were fed salt (Figure 4) or when one-kidney, one-clip hypertension was induced in the sensitive strain (Figure 5). Something crossed from one animal to the other. The authors speculated that a common pathogenic mechanism exists in both salt and renal hypertension, and suggested that many of the apparent anomalies of the angiotensin-aldosterone

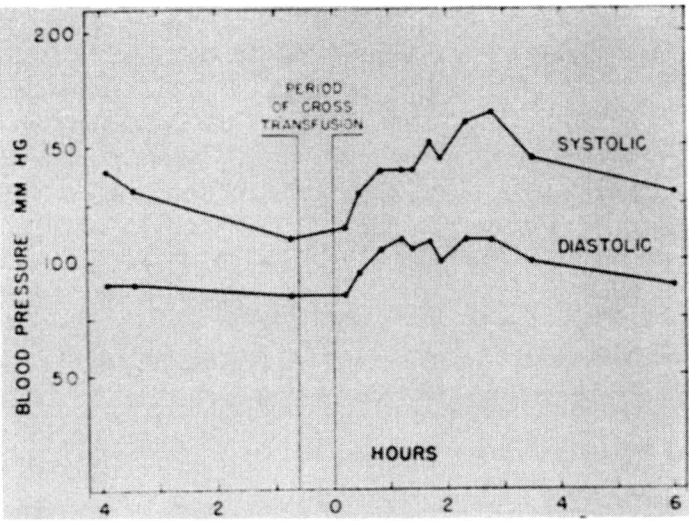

Figure 3. Blood pressure response in bioassay rabbit following cross circulation of blood from a rabbit with one-kidney, one-clip hypertension. Note that the pressor response was delayed in onset and prolonged. From Gordon et al. [27].

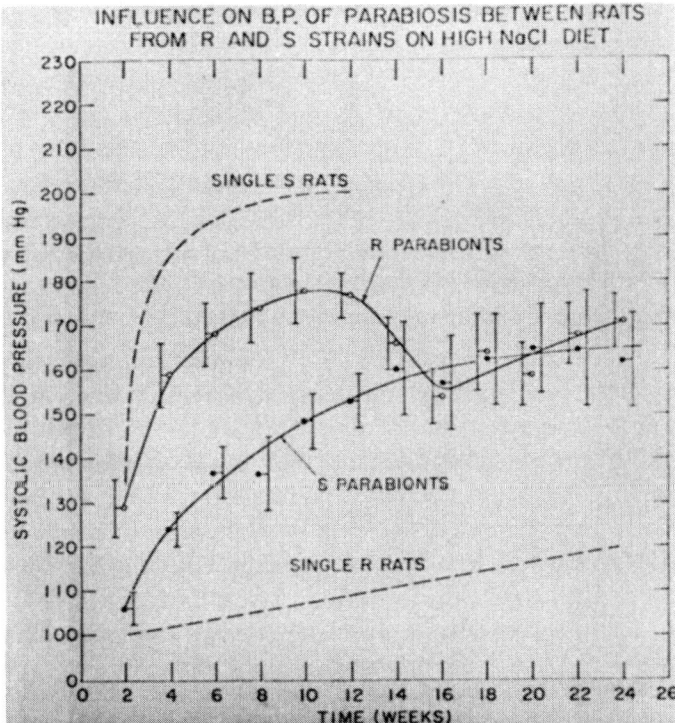

Figure 4. Effect of salt feeding on blood pressure of the Dahl salt-resistant rat (R) when in parabiosis with the Dahl salt-sensitive rat (S). Both rats were fed salt. Taken from Dahl et al. [19].

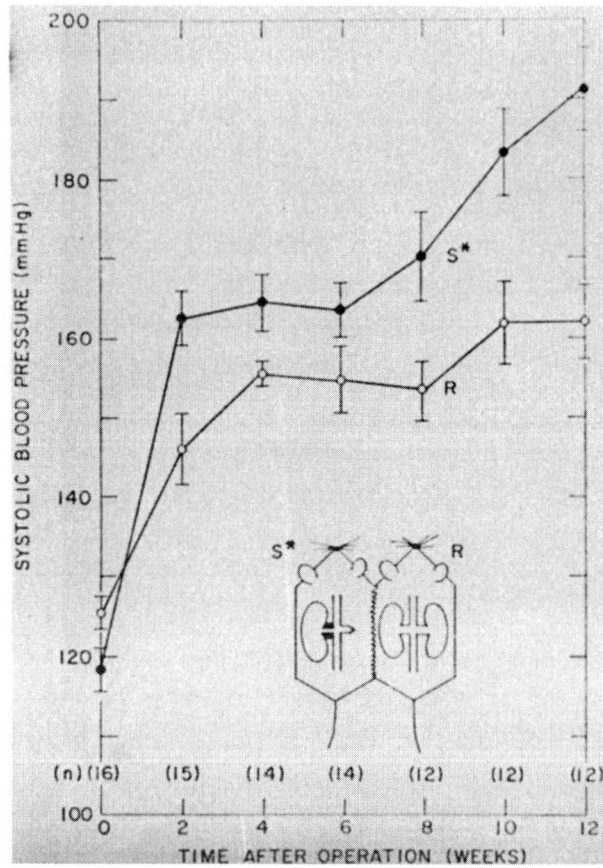

Figure 5. Effect of one-kidney, one-clip hypertension in the Dahl S rat on blood pressure in the Dahl R rat during parabiosis. Taken from Dahl et al. [19].

system in hypertension could be explained if a sodium-excreting hormone were postulated that had the capacity of also inducing hypertension when produced by a hypertension-prone subject.

In 1972, Mizukoshi and Michelakis [63] reported that plasma from hypertensive subjects, particularily those with low-renin essential hypertension, slowly raised the blood pressure and increased the pressor responses to angiotensin and norepinephrine in an assay rat. In 1975, their group [62] showed that the same was the case for plasma from dogs with one-kidney, one-clip hypertension, and that the active plasma factor appeared to be a polypeptide or a small protein. Injection of 15 μl of hypertensive plasma into the pentolinium-treated, nephrectomized rat produced a slow, prolonged increase in pressure and also increased the pressor response to angiotensin (Figure 6). More recently, they [39] extended their studies to rats with one-kidney, one-clip hypertension and to dogs with one-kidney, one wrapped hypertension, and showed that plasma from the rats also

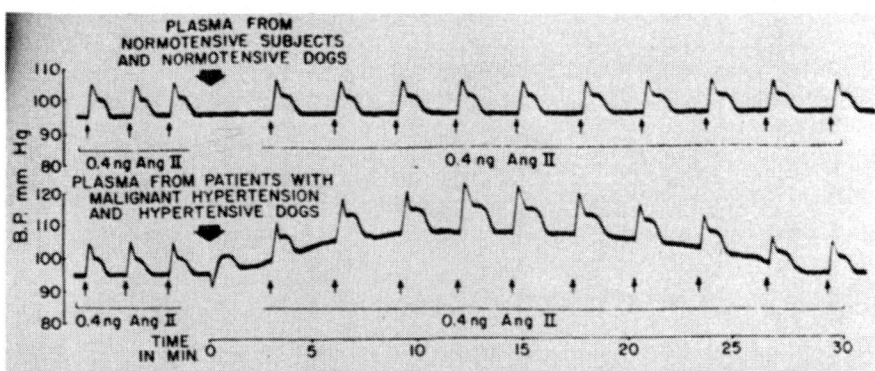

Figure 6. Effect of plasma from a dog with one-kidney, one-clip hypertension on the blood pressure and pressor response to angiotension in a bioassay rat. Taken from Michelakis et al. [62].

contains a factor with slow pressor and sensitizing activity. Plasma from the dogs increased the vasoconstrictor response to norepinephrine in small mesenteric arteries isolated from rats. Fractionation of the plasma showed the active substance to have a molecular weight of about 1000. While it is not easy to understand how the activity in 15 μl plasma, when injected intravenously in a whole rat, could produce a rise in blood pressure and an increase in pressor sensitivity, the findings have been confirmed by another group of investigators using plasma from other models of hypertension.

Meneely's group [83] used the Michelakis technique to show that serum from rats with salt hypertension also contains a factor that enhances the pressor sensitivity to norepinephrine (Figure 7). The activity of the agent is slow in onset and continues for at least three hours. It is heat-stable and active after repeated freezing and thawing. More recently, the group showed that 20 μl serum from SHR fed a diet containing 1.0 to 1.25% sodium chloride potentiates the pressor effect of norepinephrine when injected into the bioassay animals [2].

Bloom et al. [5] reported a similar effect of plasma from patients with normal renin essential hypertension, i.e., plasma perfused through an isolated femoral artery from a rabbit increased the vasoconstrictor response to norepinephrine. Kurz et al. [47] found a similar effect of blood from rabbits with 3-day old one-kidney, one-clip hypertension, i.e., infusion of 41 ml blood from these animals into bioassay rabbits made the bioassay animals more sensitive to the pressor action of intravenously injected norepinephrine (blood from control animals did not).

Finally Tobian et al. [89] recently reported that perfusion of kidneys from normal rats with blood from Dahl salt-sensitive rats results in 16% higher renal vascular resistance than perfusion with blood from Dahl salt-resistant rats.

Thus it appears that we must seriously consider the possible role of an unknown slowly acting humoral pressor, vasoconstrictor, and sensitizing agent in the genesis of salt and other varieties of low renin hypertension.

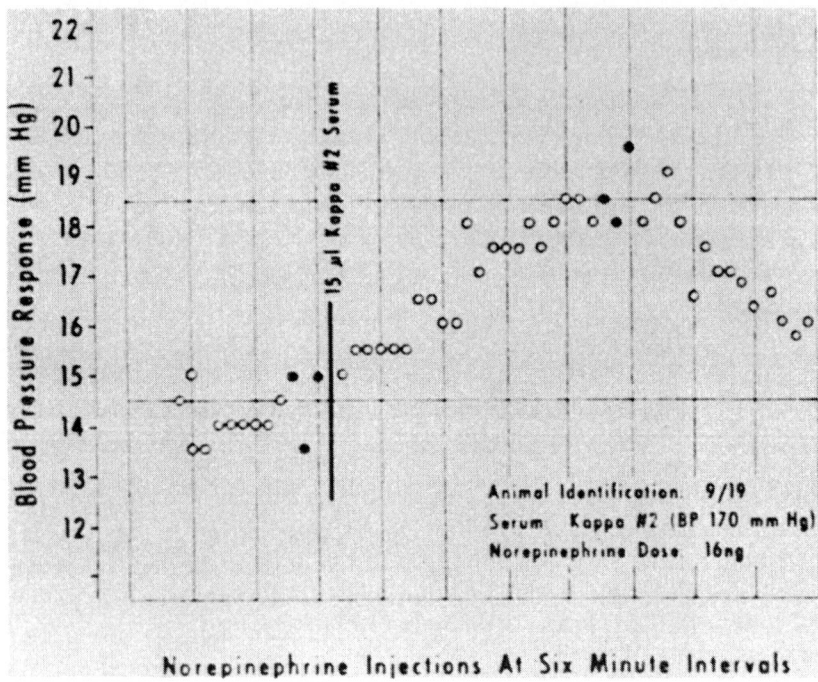

Figure 7. Effect of plasma from a common laboratory rat with salt hypertension on the blood pressure response to norepinephrine in a bioassay rat. Each point represents the response to injection of norepinephrine. Taken from Self et al. [83].

SUPPRESSED SODIUM-POTASSIUM PUMP

Other studies suggest that the cellular sodium-potassium pump is suppressed in cardiovascular muscle, again by a humoral agent, and that this suppression can at least in part explain the increased pressure and pressor sensitivity to vasoactive agents. The evidence for pump suppression comes from three sources. First, potassium vasodilation, which we showed results from stimulation of the sodium-potassium pump [9, 10], is suppressed in the forelimb of the dog with one-kidney, one wrapped hypertension [67, 68, 69]. Second, ouabain-sensitive rubidium uptake (Figure 8), a measure of sodium-potassium pump activity, is suppressed in arteries from dogs with one-kidney, one wrapped hypertension [70] (Figure 9), rats with one-kidney, one clip hypertension [75], rats with one-kidney, DOCA, salt hypertension [73] (Figure 10), and rats with reduced renal mass hypertension [75]. Third, the activity of Na^+, K^+-ATPase (Figure 11), the enzyme that drives the sodium-potassium pump, is suppressed in microsomes prepared from the left ventricle of rats with one-kidney, one clip hypertension [15, 16] (Figure 12), one kidney, DOCA, salt hypertension [13] (Figure 13), reduced renal mass hypertension [14], and acute renoprival hypertension [65].

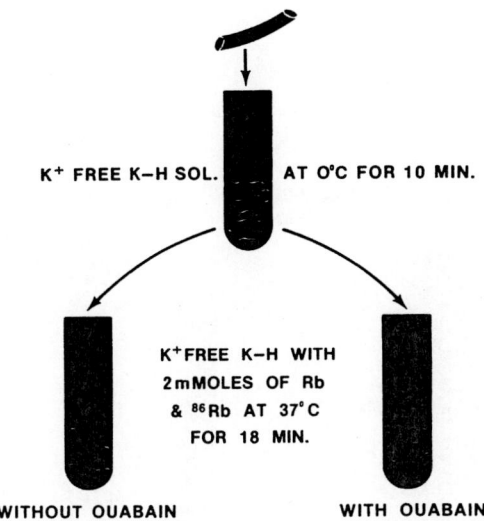

K+ FREE K–H SOL.   AT O°C FOR 10 MIN.

K+FREE K–H WITH
2mMOLES OF Rb
& 86Rb AT 37°C
FOR 18 MIN.

WITHOUT OUABAIN   WITH OUABAIN

TOTAL UPTAKE — NONSPECIFIC UPTAKE = SPECIFIC UPTAKE

(OUABAIN ABSENT) (OUABAIN PRESENT)   (OUABAIN SENSITIVE)

Figure 8. 86Rb uptake method used to estimate Na+-K+ pump activity in arteries and veins of hypertensive and normotensive animals. From Overbeck et al. [70]; Pamnani et al. [73].

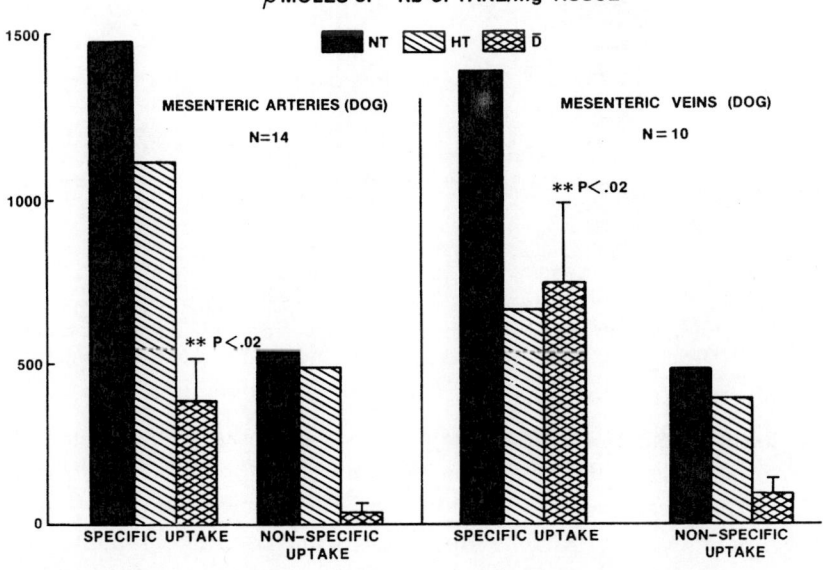

ρ MOLES of 86Rb UPTAKE/mg TISSUE

NT HT D̄

MESENTERIC ARTERIES (DOG)

N=14

MESENTERIC VEINS (DOG)

N = 10

** P<.02

** P<.02

SPECIFIC UPTAKE   NON–SPECIFIC UPTAKE   SPECIFIC UPTAKE   NON–SPECIFIC UPTAKE

Figure 9. 86Rb uptake by mesenteric arteries (left panel) and veins (right panel) in dogs with one-kidney, one-wrapped hypertension. Specific uptake: ouabain sensitive uptake; non-specific uptake: ouabain insensitive uptake; NT: normotensive control animals; HT: hypertensive animals; d: difference. Adapted from Overbeck et al., [70].

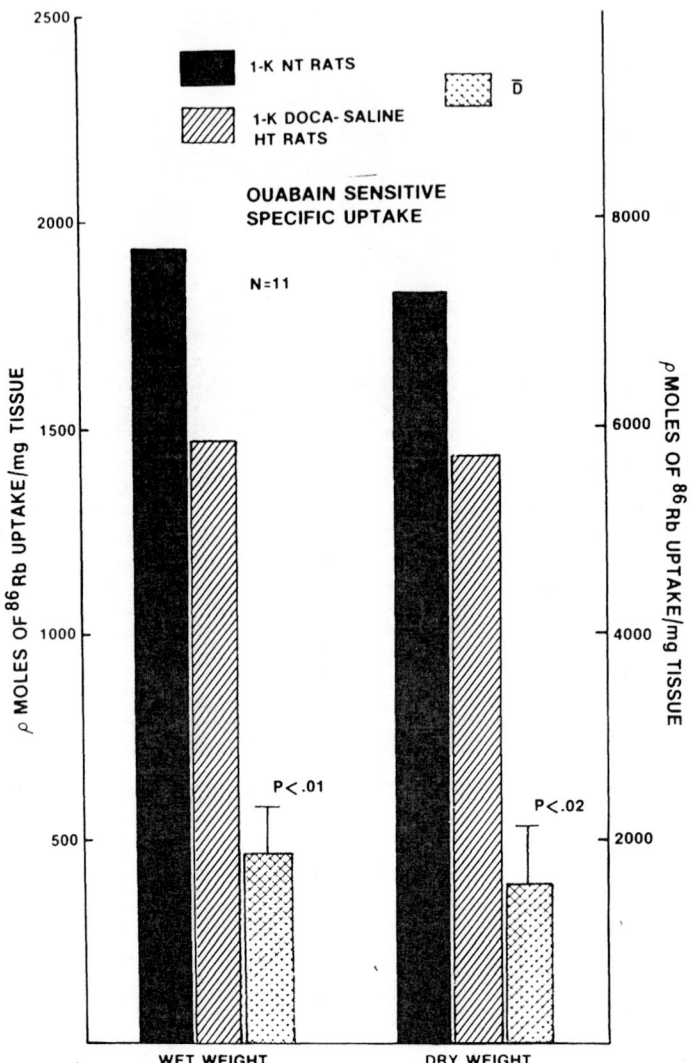

Figure 10. Ouabain-sensitive ^{86}Rb uptake by tail arteries in one-kidney, DOCA, salt hypertension, expressed both on a wet weight and dry weight basis. In both cases, left-hand bar: normotensive control animals; middle bar: hypertensive animals; right-hand bar: difference. From Pamnani et al. [73].

Several studies suggest that the pump suppression is not secondary to the elevated arterial pressure. Ouabain-sensitive rubidium uptake is also suppressed in the veins of the dog with one-kidney, one wrapped hypertension [70] (Figure 9) and Na^+, K^+-ATPase activity is also suppressed in microsomes obtained from the right ventricle of rats with one-kidney, one clip hypertension [16] (Figure 14). Efflux of radioactive potassium is increased in the portal vein of the rat with one-kidney, DOCA, salt hypertension [90], just as it is in the arteries [40, 41].

Other studies suggest that the pump suppression results from the volume

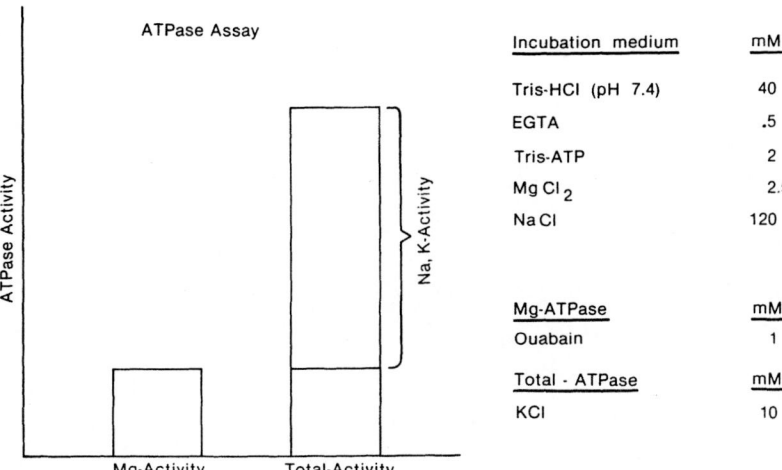

Figure 11. Method used by Clough to estimate Na⁺ K⁺-ATPase activity in left and right ventricular microsomes from hypertensive and normotensive animals. Na⁺, K⁺-ATPase activity is the difference in activity in the presence of potassium and with ouabain substituted for potassium.

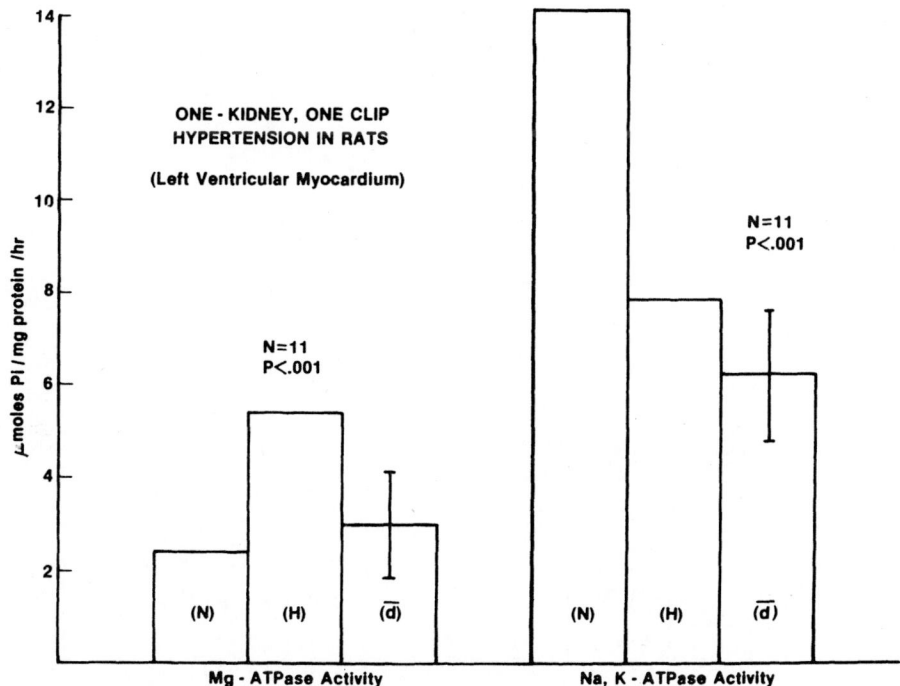

Figure 12. Na⁺, K⁺-ATPase activity in left ventricular microsomes of rats with one-kidney, one-clip hypertension. N: normotensive control animals; H: hypertensive animals; d: difference. Taken from Clough et al. [15]

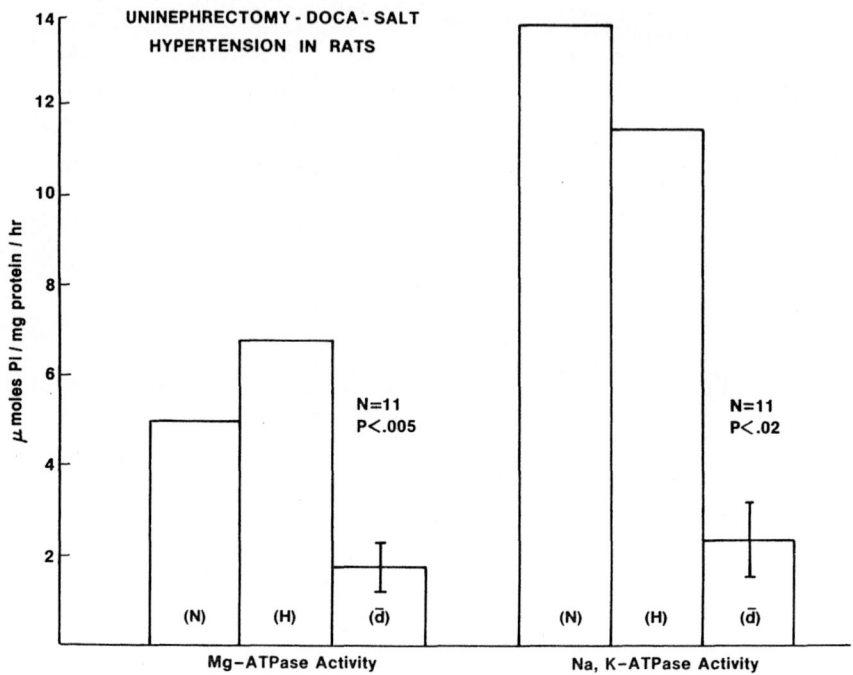

Figure 13. Na$^+$, K$^+$-ATPase activity in left ventricular microsomes of rats with one-kidney, DOCA, salt hypertension. Symbols as in Fig. 12. Taken from Clough et al. [13].

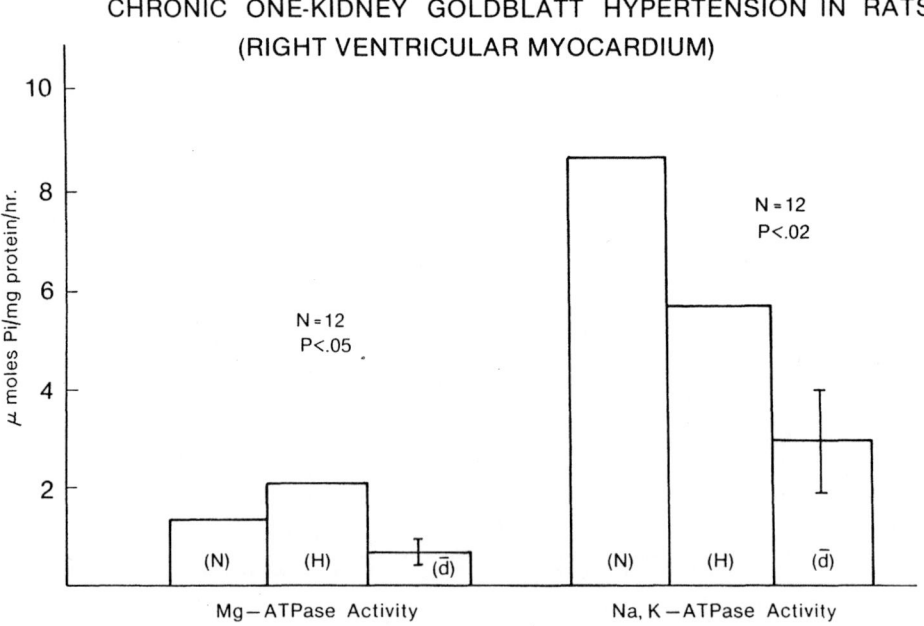

Figure 14. Na$^+$, K$^+$-ATPase activity in right ventricular microsomes of rats with one-kidney, one-clip hypertension. Symbols as in Fig. 12. Taken from Clough et al. [16].

expansion. Suppressed ouabain-sensitive rubidium uptake by arteries is not seen in two models of rat hypertension not considered to be volume expanded, namely SHR [72] and dexamethasone hypertension [73]. Furthermore, acute volume expansion per se mimics the pump changes seen in volume expanded hypertension i.e., saline loading reduces ouabain sensitive rubidium uptake by arteries of normal rats to roughly the same extent as seen in one-kidney, one clip and one-kidney, DOCA, salt hypertension [74] (Figure 15).

This pump suppression appears to result from a humoral agent. Supernatants of boiled plasma from these volume expanded animals reduce rubidium uptake when applied to arteries from another untouched rat [74] (Figure 16). The same is true of plasma from volume expanded dogs, i.e., rubidium uptake by rat arteries is decreased when exposed to supernatants of boiled plasma from volume expanded dogs (Figure 17). Furthermore, serum from rats with one-kidney, one wrapped hypertension increases the sodium content of rabbit aortic media explants [84] and supernates of boiled plasma from dogs with one-kidney, one wrapped hypertension and rats with one-kidney, one clip and reduced renal mass hypertension reduce rubidium uptake when applied to arteries from an untouched rat [75].

EFFECTS OF PUMP SUPPRESSION

Suppression of the sodium-potassium pump in cardiovascular muscle has long

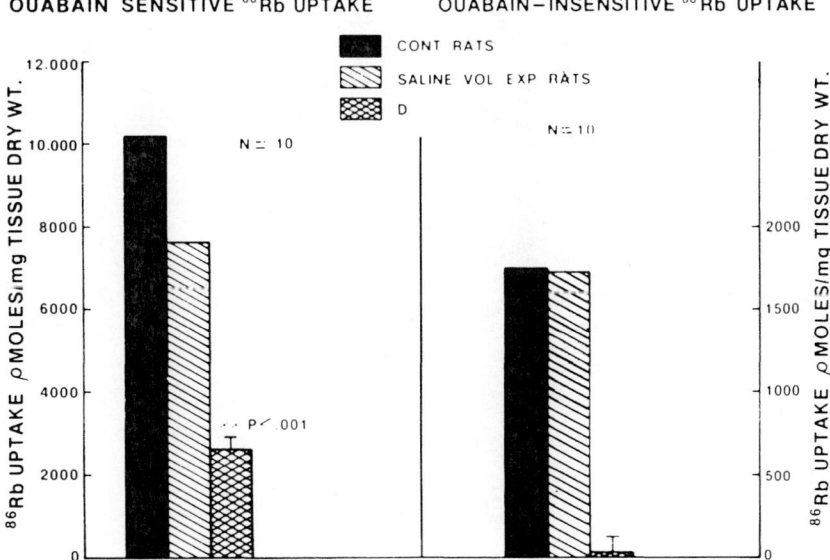

Figure 15. Effect of acute volume expansion with saline on ^{86}Rb uptake by the rat tail artery. Taken from Pamnani et al. [74].

98

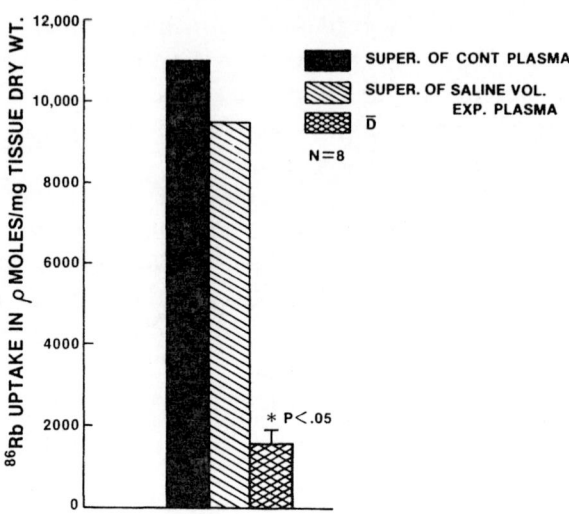

TAIL ARTERIES INCUBATED IN SUPERNATANTS OF BOILED PLASMA

Figure 16. Effect of supernates of boiled plasma from acutely volume-expanded rats on ^{86}Rb uptake by tail arteries from normal rats. Taken from Pamnani et al. [74].

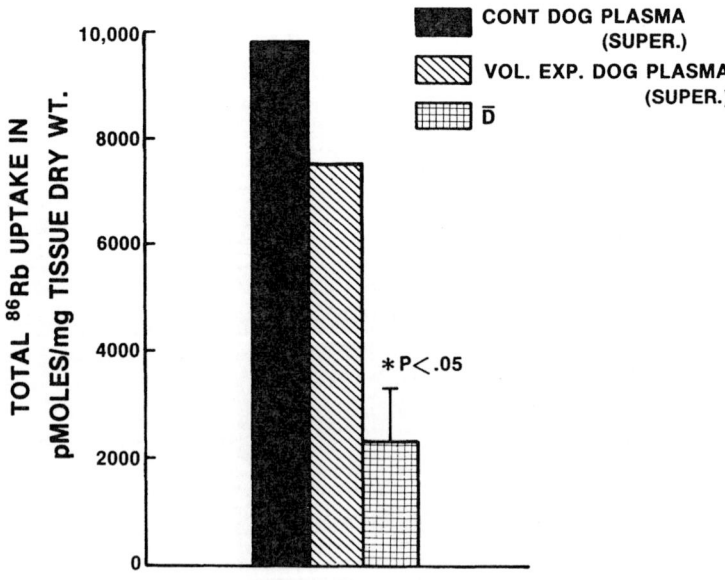

Figure 17. Effect of supernates of boiled plasma from acutely volume-expanded dogs on ^{86}Rb uptake by tail arteries from normal rats. Taken from Pamnani et al. [74].

been known to produce a positive inotropic effect in heart and constriction of arteries and veins. Two well-known methods of suppressing the pump are to administer cardiac glycosides or lower the extracellular potassium concentration. Both of these maneuvers also increase myocardial contractility and constrict blood vessels [32, 82].

They also increase the responsiveness of blood vessels to vasoactive agents. Arteries and veins isolated in a bath respond to electrical stimulation and vaso-active agents more vigorously when exposed to ouabain or low potassium [6, 7, 22, 51]. This effect is seen very quickly and presumably before the ion gradients run down.

These same abnormalities are seen in experimental volume expanded hyper-tension. Increased total peripheral resistance, decreased venous compliance, and increased cardiac contractility (at least initially) have been demonstrated by a number of investigators (see references in Haddy et al. [34]). Furthermore, blood vessels from these animals seem to be more sensitive to vasoactive agents.

The means whereby pump suppression causes increased cardiac contractility, vasoconstriction, and increased vessel sensitivity to vasactive agents is not yet clear. It is now known that the pump is electrogenic i.e., it directly affects the membrane potential [86]. Exposure of blood vessels to ouabain or low potassium depolarizes the membrane [1, 37] in association with increased contractile activity and increased sensitivity to vasoactive agents. Depolarization has in fact been observed in one low renin model of hypertension [76]. Thus, one possibility is that depolarization increases the permeability of the cell membrane to calcium result-ing in contraction. The cell is more sensitive to vasoactive agents because the membrane potential is closer to the threshold potential. It is however, difficult to use this explanation for the positive inotropic effect in heart because electrogenic effects of the pump are less prominent in heart than in blood vessels. For this and other reasons, some investigators favor an explanation based on the Na-Ca exchange mechanism [78]. Here the pump suppression raises intracellular sodium concentration, resulting in a lowered sodium gradient for calcium extrusion from the cell. The intracellular calcium concentration therefore rises.

AUTONOMIC NERVOUS SYSTEM

There also seems to be a defect in the autonomic nervous system in volume expanded hypertension. Patients with primary aldosteronism have impaired cardiovascular reflexes, i.e., they appear to have a functional sympathectomy (see references in Haddy et al. [34]). Animals with volume expanded hyperten-sion have reduced levels of endogenous norepinephrine in the cardiovascular tissues (see references in Haddy et al. [34]). Thus, as pointed out previously [34], consideration should be given to the possibility that the pump defect extends to the sympathetic nerve endings and baroreceptors. Were this the case, reflex compensation would be impaired and the humoral agent would therefore result in higher pressure.

NATURE OF THE HUMORAL AGENT

What humoral agent suppresses the sodium-potassium pump in heart and blood vessels? In our previous reviews [33, 34, 35], we tended to favor the natriuretic factor because its level in blood rises with volume and because it suppresses sodium pump activity in the renal tubule. Blaustein [4] also considers the natriuretic factor to be a good possibility. The factor is heat stable and has been partially purified [30]. It appears to have a low molecular weight, but its chemical structure is still unknown. It probably comes from the brain [3, 75] and may be released in response to pulmonary distention (see references in Haddy et al. [34[). Its relation to the slowly acting humoral pressor and sensitizing agent observed in bioassay studies (see above) and to the humoral pump suppressor seen on acute volume expansion and in animals with low renin hypertension (see above) merits study.

SUMMARY

A high salt intake can increase arterial pressure, particularly when the ability to excrete salt is impaired. The mechanism of this effect is not clear. Certain studies suggest that the salt retention increases extracellular fluid volume which in turn evokes the release of a humoral agent which, like ouabain, suppresses the cellular sodium-potassium pump in cardiovascular muscle. The pump suppression somehow increases contractile activity in arteries, veins and heart, thereby contributing to the elevated arterial pressure.

REFERENCES

1. Anderson DK: Cell potential and sodium potassium pump in vascular smooth muscle. Fed Proc 35: 1294–1297, 1976
2. Battarbee HD, Self LE: A vasopressor potentiator for norepinephrine in the serum of spontaneously hypertensive rats. Fed Proc 38: 1259, 1979
3. Bealer S, Haywood JR et al.: Impaired natriuresis and secretion of natriuretic hormone in rats with lesions of the anteroventral 3rd ventricle. Fed Proc 38: 1232, 1979
4. Blaustein M: Sodium ions, calcium ions, blood pressure regulation, and hypertension: a reassessment and a hypothesis. Am J Physiol 232: c165–c173, 1977
5. Bloom DS, Stein MB, Rosendorff C: Effects of hypertensive plasma on the responses of an isolated artery preparation to norepinephrine. Cardiovasc Res 10: 268–274, 1976
6. Brender D, Strong CG, Shepherd JT: Effects of acetylstrophanthidin on isolated veins of the dog. Circulation Res 26: 647–655, 1970

7. Brender D, Vanhoutte PM, Shepherd JT: Potentiation of adrenergic venomotor responses in dogs by cardiac glycosides. Circ Res 25: 597–606, 1969
8. Carretero OA, Amin VM et al.: Urinary kallikrein in rats bred for their susceptibility and resistance to the hypertensive effect of salt. Circ Res 42: 727–731, 1978
9. Chen WT, Anderson DK et al.: The mechanism of the vasodilator effects of potassium. J Lab Clin Med 78: 797, 1971
10. Chen WT, Brace RA et al.: The mechanism of the vasodilator action of potassium. Proc Soc Expt Biol Med 140: 820–824, 1972
11. Cherchovich GM, Capek K et al.: High salt intake and blood pressure in lower primates. J Appl Physiol 40: 601–604, 1976
12. Chrysant SG, Danisa K et al.: Racial differences in pressure, volume and renin interrelationships in essential hypertension. Hypertension 1: 136–141, 1979
13. Clough DL, Pamnani MB, Haddy FJ: Decreased Na,K-ATPase activity in left ventricular myocardium of rats with one-kidney DOCA-saline hypertension. Clin Res 26: 361, 1978
14. Clough D, Pamnani M et al.: Left ventricular Na,K-ATPase activity in rats with reduced renal mass hypertension and spontaneous hypertension. Physiologist 23: 91, 1980
15. Clough DL, Pamnani MB et al.: Decreased myocardial Na,K-ATPase in rats with one-kidney Goldblatt hypertension. Fed Proc 36: 491, 1977
16. Clough DL, Pamnani MB et al.: Decreased Na,K-ATPase in right ventricular myocardium of rats with one-kidney Goldblatt hypertension. Physiologist 20: 18, 1977
17. Dahl LK: Salt and hypertension. Am J Clin Nutr 25: 231–244, 1972
18. Dahl LK: Salt intake and hypertension. In: Genest J, Koiw E, Kuchel O (eds), Hypertension: Physiopathology and Treatment. McGraw-Hill Book Company, New York, 1977, pp 548–559
19. Dahl LK, Knudsen KD, Iwai J: Humoral transmission of hypertension: evidence from parabiosis. Circ Res 24 and 25 (Suppl. 1): 21–33, 1969
20. Davidson AJ, Talner LB, Downs WM: A study of the angiographic appearance of the kidney in an aging normotensive population. Radiology 92: 975–983, 1969
21. Finnerty FA, Davidov M et al.: Influence of extracellular fluid volume on response to antihypertensive drugs. Circ Res 26 and 27 (Suppl. 1): 71–82, 1970
22. Flaim SF, DiPette DJ: Digoxin-norepinephrine response and calcium blocker effects in vascular smooth muscle. Am J Physiol 236: H613–H619, 1979
23. Freis ED: Salt, volume and the prevention of hypertension. Circulation 53: 589–595, 1976
24. Freis ED: Salt in hypertension and effects of diuretics. Ann Rev Pharmacol Toxicol 19: 13–23, 1979
25. Fukada TR: L'hypertension par le sel chez les lapins et ses relations avec la glande surrenale. Union Med Can 80: 1278–1281, 1951
26. Ganguli M, Tobian L, Dahl L: Low renal papillary plasma flow in both Dahl and Kyoto rats with spontaneous hypertension. Circ Res 39: 337–341, 1976
27. Gordon DB, Drury DR, Schapiro S: The salt-fed animal as a test object for pressor substances in the blood of hypertensive animals. Am J Physiol 175: 123–128, 1953
28. Grim CE, McDonough JR, Dahl LK: Dietary sodium, potassium and blood pressure: racial differences in Evans County, Georgia. Circulation 42 (Suppl 3): 85, 1970
29. Grim CE, Weinberger MH et al.: Biochemical correlates of the increase in blood pressure with age. Abstracts of the 5th Meeting of the Int Soc Hypertension, p 102, 1978
30. Gruber KA, Buckalew VM Jr: Further characterization and evidence for a precursor in the formation of plasma antinatriferic factor. Proc Soc Exptl Biol Med 159: 463–467, 1978

31. Haddy FJ: Local control of vascular resistance in relation to hypertension. Arch Intern Med 133: 916–931, 1974
32. Haddy FJ: Potassium and blood vessels. Life Sci 16: 1489–1498, 1975
33. Haddy FJ, Overbeck HW: The role of humoral agents in volume expanded hypertension. Life Sci 19: 935–948, 1976
34. Haddy FJ, Pamnani M, Clough D: The sodium-potassium pump in volume expanded hypertension. Clin Exp Hypertension 1: 295–336, 1978
35. Haddy FJ, Pamnani MB, Clough DL: Humoral factors and the sodium-potassium pump in volume expanded hypertension. Life Sci 24: 2105–2118, 1979
36. Haddy FJ, Scott JB: The mechanism of the acute effect of sodium chloride on blood pressure. Proc Soc Exptl Biol Med 136: 551–554, 1971
37. Hendrickx H, Casteels R: Electrogenic sodium pump in arterial smooth muscle cells. Pflügers Arch 346: 299–306, 1974
38. Hinke JAM: In vitro demonstration of vascular hyperresponsiveness in experimental hypertension. Circ Res 17: 359–371, 1965
39. Huang CT, Cardona R, Michelakis AM: Existence of a new vasoactive factor in experimental hypertension. Am J Physiol 234: E25–E31, 1978
40. Jones AW, Hart HG: Altered ion transport in aortic smooth muscle during deoxycorticosterone acetate hypertension in the rat. Circ Res 37: 333–341, 1975
41. Jones AW, Sander PD, Kampschmidt DL: The effect of norepinephrine on aortic ^{42}K turnover during deoxycorticosterone therapy in the rat. Circ Res 41: 256–260, 1977
42. Kaplan C, Paternack B et al.: Age-related incidence of sclerotic glomeruli in human kidneys. Am J Pathol 80: 227–234, 1975
43. Kawasaki T, Delia CS et al.: The effect of high sodium and low-sodium intakes on blood pressure and other related variables in human subjects with idiopathic hypertension. Am J Med 64: 193–198, 1978
44. Kirkendall AM, Connor WE et al.: The effect of dietary sodium chloride on blood pressure, body fluids, electrolytes, renal function, and serum lipids of normotensive man. J Lab Clin Med 87: 411–434, 1976
45. Koletsky S: Hypertensive vascular disease produced by salt. Lab Invest 7: 377–386, 1958
46. Koletsky S: Role of salt and renal mass in experimental hypertension. AMA Arch Pathol 68: 11–22, 1959
47. Kurz KD, Johnson JA et al.: Pressor responses to norepinephrine following expansion with blood from rabbits with renal artery stenosis. Fed Proc 38: 1375, 1979
48. Langford HC, Watson RL: Electrolytes, environment and blood pressure. Clin Sci Mol Med 45(Suppl) 1: 111, 1973
49. Langston JB, Guyton AC et al.: Effect of changes in salt intake on arterial pressure and renal function in partially nephrectomized dogs. Circ Res 12: 508–513, 1963
50. Lenel R, Katz LN, Rodbard S: Arterial hypertension in the chicken. Am J Physiol 152: 557–562, 1948
51. Leonard E: Alteration of contractile response of artery strips by a potassium-free solution, cardiac glycosides and changes in stimulation frequency. Am J Physiol 189: 185–190, 1957
52. Levy SB, Lilley JJ et al.: Urinary kallikrein and plasma renin activity as determinants of renal blood flow. J Clin Invest 60: 129–138, 1977
53. Luft F, Block R et al.: Cardiovascular responses to extremes of salt intake in man. Clin Res 26: 365, 1978
54. Luft FC, Grim CE et al.: Effects of volume expansion and contraction in normotensive whites, blacks, and subjects of different ages. Circulation 59: 643–650, 1979
55. Luft FC, Grim CE et al.: Differences in response to sodium administration in normotensive white and black subjects. J Lab Clin Med 90: 555–562, 1977

56. Luft FC, Rankin LI et al.: Plasma and urinary norepinephrine values at extremes of salt intake in normal man. Hypertension 1: 261–266, 1979
57. McDonough J, Wilhelmj CM: The effect of excessive salt intake on human blood pressure. Am J Digest Dis 21: 180–181, 1954
58. McQuarrie I, Thompson WH, Anderson JA: Effects of excessive ingestion of sodium and potassium salts on carbohydrate metabolism and blood pressure in diabetic children. J Nutr 11: 77–101, 1936
59. Meneely GR, Ball COT, Youmans JB: Chronic sodium chloride toxicity: The protective effect of added potassium chloride. Ann Int Med 47: 263–273, 1957
60. Meneely GR, Battarbee HD: The high sodium-low potassium environment and hypertension. Am J Cardio 38: 768–786, 1976
61. Meneely GR, Dahl LK: Electrolytes in hypertension: The effects of sodium chloride. Med Clin N Am 45: 271–283, 1961
62. Michelakis AM, Mizukoshi H et al.: Further studies on the existence of a sensitizing factor to pressor agents in hypertension. J Clin Endo Met 41: 90–96, 1975
63. Mizukoshi H, Michelakis AM: Evidence for the existence of a sensitizing factor to pressor agents in the plasma of hypertensive patients. J Clin Endocrinol 34: 1016–1024, 1972
64. Murray RH, Luft FC et al.: Blood pressure responses to extremes of sodium intake in normal man. Proc Soc Exptl Biol Med 159: 432–436, 1978
65. Nivatpumin T, Scheuer J et al.: Effects of acute uremia on myocardial function in rats. Clin Res 21: 952, 1973
66. Norman RA Jr, Coleman TG et al.: Separate roles of sodium ion concentration and fluid volumes in salt-loading hypertension in the dog. Am J Physiol 229: 1068–1072, 1975
67. Overbeck HW: Peripheral vascular responses to potassium and magnesium in experimental hypertensive dogs. J Lab Clin Med 68: 1003, 1966
68. Overbeck HW: Vascular responses to cations, osmolality and angiotensin in renal hypertensive dogs. Am J Physiol 223: 1358–1364, 1972
69. Overbeck HW, Haddy FJ: Forelimb vascular responses in renal hypertensive dogs. Physiologist 10: 270, 1967
70. Overbeck HW, Pamnani MB et al.: Depressed function of a ouabain-sensitive sodium-potassium pump in blood vessels from renal hypertensive dogs. Circ Res 38 (Suppl. 2): 48–52, 1976
71. Page LB, Danion A, Moellering RC Jr: Antecedents of cardiovascular disease in six Solomon Island societies. Circulation 49: 1132–1146, 1974
72. Pamnani MB, Clough DL, Haddy FJ: Na^+-K^+ pump activity in tail arteries of spontaneously hypertensive rats. Jap Heart J 20 (Suppl. 1): 228–230, 1979
73. Pamnani MB, Clough DL, Haddy FJ: Altered activity of the sodium-potassium pump in arteries of rats with steroid hypertension. Clin Sci and Mol Med 55: 41s–43s, 1978
74. Pamnani MB, Clough DL et al.: Sodium-potassium pump activity in experimental hypertension. In: Vanhoutte PM, Leusen I (eds), Vasodilatation, Raven Press, New York, 1981, pp 391–403
75. Pamnani M, Huot S et al.: Demonstration of a humoral inhibitor of the Na^+-K^+ pump in some models of experimental hypertension. Hypertension 3 (Suppl. 2): 96–101, 1981
76. Pamnani MB, Harder DR et al.: Vascular smooth muscle membrane potentials and the influence of a ouabain-like humoral factor in rats with one-kidney, one clip hypertension. Physiologist 24: 6, 1981
77. Pratt JH, Luft FC: The effect of extremely high sodium intake on plasma renin activity, plasma aldosterone concentration, and urinary excretion of aldosterone metabolites. J Lab Clin Med 93: 724–729, 1979
78. Reuter H, Blaustein MP, Haeusler G: Na-Ca exchanged and tension development in

arterial smooth muscle. Phil Trans R Soc B 265: 87–94, 1973

79. Romoff MS, Keusch G et al.: Effect of sodium intake on plasma catecholamines in normal subjects. J Clin Endo Met 48: 26–31, 1979
80. Rowe JW, Andres R et al.: The effect of age on creatinine clearance in man: A cross-sectional and longitudinal study. J Gerontol 31: 155–163, 1976
81. Sapirstein LA, Brandt WL, Drury DR: Production of hypertension in the rat by substituting hypertonic sodium chloride for drinking water. Proc Soc Exptl Biol Med 73: 82–85, 1950
82. Schwartz A, Lindenmayer GE, Allen JC: The sodium-potassium adenosine triphosphatase: Pharmacological, physiological and biochemical aspects. Pharmacol Rev 27: 3–134, 1975
83. Self LE, Battarbee HD et al.: A vasopressor potentiator for norepinephrine in hypertensive rats. Proc Soc Exptl Biol Med 153: 7–12, 1976
84. Simon G: Angiopathic serum factor in perinephritic hypertensive dogs. Hypertension 1: 197–201, 1979
85. Solandt DY, Nassim R, Cowan CR: Hypertensive effect of blood from hypertensive dogs. Lancet 1: 873–874, 1940
86. Thomas RC: Electrogenic sodium pump in nerve and muscle cells. Physiol Rev 52: 563–594, 1972
87. Tobian L: Interrelationship of electrolytes, juxtaglomerular cells and hypertension. Physiol Rev 40: 280–312, 1960
88. Tobian L, Lange J et al.: Reduction of natriuretic capacity and renin release in isolated, blood-perfused kidneys of Dahl hypertension-prone rats. Circ Res 43 (Suppl. 1): 92, 1978
89. Tobian L, Lange J et al.: Prevention with thiazide of NaCl-induced hypertension in Dahl 'S' rats. Hypertension 1: 316–323, 1979
90. Tsay SL, Jones AW: Effect of pressure vs DOCA on ^{42}K efflux in vascular smooth muscle from the rat. Fed Proc 37: 902, 1978
91. Vogel JA: Salt-induced hypertension in the dog. Am J Physiol 210: 186–190, 1966

8. MILL'S DISEASE AMONGST MEDICAL SPECIALISTS IN HYPERTENSION

P. Mason, D.G. Beevers, C. Beretta-Piccoli, J.J. Brown,
A.M.M. Cumming, D.L. Davies, R. Fraser, A.F. Lever, J.J. Morton,
P.L. Padfield and Y. Young

INTRODUCTION

> The tendency has always been strong to believe that what-
> ever receives a name must be an entity or being having an
> independent existence of its own; and if no real entity an-
> swering to the name could be found man did not for that
> reason suppose that none existed, but imagined that it was
> something peculiarly abstruse and mysterious, too high to be
> an object of sense.

This remarkable statement is attributed to John Stuart Mill, the Nineteenth
Century political economist [20]. The idea deserves wider currency. It is certainly
relevant to the ways in which 20th Century doctors classify disease. Accordingly,
we shall describe as Mill's disease the mistaken belief that whatever receives a
name must be an entity. Though this is the first description of Mill's disease the
tendency for doctors to reason in this fashion has been commented on previously,
by Pickering [22] in relation to the false classification of hypertension, by Kendell
[15] in relation to misclassification of psychiatric disorders and by Rose and
Barker [24] in relation to the process by which diagnoses are reached.

MILL'S DISEASE AMONGST THOSE WHO DEFINE HYPERTENSION

Separation of normal and high blood pressure

Hypertension is a common disorder, but population studies show no sign of it as
an entity. The distribution of blood pressures for individual members of a large
population is continuous and bell-shaped in form; there is no downward dip in the
curve, no point where a dividing line might separate normal and pathologically
high blood pressure. This means that hypertension and normotension cannot be
separated by data on prevalence [22, 23]. High blood pressure is also lethal, it kills
by increasing the risk of vascular disease in the heart, kidneys and brain; the
higher the pressure the greater these risks. Systolic pressure and risk and related
in a graded manner, but the gradient of risk extends throughout the normal range

Sambhi, M.P. (ed.) Fundamental fault in hypertension
© *1984, Martinus Nijhoff Publishers. Boston/The Hague/Dordrecht/Lancaster.*
ISBN 978-94-010-9006-3

of pressure [13, 18]. There is no kink or dip in the gradient, no point at which a dividing line could be drawn. Thus, hypertension and normotension cannot be separated by data on risk. Apart from recent observations on intracellular electrolytes [17] we know of no other way in which the separation can be made and perhaps this means there is no basis for separation [22]. It does not necessarily follow that the term 'hypertension' should be avoided. The objection is not to the name, but to the notion 'that whatever receives a name must be an entity or being'.

The problem can be illustrated as follows: Four 40-year old men, A,B,C and D have respectively diastolic pressures of 60, 80, 100, and 120 mm Hg; each measurement is the average of a large number. Each man has a different prognosis: D worse than C; C worse than B; B worse than A. All doctors agree on the need to treat D and most would refer to him as 'hypertensive', but where should the aetiological dividing line be drawn? The weakness of placing it between C and D is that the features which separate these men (different pressure and different risk) also separate B and C and A and B. Nevertheless, physicians must decide on the level of pressure above which treatment is worthwhile and below which it is not. This level is a therapeutic, not an aetiological dividing line. Its position will vary with evidence on benefit. By 1970 it was clear that patient D would benefit [11, 28]. Trials are currently underway to determine whether patient C will benefit [19]. Thus, individuals with blood pressure above a therapeutic dividing line will benefit from reduction of blood pressure, but it does not follow that they are qualitatively different from individuals below the line.

Is this man hypertensive?

We have assumed above that the blood pressure of subjects A, B, C and D remains relatively constant. In fact it is likely to vary widely and the variability itself may differ in individuals. A great deal has been written on the way in which this can compromise the diagnosis of hypertension [3, 22]. The following is an extreme example:

The patient, a medical practitioner, aged 43 was seen in 1979 by a colleague (Dr X in Figure 1) for an insurance examination. The patient's blood pressure was raised. He was referred to one of us (Dr Y) who, using a conventional sphygmomanometer, recorded pressures of 210/126 sitting and 196/116 after a period of rest. The patient was removed to a quiet room where blood pressure was recorded automatically, no other person being present. His blood pressure fell (Figure 1). Dr Y entered the room and pressure rose; the rise was confirmed (and probably provoked) by measurement of pressure in the patient's opposite arm using a conventional sphygmomanometer. Dr Y left the room and pressure again fell. The patient was seen later, reassured that all was well and sent home. Next morning a junior doctor

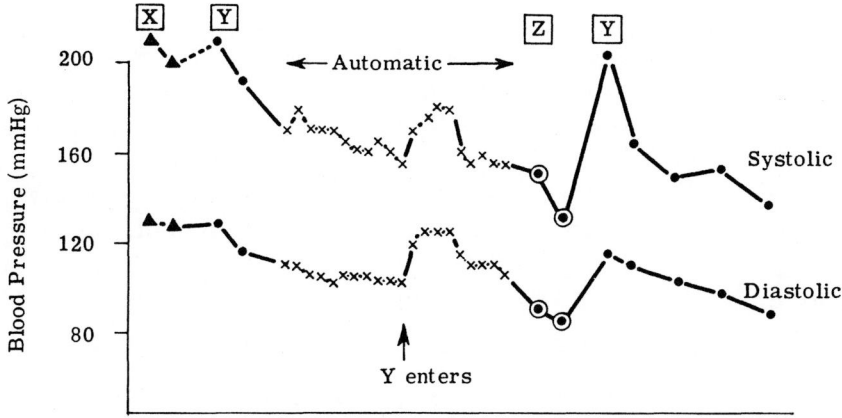

Figure 1. Measurements of blood pressure by Dr X (▲), Dr Y (●) and Dr Z (○) using conventional sphygmomanometer and by Bosomat automatic recorder at 2-minute intervals in a man referred with hypertension.

recorded a pressure of 152/90 mm Hg falling to 132–84. When the patient was seen a few minutes later by Dr Y his pressure had risen markedly (Figure 1). In the weeks that followed progressively lower values were obtained by Dr Y using the same sphygmomanometer – 150/104, 154/96 (138/82 measured by Dr Z on the same day) and 136/96 on different occasions. All investigations in this patient, including intravenous pyelogram, urea and electrolytes and electrocardiogram were normal.

The following points arise from these observations:

1) Whatever arbitrary dividing line is used, the patient had 'hypertension' and 'normotension' on the same day, crossing every dividing line at least twice in 24 hours.

2) Had automatic recordings not been made and had he been seen by Drs X and Y only, hypertension would have been diagnosed and treatment begun. On the other hand, if he had been assessed by Dr Z only his blood pressure would have been normal and no treatment would have been given. It is unusual for patients to have blood pressure recorded by three doctors and by an automatic machine before the decision on treatment is made. Thus, the changes seen in this man may be commoner than we think.

3) Drs X and Y elicited more marked pressor responses than did Dr Z, but we do not know if Drs X and Y generally elicit greater effects in their patients. The response produced by Dr Y seems to diminish with time. If pressor responses of this sort are common and if they gradually diminish, there may be another explanation for the well-known tendency of blood pressure to decrease when serial measurements are made without treatment [22]. This is usually thought to represent a genuine fall of blood pressure. The alternative is that blood pressure tends to rise less as patients become more familiar with their doctors.

4) Should this particular patient be treated? On the evidence of single measure-

ments of blood pressure [13] perhaps he should. However, other studies [25] suggest that the best indication of prognosis in hypertension is given by blood pressure measured in the basal and rested state. However, data of both sorts relate to blood pressure and risk, not to the reduction of risk by reduction of blood pressure. Successful treatment does not reduce all risks [28].

5) Doctors not committed to the concept of a dividing line will have little difficulty accepting the observations in this patient, probably attributing them to the greater than usual variation of blood pressure. Victims of Mill's disease committed to the line will have an embarrassing dilemma.

MILL'S DISEASE AMONGST THOSE WHO INVESTIGATE HYPERTENSION

Figure 2 illustrates the process by which we and others reach the diagnosis of essential hypertension. First, known causes of hypertension, such as renal artery stenosis and Conn's syndrome are excluded. Essential hypertension remains after this process of exclusion; it is a 'disease' characterised by negative features, by what it is not, rather than by what it is.

Most patients have an intravenous pyelogram. A normal result favours essential hypertension, an abnormal result suggests kidney disease which may or may not be the cause of the hypertension. How are patients to be classified if the renal lesion is demonstrable but unlikely to be the cause of the hypertension (a renal stone, for example)? Few doctors would accept such patients as having essential

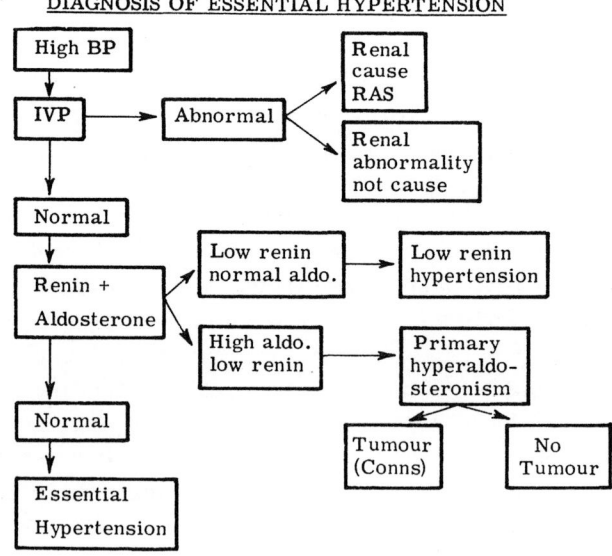

DIAGNOSIS OF ESSENTIAL HYPERTENSION

Figure 2. Schematic illustration of the manner in which the diagnosis of essential hypertension is reached.

hypertension because their pyelogram is abnormal. Few would accept them as real hypertension either, because the stone is an unlikely cause of their high blood pressure. Thus, an intermediate diagnostic group is formed, characterised by a renal lesion which is not the cause of hypertension. It is separated from essential hypertension, a condition in which the cause of hypertension is not known and from renal hypertension in which the cause lies within the kidney. This is a poor basis for classification by cause.

Low renin hypertenion

As Figure 2 shows, a similar problem probably exists in the diagnosis of low-renin hypertension. The condition was originally separated from essential hypertension because low renin is a feature of Conn's syndrome, a treatable disease once thought to be a common cause of high blood pressure. In fact, Conn's syndrome is rare; but low-renin hypertension is common, most patients with low renin having no aldosterone excess [21, 14]. Why is renin low in these patients and what is the basis of their separation from essential hypertension? Two very different explanations have been proposed. In one, the renin is thought to be depressed by sodium retention caused by excess of a mineralocorticoid other than aldosterone. In fact, there is no sodium retention as judged by measurements of exchangeable sodium (NaE); similar values are found in essential hypertension and in low-renin hypertension contrasting with the expansion of NaE seen in Conn's syndrome [7, 8]. Nor has excess of other mineralocorticoids been demonstrated except in a very small proportion of cases [14].

The second explanation is that separation of low-renin hypertension is a diagnostic artefact, another example of Mill's disease. This seems much the most likely to us since, apart from renin, there is little to distinguish the disorder from essential hypertension (Table 1). Frequency-distribution curves for renin, renin activity and angiotensin in hypertensive patients suggest that separation of normal and low renin individuals is a division of two parts of the same population, rather than a separation of different populations [21, 2, 26, 27]. A broader than normal distribution of data does not necessarily imply the existence of separate entities.

Non-tumorous primary hyperaldosteronism

Primary hyperaldosteronism is recognised by the combination of low renin and increased aldosterone (Figure 2). Some of these patients have Conn's syndrome with an adrenal adenoma, the rest having no tumour, are described as having non-tumorous primary hyperaldosteronism. Conn's syndrome is a genuine entity distinct from essential hypertension, from low-renin hypertension and from non-

Table 1. Primary hyperaldosteronism

	Conn's	Non-tumour	Essential Hypertension	Low-renin Hypertension	Source
Pathology	Tumour	usually nodules	often nodules	often nodules	Dobbie 1969, J Path 99,1; Grim 1974, J Clin Endo Metab 39,247; Neville 1978, Invest Cell Path 1,99.
Exchangeable Na	↑	insignificantly different from normal (N)	N	N	Davies et al., 1979a and b.
Exchangeable K	↓	N	N	N	Davies et al., 1979a and b.
Response of aldosterone to angiotensin II.	↓	↑	↑	↓	Brown et al., 1979 (Figure 5) Wisgerhof & Brown 1978.

tumorous primary hyperaldosteronism on pathological, clinical and biochemical grounds (Table 1 and Figure 3). However, the distinction of essential hypertension and non-tumorous hyperaldosteronism is much less clear. Our interest here is that those who assume a difference to exist (including ourselves on earlier occasions) may be suffering from Mill's disease.

Aldosterone excess in Conn's syndrome is primary in the sense that it is caused by autonomous overproduction of aldosterone from the adrenal cortex. Correlation of angiotensin II and aldosterone is negative (Figure 4): angiotensin II is low because aldosterone is high. In non-tumorous hyperaldosteronism, on the other hand, the correlation is positive. This suggests that hyperaldosteronism in the non-tumorous form is not primary. What led to the idea that it might be primary? Increased aldosterone in the presence of low renin and low angiotensin II is certainly a feature of genuine primary hyperaldosteronism but not all patients with the combination have primary hyperaldosteronism. There may be other explanations for the combination, therefore. One is that the response of aldosterone to its stimuli is enhanced. In these circumstances, normal or low angiotensin II would maintain relatively high aldosterone. There is evidence that this is the state of affairs in essential hypertension where infusion of angiotensin II produces a greater than normal response of aldosterone ([16, 29], and Figure 5). In patients with Conn's syndrome, on the other hand, the response to angiotensin is subnormal (Figure 5). It is of some interest to compare these responses with those in three patients with non-tumorous hyperaldosteronism. All show the pattern found in essential hypertension (Figure 5). Wisgerhof et al. [30] have also demonstrated an increased response in such patients during sodium loading and during dexamethasone suppression.

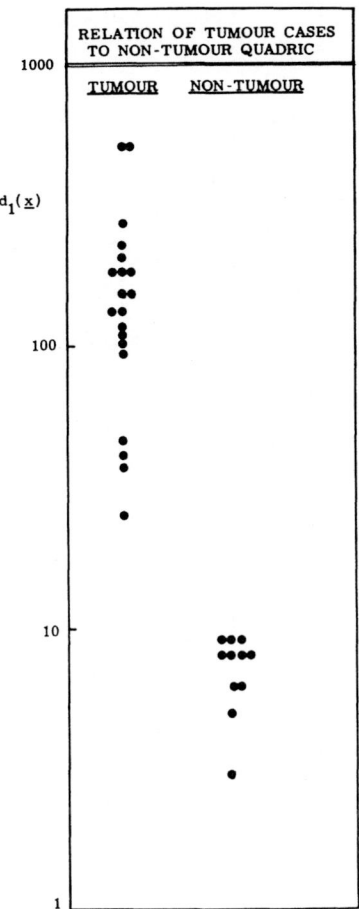

Figure 3. Distribution of data from patients with tumorous and non-tumorous primary hyper-aldosteronism using quadric analysis. Each point is the product of the analysis of eight features from one patient. The technique of quadric analysis as applied to these data is outlined in Aitchison et al., Amer Heart J 82:660–671, 1971. We thank the editors of the American Heart Journal for permission to publish the figure.

We have also measured the plasma concentration of 18 OH-corticosterone, a possible precursor of aldosterone. This too showed a similar pattern of response to angiotensin II – greater than normal in essential hypertension and non-tumorous hyperaldosteronism (Figure 5), and a less marked response in Conn's syndrome. It can also be seen that the plasma concentrations of 18 OH-cor-ticosterone before infusion were higher in Conn's syndrome than in essential hypertension and non-tumorous hyperaldosteronism, a further resemblance of the two conditions and a contrast with Conn's syndrome. Biglieri and his colleagues [4] have previously noted clear separation of Conn's syndrome and non-tumorous hyperaldosteronism measuring plasma 18 OH-corticosterone. The direction of the diurnal changes of the steroid was also different.

112

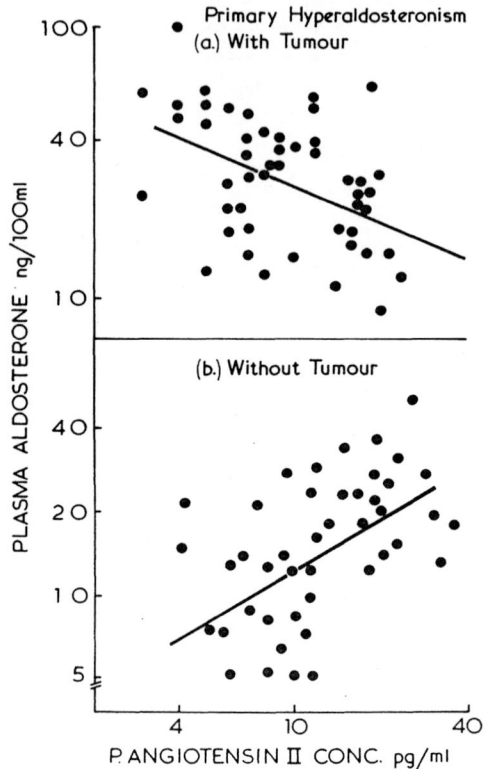

Figure 4. Correlation of plasma angiotensin II concentration and plasma aldosterone concentration in (a) untreated Conn's syndrome and (b) primary hyperaldosteronism without tumour, or idiopathic hyperaldosteronism.

Other points of difference and resemblance are given in Table 1. There is much to distinguish Conn's syndrome and non-tumorous hyperaldosteronism, but little to distinguish non-tumorous hyperaldosteronism and essential hypertension. We have suggested that these are different parts of the same condition rather than different conditions [7, 5].

Conn's syndrome usually presents with hypokalaemia. One method of screening for the disease is to measure plasma potassium. This was done in a group of unselected patients found to be hypertensive in a screening survey. Hypokalaemia was common, but after further testing no patient with hypokalaemia was found to have Conn's syndrome [1]. Another method of screening is to measure plasma aldosterone concentration. This was also done in the same study and results in hypertensive patients were compared with those in normal subjects of the same age and from the same population. Figure 6 shows the results. Eleven patients in the hypertensive group had plasma aldosterone concentrations above the upper limit of normal. In three it resulted from secondary hyperaldosteronism, two having renal artery stenosis; in the remainder, excess aldosterone did not persist: in none was Conn's syndrome the explanation. This suggests that

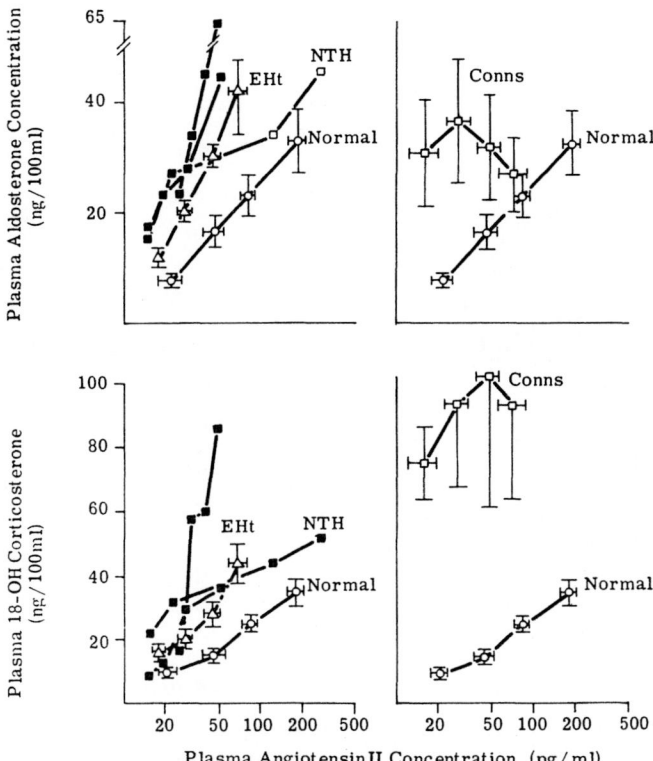

Figure 5. Intravenous infusion of angiotensin at three incremental rates (from 0.5, 1, 2, 4, 8 ng/kg/min) were given to 7 normal subjects, 8 patients with essential hypertension and 4 patients with Conn's syndrome. Plasma samples were taken before and at the end of each period of infusion and angiotensin II, 18 OH-corticosterone and aldosterone were measured in all samples. Dose-response curves were then constructed as above. Data for three patients with non-tumorous hyperaldosteronism studied in the same way are shown individually.

Conn's syndrome is a very rare cause of hypertension and that occasional aldosterone excess is relatively common in patients who would otherwise be classified as essential hypertension.

If the finding of aldosterone excess in a hypertensive patient is a reason for abandoning the diagnosis of essential hypertension it is hardly surprising that essential hypertension is 'characterised' by normal aldosterone. If, on the other hand, occasional aldosterone excess is accepted as a feature of essential hypertension several other observations become easier to explain: the brisker than normal response of aldosterone is angiotensin (Figure 5) and ACTH [12]; the failure of aldosterone to suppress normally in essential hypertension [6] and the higher than normal mean plasma aldosterone concentration, sometimes reported for groups of patients with essential hypertension [10]. It also follows that the diagnostic separation of essential hypertension and non-tumorous primary hyperaldosterone is less necessary.

114

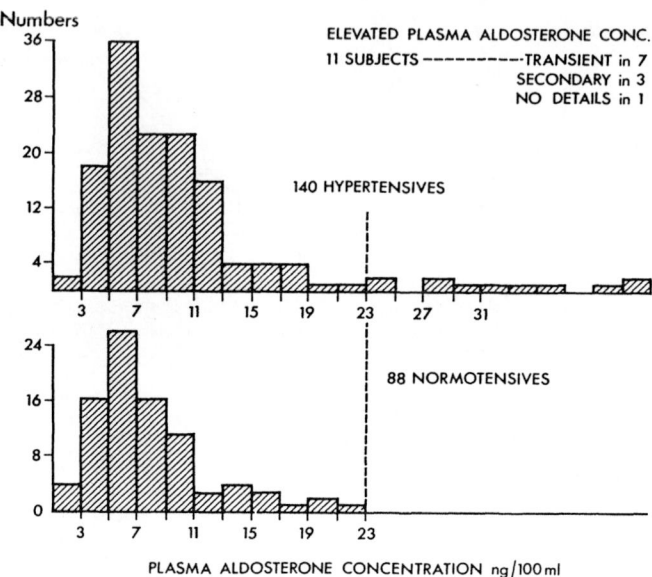

ALDOSTERONE

Figure 6. Frequency distributions of plasma aldosterone concentration in 140 unselected hypertensives and 88 normal subjects of the same age.

One primary hyperaldosteronism is diagnosed there usually follow investigations to distinguish the tumorous from the non-tumorous form. It is fortunate that the distinction can be made so easily (Figure 3). In the past several groups of workers, including ourselves, have subjected patients with the non-tumorous form to sub-total adrenalectomy. Blood pressure fell in most, much as it does in Conn's syndrome [9]. The operation was not, therefore, a failure, but the need for it was not that the excess of aldosterone was primary.

CONCLUSION

John Stuart Mill described a state of mind which is probably common: a belief that 'whatever receives a name must be an entity'. Some disorders are genuine entities and Conn's syndrome is probably one. Others have been granted the status of entity on inadequate evidence. In our view, essential hypertension itself, low-renin hypertension and non-tumoros primary hyperaldosteronism are three examples.

REFERENCES

1. Beevers DG, Nelson CS, Padfield PL, Barlow DH, Duncan S, Hawthorne VM, Morton JJ, Young GAR, Young J: The prevalence of hypertension in an unselected population, and the frequency of abnormalities of potassium, angiotensin II and aldosterone in hypertensive subjects. Acta Clin Bel 29: 276–280, 1974
2. Beevers DG, Morton JJ, Nelson CS, Padfield PL, Titterington M, Tree M: Angiotensin II in essential hypertension. Bri Med J 1: 415, 1977
3. Bevan AT, Honour AJ, Stott FH: Direct arterial pressure recording in unrestricted man. Clin Sci 36: 329–344, 1969
4. Biglieri EG, Schambelan M, Hirai J, Chang B, Brust N: The significance of elevated levels of 18-hydroxycorticosterone in patients with primary hyperaldosteronism. J Clin Endo & Metab 49: 87–91, 1979
5. Brown JJ, Lever AF, Robertson JIS, Beevers DG, Cumming AMM, Davies DL, Fraser R, Mason P, Morton JJ, Tree M: Are idiopathic hyperaldosteronism and low renin hypertension variants of essential hypertension? Ann of Clin Biochem 16: 380–388, 1979
6. Collins RD, Weinberger MH, Dowdy AJ, Nokes GW, Gonzalez CM, Leutcher JA: Abnormally sustained aldosterone secretion during salt loading in patients with various forms of benign hypertension; relation to plasma renin activity. J Clin Invest 49: 1415–1426, 1970
7. Davies DL, Beevers DG, Brown JJ, Cumming AMM, Fraser R, Lever AF, Mason PA, Morton JJ, Padfield PL, Robertson JIS, Titterington M, Tree M: Aldosterone and its stimuli in normal and hypertensive man: are essential hypertension and primary hyperaldosteronism without tumour different parts of the same condition? J Endocrin 18: 79P–91P, 1979
8. Davies DL, McElroy K, Atkinson AB, Brown JJ, Cumming AMM, Fraser R, Leckie BJ, Lever AF, Mackay A, Morton JJ, Robertson JIS: Relationship between exchangeable sodium and blood pressure in different forms of hypertension in man. Clin Sci 57: 69s–75s, 1979
9. Ferriss JB, Beevers DG, Boddy K, Brown JJ, Davies DL, Fraser R, Kremer D, Lever AF, Robertson JIS: The treatment of low-renin (primary) hyperaldosteronism. Amer Heart J 96: 97–109, 1978
10. Genest J, Nowaczynski W, Boucher R, Rojo-Ornega JM: The role of the adrenal cortex in human essential hypertension. Mayo Clin Proc 52: 191–307, 1977
11. Hamilton M, Thompson EN, Wisniewski TKM: The role of blood pressure control in preventing complications of hypertension. Lancet 1: 235–238, 1964
12. Honda M, Nowaczynski W, Guthrie GP, Messeri FN, Tolis G, Kuchel O, Genest J: Response of several adrenal steroids to ACTH stimulation in essential hypertension. J Clin Endo and Metab 44: 264–272, 1977
13. Kannel WB, Gordon T, Schwartz MJ: Systolic versus diastolic blood pressure and risk of coronary heart disease. Amer J of Cardiology 27: 335–346, 1971
14. Kaplan NM, Lieberman E: Clinical hypertension. Williams & Wilkins, 1978
15. Kendell RE: The role of diagnosis in psychiatry. Blackwell, 1975
16. Kisch ES, Dluhy RG, Williams GH: Enhanced aldosterone response to angiotensin II in human hypertension. Circ Res 38: 502–505, 1976
17. Essential hypertension – another defect? Lancet i: 1227–1229, 1980
18. Lew EA: High blood pressure. Other risk factors and longevity. Amer J Med 55: 281–294, 1973
19. Miall WE, Brennan PJ, Mann AH: Medical Research Council's treatment trial for mild hypertension: an interim report. Clin Sci & Mol Med 51: 563s–565s, 1976

116

20. Ogden & Richards: The meaning of meaning. 10th Edition. Routledge & Kegan Paul, London, 1972
21. Padfield PL, Beevers DG, Brown JJ, Davies DL, Lever AF, Robertson JIS, Schalekamp MAD, Tree M: Is low-renin hypertension a stage in the development of essential hypertension or a diagnostic entity? Lancet 1: 548–564, 1975
22. Pickering GW: High blood pressure. 2nd Edition. J & A Churchill Ltd, London, 1968
23. Pickering GW: Normotension and hypertension: the mysterious viability of the false. Amer J Med 65: 561–563, 1978
24. Rose GL, Barker DJP: Epidemiology for the uninitiated. Publ Brit Med Assoc, London, 1979
25. Smirk, H: Casual, basal and supplemental blood pressure in 519 first degree relatives of substantial hypertensive patients in 530 population controls. Clin Sci & Mol Med 51: 13s–17s, 1976
26. Thomas GW, Ledingham JGG, Beilin LJ, Stott AN, Yates KM: Reduced renin activity in essential hypertension. A reappraisal. Kidney Internat 13: 513–518, 1978
27. Thurston H, Bing RF, Pohl JEF, Swales JD: Renin subgroups in essential hypertension: an analysis and critique. Q J Med 47: 325–337, 1978
28. Veterans Administration Cooperative Study Group on antihypertensive compounds: Effects of treatment on morbidity in hypertension: results in patients with diastolic blood pressures averaging 115 through 129 mm Hg. Veterans Admin Cooop Study Group on anti-hypertensive agents. J A M A 202: 1028–1034, 1967
29. Wisgerhof M, Brown RD: Increased adrenal sensitivity to angiotensin II in low renin essential hypertension. J Clin Invest 61: 1456–1462, 1978
30. Wisgerhof M, Carpenter PC, Brown RD: Increased adrenal sensitivity to angiotensin II in idiopathic hyperaldosteronism. J Clin Endocrin & Metab 47: 938–943, 1978

IV. A DEFECT IN CELL MEMBRANE PERMEABILITY

9.   CELL MEMBRANE PERMEABILITY AND HYPERTENSION

DAVID F. BOHR

In recent decades, investigators grappling with the mechanism responsible for hypertension have been confronted with the evidence that this disease may be a product of the dysfunction of numerous body systems: Guyton and his collaborators [23] have emphasized the role of an inadequate renal excretory system for salt and water. Folkow [17] has supported the view that structural changes in the wall of the resistance vessels play a major role in the increase in vascular reactivity and resistance that causes hypertension. Brody and his collaborators [10] have presented evidence that suggests that a specific hypothalamic nucleus may be involved in the origin of this disease. At Michigan, we [7, 4], have stressed the possibility that an altered vascular smooth muscle function may be involved.

Actually, it has been three decades since Irvine Page [35] lucidly articulated the involvement of multiple systems in the 'Mosaic Theory' for hypertension. This theory recognized that various mechanisms regulate tissue perfusion and hence regulate arterial pressure. These regulatory mechanisms act in consort, so that changes in one may alter the performance of the other. For instance, a change in the nervous system that regulates vascular resistance may induce an altered renal endocrine function. Because of this type of interdependence of the vascular regulatory systems, it has been difficult to identify the 'prime mover' in hypertension – to sort out cause and effect.

One rationale for establishing the primacy of a specific defect in the etiology of hypertension involves the appearance of the defect in a system not related to the regulation of arterial pressure. This avoids the problem of cause and effect of interacting blood pressure regulating systems.

The red blood cell membrane is a case in point. Recently, several laboratories have reported an abnormality in the permeability of this membrane in hypertensive humans and animals. This parameter is not directly involved with the systems that interact in the regulation of blood pressure – it is not a component of Dr. Page's Mosaic.

Although it is unlikely that the altered membrane of the red blood cell has any effect at all on arterial blood pressure, there is evidence that similar membrane changes occur in the vascular smooth muscle cell in hypertension. The hypothesis to be supported in this review is that genetic hypertension, both clinically and in the experimental animal, is caused by a primary fault in cell membranes. This

Sambhi, M.P. (ed.) Fundamental fault in hypertension
© *1984, Martinus Nijhoff Publishers. Boston/The Hague/Dordrecht/Lancaster.*
ISBN 978-94-010-9006-3

fault may be most readily studied in the red blood cell. When it occurs in the vascular smooth muscle cell, this membrane changes causes an increase in excitability of the cell, hence its contraction is increased, resulting in an increase in total peripheral resistance and hypertension.

This review will deal first with evidence that there is an alteration in the cell membrane of vascular smooth muscle and hypertension. Indirect evidence supporting this hypothesis is to be found in the observations that vascular smooth muscle sensitivity is increased. More direct evidence has been reported indicating that vascular smooth muscle membrane permeability to ions is increased in hypertension. The mechanism by which this alteration in membrane permeability may alter the vascular response is then presented. Evidence is presented that similar changes occur in the membrane of the red blood cell in hypertension. Finally, the reader is reminded of the general significance of alterations in electrolyte metabolism in the etiology of hypertension.

VASCULAR SMOOTH MUSCLE SENSITIVITY

The major cause of the increased arterial pressure in both clinical and experimental hypertension is an elevation in vascular resistance. Vascular reactivity, which is a measure of the increase in vascular resistance produced by a constrictor agent, is also elevated in hypertension. These changes could be caused by a structural thickening of the wall of the resistance vessel or by functional changes in the vascular smooth muscle. Changes of the latter type could be mediated neurogenically, humorally, or myogenically. This review will focus on evidence that intrinsic changes in the smooth muscle cell (myogenic changes) may make the cell more sensitive to external stimuli.

The sensitivity of vascular smooth muscle may be evaluated by determining the concentration of the stimulating agent necessary to produce a threshold response, or the concentration of the agent necessary to produce a half maximal response (ED_{50}). Information regarding vascular smooth muscle sensitivity may be obtained by wholebody vascular reactivity studies, by perfusion of an isolated vascular bed, or by isolated vascular strip studies in the muscle bath. Studies in the isolated muscle bath may have the disadvantage of being carried out in a unnatural environment; however, if differences between vascular smooth muscle from normotensive and hypertensive animals persist in this environment, it must be concluded that there are intrinsic differences in the muscles being studied. Although some investigators [33] have found no evidence for increased vascular smooth muscle sensitivity in hypertension, many reports present evidence supporting such an increase. The basis for this discrepancy is not evident, but may reside in differences in experimental animals, types of hypertension, measurement techniques, or sources of vessels.

An example of the type of evidence available in support of a greater vascular sensitivity in hypertension is presented in Figure 1. Concentration-response curves of rat femoral artery from controls and from animals with one of three different types of hypertension indicate that there is a shift to the left in the concentration-response curve in the hypertensive animals. The increase in sensitivity to epinephrine appears to be much more prominent in DOCA and renal hypertensive rats than it does in spontaneously hypertensive rats. The reverse is true following stimuation by strontium or lanthanum [28, 41].

Another mechanical index of the increase in vascular smooth muscle sensitivity is the degree of spontaneous rhythmicity displayed by the isolated muscle. Smooth muscle from femoral arteries of normotensive rats usually remains relaxed and quiescent unless stimulated by specific constrictor agents. In contrast, spontaneous rhythmicity is common in rats with spontaneous, DOCA, or renal hypertension [28, 9, 2]. Figure 2 documents this rhymicity, which is evidence of plasma membrane lability. This figure also demonstrates the effect of an increase in calcium concentration on this spontaneous activity.

Two types of evidence may be cited that indicate that the changes in vascular smooth muscle sensitivity are primary and not secondary to the increase in wall stress produced by the elevated arterial pressure. In the first place, these changes in sensitivity have been observed to occur prior to the increase in arterial pressure [13, 4]. Additional evidence supporting the hypothesis that this vascular change is not secondary to increased wall stress comes from experiments in which one

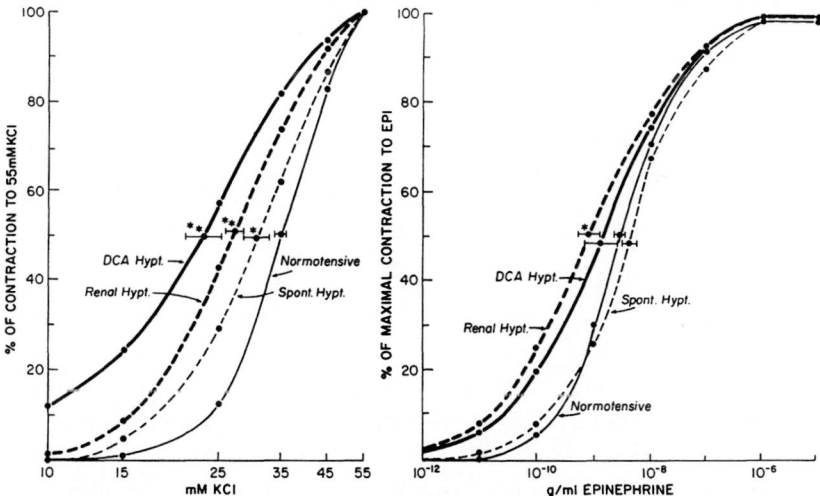

Figure 1. Normalized cumulative concentration-response curves. *Left*: KCl as agonist. Curves for all hypertensive groups (ten in each group) are shifted to the left. The difference of these curves from that of the normotensive rats is greatest for DCA-hypertensive rats and successively less for renal and spontaneously hypertensive rats. The values of ED_{50} for the first two groups are significantly different from that of the normal group (P<0.001, double asterisks) and that for the spontaneously hypertensive group (P = 0.05, asterisk). Brackets indicate SE. *Right*: Epinephrine as agonist. Curves for DCA– and renal hypertensive groups (ten in each group) are shifted somewhat to the left. Only the ED_{50} of the renal hypertensive rats is significantly different (P <0.05) from that of the normotensive control. (From Holloway and Bohr, [28]. Reproduced by permission.)

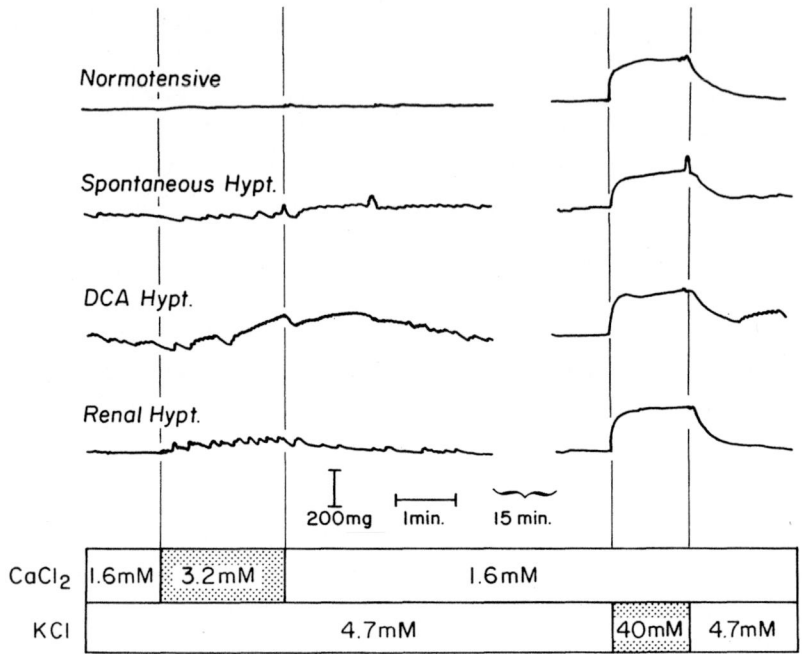

Figure 2. Responses of four femoral artery strips to 3.2 mM CaCl$_2$ and to 40 mM KCl. Spontaneous rhythmic contractions are seen in strips from the three types of hypertensive rats but not in the normotensive rat strips. Strips from DCA- and renal hypertensive rats contracted in response to 3.2 mM CaCl$_2$, but strips from normotensive and spontaneously hypertensive rats did not. All strips responded to the KCl stimulus. (From Holloway and Bohr [28]. Reproduced by permission.)

femoral artery of a DOCA hypertensive rat has been protected from the increase in wall stress by iliac artery ligation [25]. In this experiment there were equivalent increases in smooth muscle sensitivity in both the protected and unprotected femoral arteries.

VASCULAR SMOOTH MUSCLE CELL MEMBRANE IN HYPERTENSION

Although an increase in sensitivity of vascular smooth muscle is taken as evidence for an aberration in the excitatory process of the plasma membrane of this muscle, this evidence is very indirect. Altered water and electrolyte metabolism of vascular smooth muscle has long been associated with hypertension in human beings and in experimental hypertension in both dogs and rats [43, 37]. Increased water and sodium content were commonly found; increased potassium content occurred less frequently. Whether altered ionic composition was the result of the increased pressure has been questioned since some investigators found alterations above, but not below aortic coarctation in dogs [27]. In more recent studies, elevated sodium content of vessel wall has been observed in coarctation hypertension both above and below the constriction, and also in veins [36]. Aortas from spontaneously hypertensive rats (SHR), unlike those of other models, did not exhibit increased water and electrolyte contents during the early hypertensive phae [29, 34]. Increases were associated with prolonged hypertension.

Studies of ion transport indicated increased aortic turnover of ^{42}K, ^{36}Cl, and ^{24}Na in SHR and DOC/NaCl-hypertensive rats [31, 19, 20, 30]. Friedman[18] also reported increased exhange of lithium for cellular sodium and potassium in tail arteris from DOCA/NaCl rats. Figure 3 demonstrates that in smooth muscle from the control animal lithium was taken up very slowly, whereas in the smooth muscle from the SHR lithium was taken up and sodium and potassium lost at a much more rapid rate.

Evidence from two additional types of experiments has suggested that there is an important abnormality in the plasma membrane of vascular smooth muscle in hypertension. Jones [29] observed that the increased sensitivity of vascular smooth muscle from SHR to norepinephrine and to angiotensin was accompanied by a greater increase in membrane permeability to potassium produced by these agents. Hermsmeyer [26], studying membrane potential of vascular smooth muscle, noted that norepinephrine produced a greater depolarization in that from SHR than in that from normotensive controls.

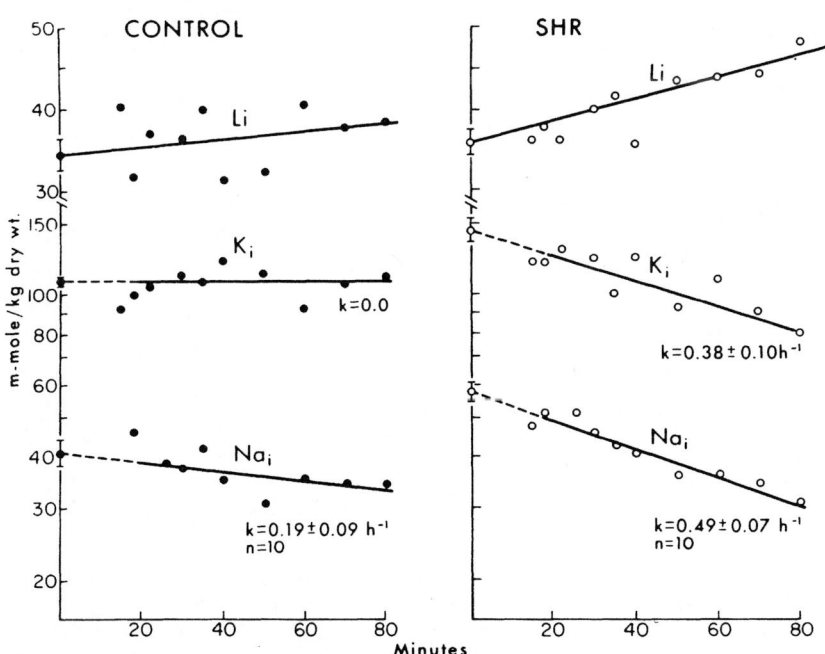

Figure 3. Cell Na and K in freshly excised tail arteries from control and spontaneously hypertensive rats (SHR) at various intervals after incubation in Li-substituted physiologic salt solution at 2°C. (From Friedman and Friedman, [19]. Reproduced by permission.)

ELECTROLYTES AND THE VASCULAR SMOOTH MUSCLE RESPONSE

For over a century, it has been recognized that shifts in electrolyte concentration have a profound effect on muscle contraction. Calcium is the essential ion for contraction of any muscle; shifts in its intracellular concentration constitute the final common pathway of the regulatory systems for the state of contraction of muscle. The amount of tension developed by the contractile protein is a direct function of the concentration of this ion. The concentration of calcium in the cell, which transforms the muscle from one with no active tension to one with maximal active tension, is extremely low [16]. It is now safe to assume that, when a shift in the concentration of any electrolyte produces an effect on muscle contraction, it does so by altering the concentration of ionized calcium in the environment of the contractile protein.

In relation to the pathogenesis of hypertension, the sodium ion is of particular interest. It is relevant, therefore, to explore the possible mechanisms by which a shift in sodium concentration or distribution may alter the concentration of ionized calcium at the intracellular site where it activates the contractile machine. All answers to this question deal with the influence that the sodium ion may have on some property of the plasma membrane or of the sarcoplasmic reticulum, where calcium is stored.

Membrane systems regulating the translocation of sodium, potassium, and calcium are illustrated in Figure 4 [8]. The sodium-potassium exchange system serves as the mechanism that maintains a concentration gradient of sodium (low on the inside) across the cell membrane. This pump is electrogenic, tending to

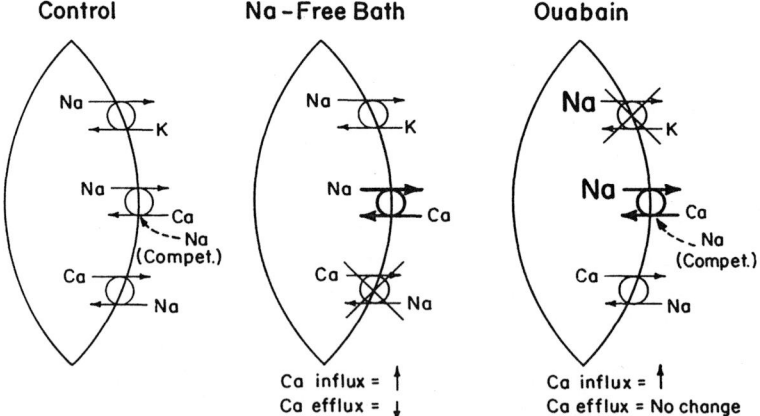

Figure 4. Schematic model illustrating hypothetical pump systems (or exchange diffusion). Three pumps are illustrated in each cell: the uppermost is a ouabain-sensitive pump which exchanges sodium for potassium; the middle pump, a sodium-calcium exchanger, may be accelerated by either removal of external sodium (which competes with calcium for a carrier) or by increasing the concentration of intracellular sodium by poisoning the ouabain-sensitive sodium-potassium pump; the lowermost exchange system, which may be driven by the transmembrane concentration gradient of sodium, is pictured as being responsible for calcium efflux. (From Bohr et al., [8]. Reproduced by permission.)

hyperpolarize the membrane. The pump system illustrated at the middle in Figure 4 exchanges sodium moving out for calcium moving in. Calcium competes with sodium for the carrier that moves it into the cell. The lowermost transfer system illustrated in this figure is a calcium extrusion system. Sodium moving down its concentration gradient into the cell is coupled to calcium extrusion. The influence of sodium on muscle contraction in these exchange systems is illustrated in Figure 5. It is evident that the absence of sodium in the bathing media causes a greater contraction and a slower relaxation. The contraction is larger because of the greater calcium influx where there is no sodium competing for influx channels; the relaxation is impaired because there is no sodium to exchange with calcium for its extrusion.

Blaustein [5] has hypothesized that altered operation of a sodium-calcium counterexchange system may contribute to increased intracellular calcium and contractile activity. According to this concept, competition between sodium and calcium occurs at the transport site. A relatively small increase in intracellular sodium decreases the transport of calcium out of the cell, thereby increasing calcium concentration available for the activation of the contractile apparatus. Only a small increase in the cellular sodium would be required significantly to affect intracellular calcium concentration.

In this context, it is relevant to point out that calcium has a dual effect on the vascular smooth muscle cell [6]. One is that of intracellular activator calcium, which is necessary for initiating the chemomechanical transduction that results in contraction. The other is the effect that calcium has on the membrane per se, 'stabilizing' it. This effect makes it more difficult to produce excitation of the cell. By this effect, an elevated concentration of extracellular calcium above physiological levels causes a reduction in the magnitude of contraction produced by various agonists.

Figure 6 illustrates the complexity and individuality of these sodium-calcium exchange systems. In these tracings it is evident that neither the rabbit aorta nor the dog mesenteric artery contracted when exposed to 120 mM Na, high Ca (25–50 mM) solution, or to a 120 mM Na, Ca-free solution. As illustrated in this figure, however, both contracted in a Na-free, high-Ca solution. If the vessels

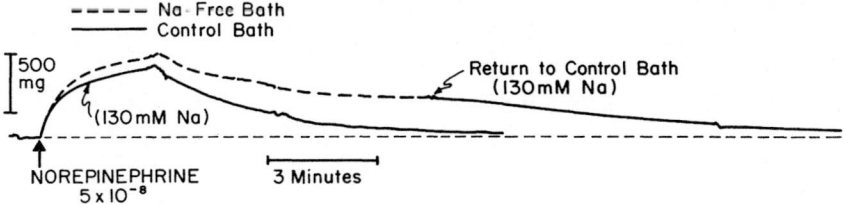

Figure 5. Effect of sodium-free (Li substituted) on norepinephrine response and on rate of relaxation in rabbit aorta. The superimposition of the response in the sodium-free bath emphasized the greater tension development and lower rate of relaxation displayed by this muscle. *R:* = bath rinsed. When the strip that had responded in a sodium-free bath was placed in the control bath, a more abrupt relaxation commenced. (From Bohr et al., [8]. Reproduced by permission.)

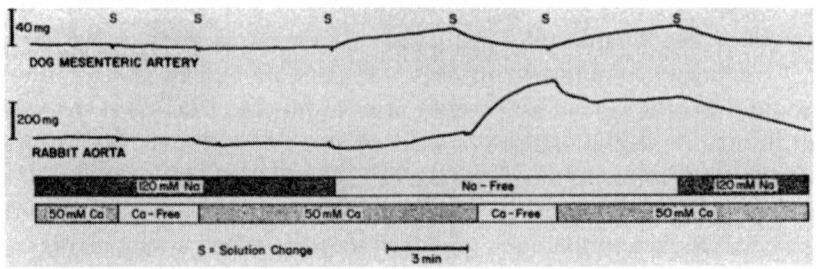

Figure 6. Effect of Na on response to 50 mM Ca, and Ca-free PSS. Neither dog mesenteric artery (upper tracing) nor rabbit aorta (lower tracing) contracts in 50 mM Ca PSS containing control, 120 mM Na. Na-free, 50 mM Ca PSS, however, causes a small contraction in both strips. Introduction of a Na-free PSS after high Ca causes relaxation of mesenteric artery but contraction of rabbit aorta. Reintroduction of 50 mM Ca causes contraction of mesenteric artery but relaxation of aorta, not, however, to tension before Ca-free solution was introduced. Further relaxation of both vessel types occurs when 120 mM Na, 50 mM Ca PSS is introduced. (From Sitrin and Bohr [42]. Reproduced by permission.)

strips were then exposed to Na-free, Ca-free solution, the dog mesenteric strip immediately relaxed, but the rabbit aorta strip underwent a large contraction. Reintroduction of the high calcium solution caused a contraction in the mesenteric artery strip, but relaxation of the aorta. When 120 mM Na, high Ca-solution was washed in, both vessels immediately relaxed to the tension maintained before treatment. Responses of the rabbit aorta are dominated by membrane excitability and calcium available from intracellular stores. Those of the dog mesenteric artery are primarily dependent on the availability of extracellular calcium. In both types of vessels the contractile response is governed by the properties of the plasma membrane.

Studies of vascular smooth muscle from rats with various types of hypertension have indicated that this muscle is not as readily stabilized by increasing concentrations of extracellular calcium as is that from normotensive control animals. Results demonstrating this difference are depicted in Figure 7. Smooth muscle from femoral arteries of a normotensive control and of three different types of hypertensive rats were mounted in the same muscle bath. All were stimulated to contract by a 40 mM concentration of KCl. Once a plateau of tension development had occurred, the concentration of calcium in the bath was increased as indicated on the horizontal axis. The amplitude of contraction of the smooth muscle from the normotensive rat was readily depressed. Smooth muscle from all three types of hypertensive animals required a much higher concentration of calcium to achieve a depression in contraction. These results were interpreted as indicating that vascular smooth muscle from hypertensive animals is not as readily stabilized by calcium as is that of the normotensive control. This results suggest that there may be fewer calcium binding sites on the plasma membrane in the smooth muscle from the hypertensive animals.

RED BLOOD CELL

Ion transport studies have indicated that there is a difference between the properties of the plasma membrane of the red blood cell from normotensive and from hypertensive humans and animals.

Early reports from two laboratories in Germany [32, 44] indicated that red blood cells from patients with essential hypertension had a slightly but significantly greater than normal intracellular sodium concentration. In 1966, von Wessels et al. reported a greater difference between red cells of normal and hypertensive patients if, instead of measuring sodium concentration, they measured ^{22}Na influx. Subsequently, these investigators [47] reported that plasma from patients with essential hypertension caused an increase in influx of sodium into normal red cells. They also noted that in hypertensive patients there was a direct correlation between the magnitude of the pressor response to norepinephrine or to angiotensin and the degree of elevation of sodium influx into the red cell [46]. In recent studies from three additional laboratories, observations have been made on sodium transport across the membranes of red blood cells from patients with essential hypertension. Although each laboratory used a different

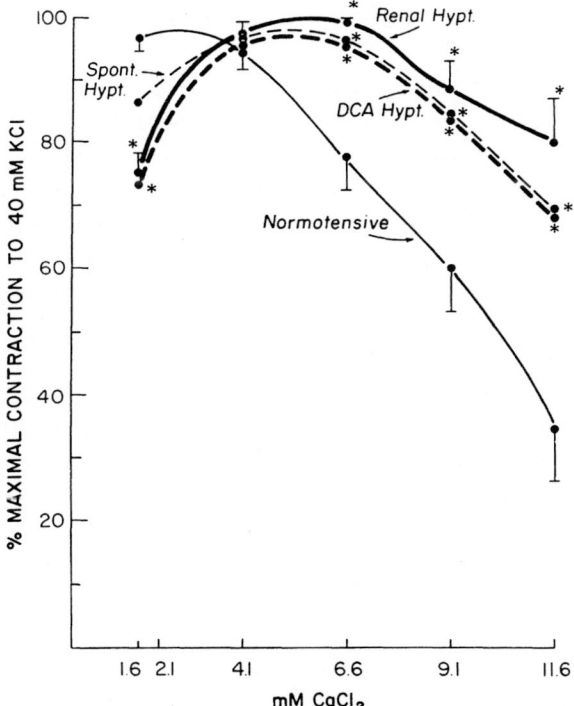

Figure 7. Normalized average of responses to 40 mM KCl at various calcium concentrations. The greatest response of strips (eight or nine each group) from normotensive rats was at 1.6 mM Ca, from the spontaneously hypertensive rats it was 4.1 mM, and from the DCA- and renal hypertensive rats it was at 6.6 mM. Brackets indicate SE, and an asterisk indicates a significant difference from normotensive value at $P < 0.05$. (From Holloway and Bohr [28]. Reproduced by permission.)

measure of electrolyte transport, all three reported differences between the red blood cell membranes from normals and those from patients with essential hypertension.

Postnov et al. [40] measured sodium influx and the rate constant for Na/Na exchange for red blood cells loaded with ^{22}Na. Cells from 20 patients with essential hypertension were compared with those from 20 normotensive patients. In the presence of 5×40^{-4} M ouabain, the average rate constant for this exchange was twice as great in red blood cells from hypertensive patients (1.52 ± 0.12 vs. 0.70 ± 0.12 10^{-5} mole/min/l of cells).

These investigators have also studied the effect of calcium concentration on the inner and outer membranes of the red blood cell in normotensive and hypertensive patients. In studies of calcium depletion from the red blood cell with EDTA, they found that more calcium ion was removed from the outer part of the red blood cell membrane of the hypertensive patient than from that of the normotensive subject (60 ± 5 vs. 41 ± 3 μEq/l of cells). They considered this to be evidence that there was an alteration of calcium binding to the outer membrane of the red blood cell in essential hypertension. In additional studies they evaluated the activity of a calcium-dependent ATPase by varying the concentration of intracellular calcium. The ATPase activity was less for the hypertensive than that for the normotensive subject (0.77 ± 0.04 vs. 0.93 ± 0.03 μM Pi/ml cell/hr). They interpreted this depression of ATPase activity as indicating that there was an alteration in the calcium binding ability of the inner part of the red blood cell.

Garay and Meyer [22] measured rate of potassium uptake and sodium loss from sodium-loaded red blood cells. The average ratio of net Na^+/K^+ flux of 18 patients with essential hypertension was less than half of this ratio for red blood cells from 17 normotensive patients. There was no overlap of these data. Five of eight young normotensive people born of parents with essential hypertension had ratios that fell among the values of those of red blood cells from patients with essential hypertension.

Canessa et al. [11] used a method previously reported by Haas, Schooler, and Tosteson [25] to measure the maximum rate of Li-Na countertransport in red blood cells. In 18 men with essential hypertension, the ouabain-resistant Li efflux was over twice that in 17 normotensive men (0.62 ± 0.03 vs. 0.26 ± 0.03 moles Li/hr).

Whereas these studies were all carried out in patients with essential hypertension, recent studies have also demonstrated a similar membrane leakiness in red blood cells from spontaneously hypertensive rats. Again, using quite different techniques for the assessment of sodium flux and two different strains of genetically hypertensive rats, this increase in leakiness has been reported in studies from at least four separate laboratories.

Ben-Ishay et al. [3] measured sodium efflux from red blood cells loaded with ^{22}Na. Red cells from the Israeli strain of hypertensive rats had a half life for ^{22}Na efflux of 30.5 ± 2.9 min; those from the normotensive strain had a half time of

40.1 ± 5 min.

Friedman et al. [21] measured the rate of lithium uptake of red blood cells placed in a medium in which Li had replaced Na. Red blood cells from spontaneously hypertensive rats (Kyoto strain) took up Li more rapidly than did those from normotensive controls (3.53 ± 0.31 vs. 3.00 ± 0.40 mole/lcell/hr). In addition, the authors observed the rate of sodium and potassium exchange between red blood cells and plasma when whole blood was stored at 2° C. After 23 hours, plasma sodium had decreased twice as much in the hypertensive as in the normotensive blood (7.2 ± 0.3 vs. 2.0 ± 0.6 in mEq/l), while plasma potassium had increased twice as much as in the blood from the normotensive control (6.54 ± 0.31 vs. 2.93 ± ;0.16 in mEq/l).

Postnov et al. [39] reported that the sodium concentrations of red blood cells of prehypertensive and early hypertensive rats (SHR) were 9.6 ± 0.4 and 9.2 ± 0.8 mEq/l of cells respectively, as compared to 7.2 ± 0.6 and 6.4 ± 0.9 mEq/l of cells from control Wistar and Sprague Dawley rats, respectively. The rate constant for Na/Na exchange (Figure 8) was over twice as great in ouabain-treated red blood cells from hypertensive animals as in those similarly treated cells from controls (2.83 ± 0.31 and 2.73 ± 0.30 vs. 1.38 ± 0.20 10^5 mole/min/lcells). Without ouabain treatment, the difference was not so great (4.81 ± 0.61 and 4.93 ± 0.70 in hypertensive compared to 3.23 ± 0.41 and 3.30 ± 0.38 10^{-5} mole/min/l cells for the two types of control rats).

Yamori et al. [48] measured the rate of ^{22}Na efflux from red blood cells in the presence of ouabain. After 75 minutes of incubation, 66.0 ± 1.6% of the original

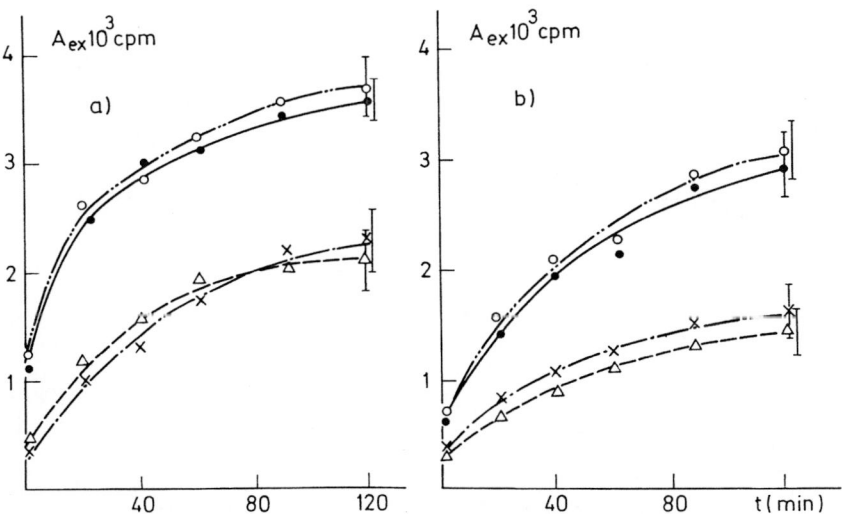

Figure 8. ^{22}Na efflux from the erythrocytes (calculated as c.p.m. of ^{22}Na). o, SHR, pre-hypertensive stage (n = 6; •, SHR, early hypertensive stage (n = 8); △, Wistar rats (n = 6); △, Sprague-Dawley rats (n = 6). (n is the number of separate rats on which an observation was made.) *a*. Medium without ouabain; *b*. medium containing ouabain (5 × 10^{-4} mol/l). (From Postnov et al., [39]. Reproduced by permission.)

^{22}Na was still present in the red blood cells of stroke-resistant (SR) spontaneously hypertensive rat (SHR), whereas only $58.1 \pm 1.9\%$ was still present in the stroke-prone SHR. This difference was significant.

GENERALIZED NATURE OF A PLASMA MEMBRANE CHANGE IN HYPERTENSION

In support of the possibility that a membrane change may be generalized in hypertension, a few observations have been reported indicating that there is an increase in membrane permeability in other tissues; these are visceral smooth muscle [1], leucocytes [15], and adipose tissue [38].

In addition to the evidence cited from vascular smooth muscle, red blood cells, and a few other tissues, there is indirect evidence from whole animal studies that may reflect membrane abnormalities. Much of this is related to the known relationship between sodium intake and blood pressure elevation in hypertension. That hypertension is made worse by a high sodium intake is well documented [14]. Renal handling of sodium is different in hypertension: a sodium load is more rapidly excreted in the urine (exaggerated natriuresis). High levels of mineralocorticoid cause hypertension that can be completely reversed by low sodium intake [12]. Since one characteristic of the membrane abnormality in hypertension is its increased permeability to sodium, this membrane characteristic may have a direct bearing on the mechanism by which sodium intake influences the blood pressure level in hypertension more than it does in the normal subject.

Finally, since the functions of all body systems are influenced by the property of their plasma membranes, a generalized abnormality in these structures would account for multiple systemic abnormalities recognized by Page in his Mosaic.

ACKNOWLEDGEMENT

Research has been supported by a Grant from the National Institute of Health HL 18575.

REFERENCES

1. Altman J, da Ponte R, Worcel M: Evidence for a visceral smooth muscle abnormality in Okamoto spontaneous hypertension. Br J Pharmac 59: 621–625, 1977
2. Bandick NR, Sparks HV: Contractile response of vascular smooth muscle of renal hypertensive rats. Am J Physiol 219: 340–344, 1970
3. Ben-Ishay D, Aviram A, Viskoper R: Increased erythrocyte sodium efflux in genetic hypertensive rats of the Hebrew University strain. Experientia 31: 660–662, 1975
4. Berecek KH, Bohr DF: Whole body vascular reactivity during the development of

deoxycorticosterone acetate hypertension in the pig. Circ Res 42: 764–771, 1978
5. Blaustein MP: Sodium ions, calcium ions, blood pressure regulation, and hypertension: a reassessment and a hypothesis. Am J Physiol 232: C165–C173, 1977
6. Bohr DF: Vascular smooth muscle: dual effect of calcium. Science 139: 597–599, 1963
7. Bohr DF: The role of altered vascular reactivity in hypertension. Hosp. Prac. 9: 107–116, 1974
8. Bohr DF, Seidel C, Sobieski J: Possible role of sodium-calcium pumps in tension development of vascular smooth muscle. Microvascular Res 1: 335–343, 1969
9. Bohr DF, Sitrin M: Regulation of vascular smooth muscle contraction: Changes in experimental hypertension. Circ Res 26 & 27, Suppl 11: 83–90, 1970
10. Brody MJ, Fink GD, Buffy J, Haywood JR, Gordon FJ, Johnson AK: The role of the anteroventral third ventricle (AV3V) region in experimental hypertension. Circ Res 43, Suppl I: 1–2 – I–13, 1978
11. Canessa M, Adragna N, Connolly T, Solomon H, Tosteson DC: Li-Na countertransport is increased in the red cells of patients with essential hypertension. Presented at the Sixth Scientific Meeting of the International Society of Hypertension, Göteborg, June 11–13, 1979
12. Cohen DM, Grekin RJ, Mitchell J, Rice WH, Bohr DF: Hemodynamic, endocrine and electrolyte changes during sodium restriction in DOCA hypertensive Pigs. Hypertension 2: 490–496, 1980
13. Collis MG, Alps BJ: Vascular reactivity to noradrenaline, potassium chloride, and angiotensin II in the rat perfused mesenteric vasculature preparation, during the development of renal hypertension. Cardiovasc Res 9: 118–126, 1975
14. Corcoran AC, Taylor RD, Page IH: Controlled observations on the effect of low sodium dietotherapy in essential hypertension. Circulation 3: 1–16, 1951
15. Edmonson RPS, Hilton PJ, Thomas RD, Patrick J, Jones NF: Abnormal leucocyte composition and sodium transport in essential hypertension. Lancet 1: 1003–1005, 1975
16. Filo RS, Bohr DF, Rüegg JC: Glycerinated skeletal and smooth muscle: calcium and magnesium dependence. Science 147: 1581–1583, 1965
17. Folkow B: Cardiovascular structural adaptation: its role in the initiation and maintenance of primary hypertension. Clin Sci Mol Med 55: 3s–22s, 1978
18. Friedman SM: An ion-exchange approach to the problem of intracellular sodium in the hypertensive process. Circ Res 34, Suppl I: 123–128, 1974
19. Friedman SM, Friedman CL: Cell permeability, sodium transport, and the hypertensive process in the rat. Circ Res 39: 433–441, 1976
20. Friedman SM, Nakashima M, Friedman CL: Cell Na and K in the rat tail artery during the development of hypertension induced by desoxycorticosterone acetate. Proc Soc Exp Biol Med 150: 171–176, 1975
21. Friedman SM, Nakashima M, McIndoe RA, Friedman CL: Increased erythrocyte permeability to Li and Na in the spontaneously hypertensive rat. Experientia 32: 476–478, 1976
22. Garay, RP, Meyer P: A new test showing abnormal net Na^+ and K^+ fluxes in erythrocytes of essential hypertensive patients. Lancet 1: 349–353, 1979
23. Guyton A, Coleman T, Granger H: Circulation: overall regulation. Ann Rev Physiol 34: 13–46, 1972
24. Haas M, Schooler J, Tosteson DC: Coupling of lithium to sodium transport in human red cells. Nature 258: 425–427, 1975
25. Hansen TR, Bohr DF: Hypertension, transmural pressure, and vascular smooth muscle response in rats. Circ Res 36: 590–592, 1975
26. Hermsmeyer K: Electrogenesis of increased norepinephrine sensitivity of arterial

vascular muscle in hypertension. Circ Res 38: 362–367, 1976

27. Hollander W, Kramsch DM, Farmelant M, Madoff IM: Arterial wall metabolism in experimental hypertension of coarctation of the aorta of short duration. J Clin Inv 47: 1221–1229, 1968
28. Holloway, ET, Bohr DF: Reactivity of vascular smooth muscle in hypertensive rats. Circ Res 33: 678–685, 1973
29. Jones AW: Altered ion transport in vascular smooth muscle from spontaneously hypertensive rats. Circ Res 33: 563–572, 1973
30. Jones AW: Functional changes in vascular smooth muscle associated with experimental hypertension. In: Bevan JA, Johansson B, Maxwell RA, Nedergaard OA (eds), Vascular neuroeffector mechanisms.. S. Karger, 1976, pp 182–189
31. Jones AW, Hart TG: Altered ion transport in aortic smooth muscle during deoxycorticosterone acetate hypertension in the rat. Circ Res 37: 333–341, 1975
32. Losse H, Wehmeyer H, Wessels F: Der Wasser- und Elektrolytgehalt von Erythrocyten bei Arterieller Hypertonie. Klin Wsch 38: 393–395, 1960
33. Lundgren Y, Hallback M, Weiss L, Folkow B: Rate and extent of adaptive cardiovascular changes in rats during experimental renal hypertension. Acta Physiol Scand 91: 103–115, 1974
34. Nagaoki A, Kituchi Y, Aramaki Y: Participation of tissue electrolytes and water in the spontaneous hypertension in rats. Jap Circ J 34: 489–497, 1970
35. Page IH: Pathogenesis of arterial hypertension. J Am Med Assoc 140: 451–457, 1949
36. Pamnani MB, Overbeck HW: Abnormal ion and water composition of veins and normotensive arteries in coarctation hypertension in rats. Circ Res 38: 375–378, 1976
37. Peterson LH: Systems behavior, feed-back loops, and high blood pressure research. Circ Res 12: 585–594, 1963
38. Postnov YV: Alteration of cell membranes in hypertension. In: Thurm RH (ed), Essential Hypertension. Symposia Specialists, Chicago, 1979, pp 293–297
39. Postnov Y, Orlov S, Gulak P, Shevchenko A: Altered permeability of the erythrocyte membrane for sodium and potassium ions in spontaneously hypertensive rats. Pflügers Arch 365: 257–263, 1976
40. Postnov YV, Orlov SN, Shevchenko A, Adler AM: Altered sodium permeability, calcium binding and Na-K-ATPase activity in the red blood cell membrane in essential hypertension. Pflügers Arch 371: 263–269, 1977
41. Shibata S, Kurahashi K, Kuchii M: Possible etiology of contractile impairment of vascular smooth muscle from spontaneously hypertensive rats. J Pharmacol Exp Ther 185: 406–417, 1973
42. Sitrin MD, Bohr DF: Ca and Na interaction in vascular smooth muscle contraction. Am J Physiol 220: 1124–1128, 1971
43. Tobian L: Interrelationship of electrolytes juxtaglomerular cells and hypertension. Physiol Rev 40: 280–312, 1960
44. von Gessler U: Intra- und extrazelluläre Elektroytveränderungen bei essentieller Hypertonie vor und nach Behandlung. Z Kreislaufforsch 51: 177–183, 1961
45. von Wessels R, Junge-Hulsing G, Losse H: Untersuchungen zur Natriumpermeabilität der Erythrozyten bei Hypertonikern und Normotonikern mit familiärer Hochdruckbelastung. Z Kreislaufforsch 56: 374–380, 1966
46. von Wessels F, Zumkley H: Untersuchungen über den Einfluss des intra- und extrazellulären Elektrolytstoffwechsels auf die Gefässreagibilität. Z Kreislaufforsch 59: 427–437, 1969
47. von Wessels F, Zumkley H, Losse H: Untersuchungen zur Frage des Zusammenhanges zwischen Kationenpermeabilität der Erythrozyten und Hochdruckdisposition. Z Kreislaufforsch 59: 415–426, 1969
48. Yamori Y, Nara Y, Horie R, Ohtaka M: Ion permeability of erythrocyte membrane in SHR. Jap Heart J 18: 604–605, 1977

10. IS BIOMEMBRANE ABNORMALITY A PATHOGENIC FACTOR OR A GENETIC MARKER OF HYPERTENSIVE DISEASES?

YUKIO YAMORI, YASUO NARA, HIROSHI IMAFUKU

SUMMARY

The establishment of the strains of spontaneously hypertensive rats (SHR) and stroke-prone SHR (SHRSP) indicates that genetic factors are important in the pathogenesis of hypertension and hypertensive diseases such as stroke. Among various characteristics observed in SHR and SHRSP, the membrane abnormality noted in erythrocytes may be related to a fundamental fault in hypertension or considered as a genetic marker of hypertensive diseases. We have therefore sought to analyze characteristics of various membranes (erythrocytes, platelets, and synaptosomes) by different methods (membrane viscosity by a microviscosimeter, membrane permeability of lipophilic ions by a newly developed biomembrane-permeability detector, osmotic fragility by a coil-planet centrifugation) in SHRSP, SHR, and their normotensive control Wistar-Kyoto (WK) strain, as well as in men with or without family history of stroke. Moreover, the changes in synaptosomal membrane potential induced by depolarization with various potassium ion concentrations were determined, using a fluorochrome as an indicator. Norepinephrine uptake into and release from synaptosomes were also quantitatively estimated.

Even before the development of severe hypertension, erythrocytes from SHRSP showed an increase in fluidity and permeability, and were proven to be more fragile to osmotic stress than those from SHR and WK. A similar increase in fluidity was also noted in SHRSP platelets.

Membrane fragility was determined in human erythrocytes. Two groups of people were selected from about 2000 inhabitants under our community health control program. Erythrocytes from the group that had stroke in their family history were proven to be more fragile than those from the corresponding group without stroke in their family history.

The response of synaptosomal membrane potential to various potassium ion concentrations was significantly different between young WK and SHRSP. Norepinephrine release by deporalization with a low potassium ion concentration was significantly accelerated in SHRSP.

Altered biomembrane characteristics noted not only in erythrocytes and platelets but also in synaptosomes may be primarily or secondarily involved in the

Sambhi, M.P. (ed.) Fundamental fault in hypertension
© *1984, Martinus Nijhoff Publishers. Boston/The Hague/Dordrecht/Lancaster.*
ISBN 978-94-010-9006-3

pathogenesis of hypertension or hypertensive diseases; such a membrane characteristic may be utilized as a marker for the detection of predisposition to these diseases.

INTRODUCTION

Recent studies on spontaneously hypertensive rats (SHR) [10, 9], and stroke-prone SHR (SHRSP) [18, 11] have brought us both good news and bad news [17]. The bad news is that hypertension and stroke are so definitely determined by genetic factors [13]. The good news is that hypertension and stroke can be prevented by modifying environmental factors or by treatment, even when genetic predisposition is strong [14, 15, 17].

As the development of these adult diseases is based on genetic predisposition and its interaction with environmental factors, it might be possible to detect the genetic predisposition before the damage is done. [17]. Such an early detection of predisposition would hopefully contribute to the prevention of hypertension and stroke. Our studies have indicated that biomembrane characteristics may be a promising measure for the detection of the genetic disposition of hypertensive diseases [19, 20, 21, 17, 23].

MECHANISMS OF HYPERTENSIVE DISEASES

Ever since SHRSP were established in 1974 we suspected that there might be some biomembrane abnormalities in hypertensive diseases, as because the cerebral hemorrhage and infarction noted in the stroke-prones were commonly caused by 'arterionecrosis.' Arterionecrosis is induced by the extensive exudation of plasma arterial walls damaged by physical (e.g., hypertension) or chemical (e.g., hypoxia, humoral factors) stress. As schematically summarized in Figure 1, severe hypertension functionally or hemodynamically reduces regional cerebral blood flow (rCBF) in the predilection sites of stroke lesions fed by recurrent arteries. Such chronic mild hypoxia due to the reduction in rCBF increases vascular permeability and finally induces arterionecrosis. Hemorrhage occurs when microaneurysms formed at necrotic arterial walls rupture; infarction occurs when arteries are occluded, with thrombosis at the site of the necrosis or microaneurysms [14, 15].

Increased vascular permeability, one of the basic processes inducing arterionecrosis, is detected by the leakage of horse-radish peroxidase or ^{131}I-labelled albumin into the brain through cerebral arteries with a tight blood-brain barrier [16].

Scanning electromicroscopic studies on arterial endothelial cells demonstrate small craters and abundant villi formations in SHRSP, not only in the advanced

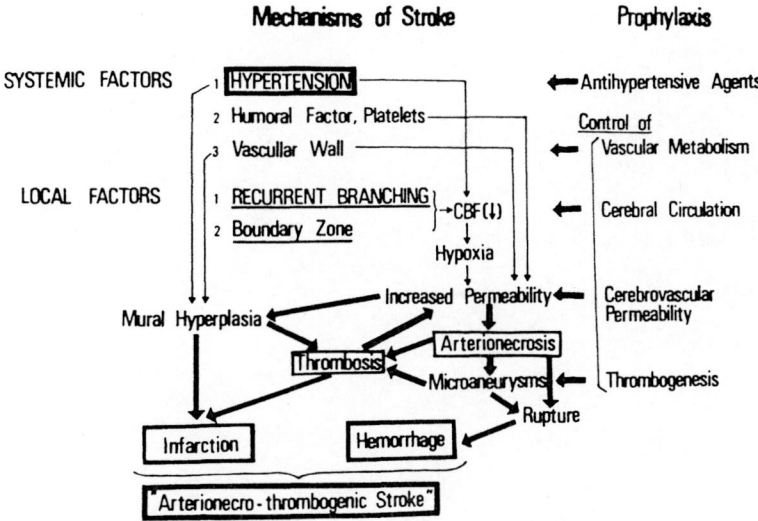

Figure 1. Mechanisms of stroke in stroke prone spontaneously hypertensive rats (SHRSP).

stage but also in relatively early stages of hypertension (Figure 2). These morphologically detectable membrane alterations may be based on a more generalized basic membrane abnormality related to the genetic pathogenesis of hypertensive diseases.

DEVIATIONS IN IONIC TRANSPORT IN SHR

Corcerning deviation in ionic transport, Jones first reported an increased potassium ion washout from arterial walls in SHR [5, 6], and Hermsmeyer further demonstrated a lower intracellular potassium ion activity in the vascular muscle cells of caudal arteries in SHR [3, 4]. Such an abnormal ionic transport is not limited to vascular muscle cells but is also found in erythrocytes. Postnov and associates and our group found it independently in SHR [12] and SHRSP [19, 20], respectively.

Hermsmeyer [3, 4] demonstrated that the membrane potential of muscle cells, measured under various extracellular potassium ion concentrations, did not change at 36° C but was significantly lower in SHR at 16° C. This means that a lesser membrane potential due to ionic gradient is present in SHR, but is compensated by the greater contribution of electrogenic ion transport in SHR at 36° C. This finding suggests that the membrane itself is different in SHR. The leakage of sodium ion from erythrocytes was actually accelerated in SHRSP as compared with SHR; this greater sodium extrusion was noted after ouabain treatment [19]. Blood cells in hypertension are recently being studied more widely in the world [2]. All these studies from different countries indicated a

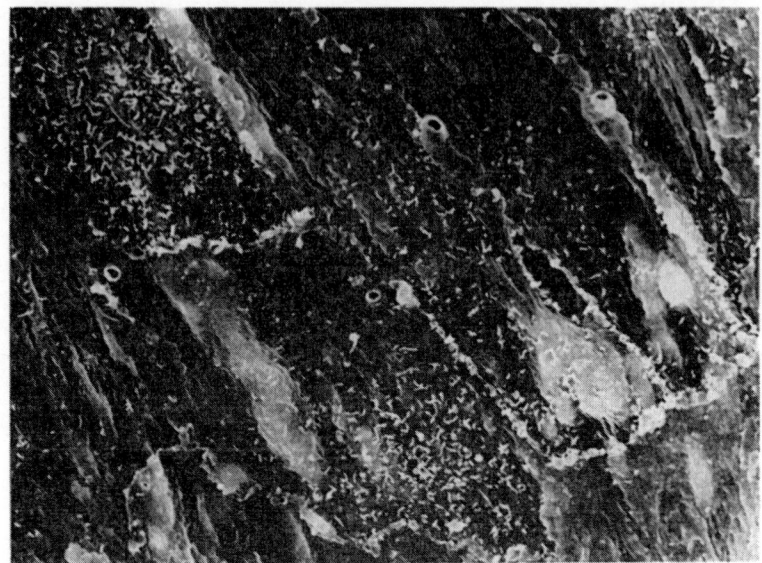

Figure 2. Scanning electronmicroscopic findings in endothelial cells of the cerebrobasal arteries from a 8-month-old SHRSP.

difference in ionic transport in hypertensive patients. Ionic transport abnormality may therefore be common in SHR and in human essential hypertension, and may be related to a fundamental fault in spontaneous or essential hypertension, as Dr. Bohr explained beautifully in the preceding paper.

CHARACTERISTICS OF ERYTHROCYTE MEMBRANE IN SHR

Biomembrane abnormalities in membrane permeability, fluidity, and osmotic fragility were further studied in SHR and SHRSP by applying various methodologies.

We recently developed a simple method to detect the permeability of erythrocytes by using a lipophilic ion, tetraphenyl phosphonium, as an indicator [17, 22, 23]. When erythrocyte membranes are more permeable, there is an increase in electric potential change rate due to the alteration in ion concentration in the solution mixed with a given amount of erythrocytes (Figure 3). The potential change rate in SHRSP erythrocytes was already higher at age 3 months than in WK rats, indicating that membrane permeability is increased in SHRSP even in the early hypertensive stage. The permeability is apparently different between aged SHRSP and WK rats.

Moreover, microviscosimetry (Elscint) was applied to erythrocyte membranes from SHRSP, and WK rats. In SHRSP and SHR, the membrane viscosity was lower [23]; in other words, the membrane fluidity was increased, and erythrocyte membranes might be more permeable in SHRSP. Since membrane fluidity is generally affected by the cholesterol concentration in biomembranes, we exam-

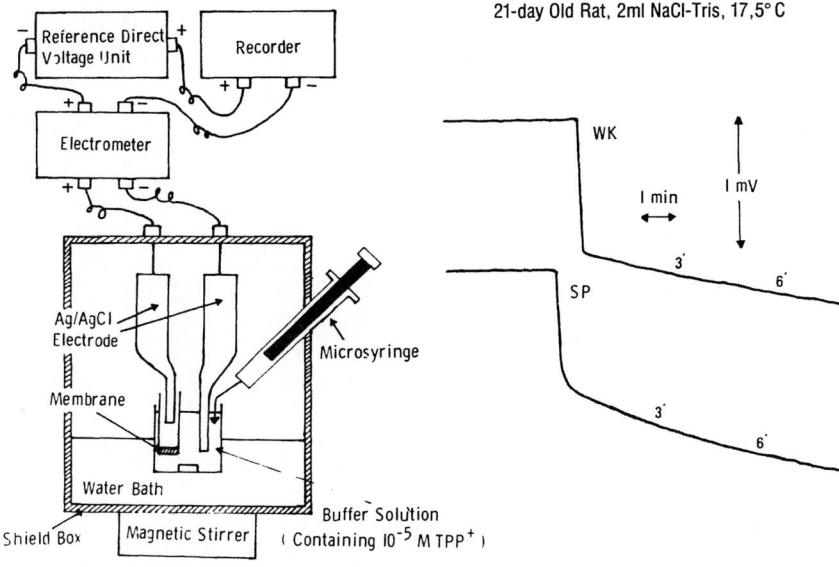

Figure 3. A new method for detecting the membrane permeability of lipophilic ion (tetraphenyl phosphonium). The potential change rates (right) of erythrocytes from a 3-month-old SHRSP $(1.00 \pm 0.08 \, \mu V/sec)$ were significantly greater than those from the age-matched WK (0.85 ± 0.04).

ined cholesterol levels of erythrocyte membranes and found them to be significantly decreased in SHRSP compared with WK rats. This reduction seems to be related to the lower plasma cholesterol level in SHRSP (Figure 4). It is interesting that the incidence of stroke, that is, 'arterionecro-thrombogenic stroke,' but not 'athero-thrombogenic stroke,' is high in SHRSP with a lower cholesterol level as well as in rural inhabitants in Japan with a relatively lower cholesterol level. A similar increase in membrane fluidity was also noted in platelets from SHRSP compared with WK rats, and the cholesterol vs. phospholipid ratio was also decreased in SHRSP. Moreover, the distribution of platelet size (analyzed by a Coulter counter) was greater in SHRSP than that in WK, and platelets from SHRSP were more easily changed into larger sizes during washing (Figure 5). Such a difference in size may reflect the altered characteristics of platelet membrane.

Since sodium permeability and membrane fluidity were different in SHRSP erythrocytes, we further tested their osmotic fragility by passing a minute amount of erythrocytes through the osmotic gradient in a thin polyethylene tube 3 m long. During coil-planet centrifugation (CPC-method), erythrocytes migrate from high to low osmotic pressure. Erythrocytes from SHRSP are hemolyzed at a higher osmotic pressure than those from SHR and WK rats (Figure 6) [19, 20]. Both starting and end points of hemolysis were higher in SHRSP, indicating that erythrocyte membranes from SHRSP were more fragile than those from other strains.

138

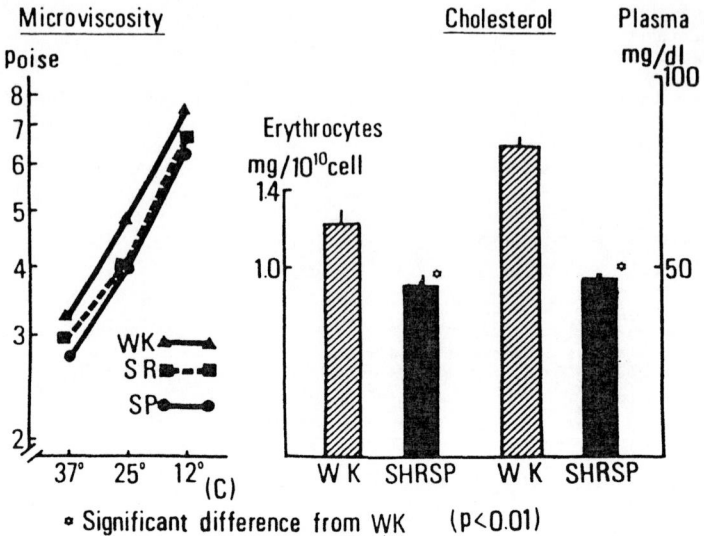

Figure 4. Microviscosity and cholesterol values for the ghosts of erythrocytes from SHRSP, SHR, and WK rats.

CHARACTERISTICS OF SYNAPTOSOMES FROM SHR

The membrane characteristics of synaptosomes were analyzed further in order to clarify whether the biomembrane abnormality noted in erythrocytes could be part of more generalized abnormalities in hypertension. We used a fluorochrome method, labelled norepinephrine uptake, and release to test the synaptosomal membrane characteristics [8].

Fluorochrome (3, 3'-dihexyloxacarbocyanine) incorporated into synaptosomes is extruded when the membrane is deporalized. The greater the membrane potentiel change, the more fluorochrome is extruded. Linear relations were found between the amount of fluorochrome extruded and the concentration of potassium ions applied to deporalize the synaptosomes. The relationship between fluorochrome and potassium ion in 2-month-old SHRSP was proven to be significantly different from that in the age-matched WK rats, indicating that synaptosomal depolarization in response to potassium ion was different in the young SHRSP.

Norepinephrine uptake into the synaptosomes, especially in the initial phase, was significantly larger in SHRSP than in WK rats, and the uptake in SHR was intermediate between the two.

On the other hand, the release of labelled norepinephrine from synaptosomes was greater in SHRSP than in WK, especially in response to lower concentrations of potassium ions (Table 1). These findings indicate the possible alteration of synaptosomal functions that might be related to autonomic nervous function in these hypertensive models.

An analysis of the present ideas on the pathogenesis of spontaneous hypertension may be summarized as follows; Spontaneous hypertension is caused by the interaction between genetic and environmental factors. Two main hypertension mechanisms currently under study involve neural and vascular factors, both of which contribute to functional and structural increases in peripheral vascular resistance to establish hypertension. Generalized biomembrane abnormalities may affect neural factors as well as vascular reactivity or metabolism. They may also affect not only ionic transport at the cellular level but also electrolyte balance in the whole body to induce salt retention or to increase circulatory volume. Such a biomembrane abnormality may be one of the basic genetic pathogenesis of hypertension, and in extreme cases such as SHRSP, even vascular endothelial cells would be also involved, so that increased vascular permeability would cause 'arterionecrosis,' the common basic cerebrovascular lesions in both hemorrhage and infarction.

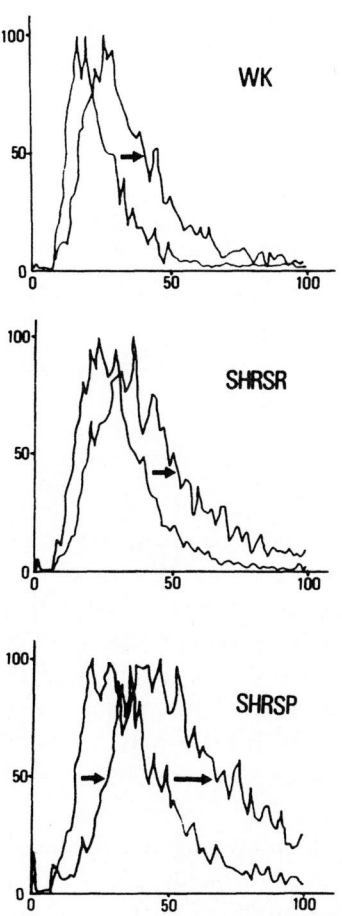

Figure 5. Size distribution and its lability of platelets from SHRSP, SHR (SR), and WK rats.

140

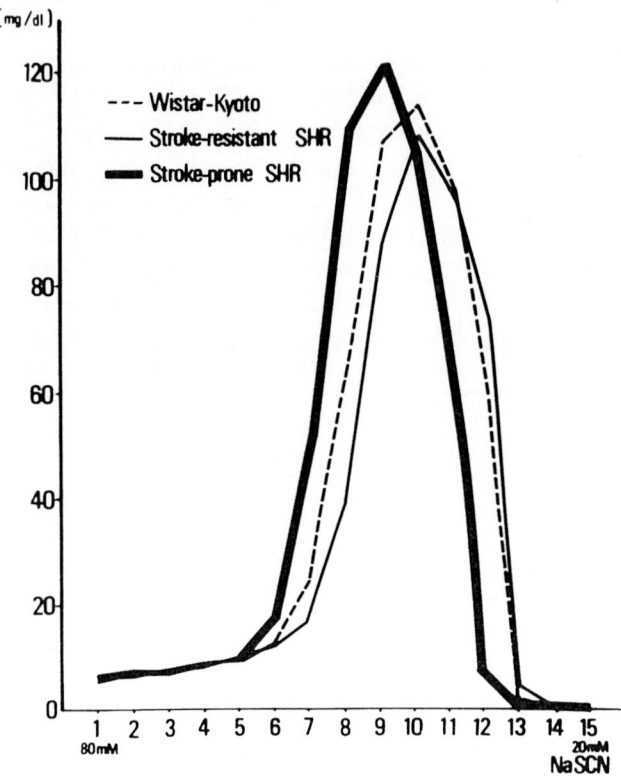

Figure 6. Hemolysis curves of erythrocytes from SHRSP (SP), SHR (SR), and WK rats.

CLINICAL AND EPIDEMIOLOGICAL APPLICATIONS

Biomembrane abnormalities may therefore be utilized to detect genetic pre-disposition to hypertension and stroke. The detection of these predisposition is very important for complete prevention of these hypertensive diseases. Garay and Meyer [1] reported that 'net sodium efflux' from erythrocytes was decreased in SHR and salt-sensitive hypertensive rats of the Sabra strain. Moreover, they found a similar reduction of 'net sodium efflux' in erythrocytes from essential hypertensive patients (but not in renal hypertensives) in comparison with the normotensives. They also reported a similar reduction in normotensive offspring from hypertensive parents.

As synaptosomes cannot be used as clinical material, platelets may be utilized instead. Mattiasson et al. [7] reported that norepinephrine efflux from platelets was highly significantly correlated to the diastolic pressure in hypertensive pa-tients. Comparative studies on platelets and synaptosomes in SHR would be a

Table 1. Effect of various concentration of K⁺ on norepinephrine (NE) release from synaptosomes

K⁺ Concentration (mM)	10	25	35	55
Amount of NE released (p mole/mg protein)				
SHRSP	2.62 ± 0.24	4.15 ± 0.27	3.88 ± 0.39	4.20 ± 0.15
SHRSR	1.17 ± 0.38*	2.77 ± 0.67	3.38 ± 0.81	3.99 ± 0.80
WKY	1.67 ± 0.28*	2.63 ± 0.48*	2.42 ± 0.67	3.39 ± 0.51

* Significant difference from SHRSP ($p < 0.05$)

clue for the clinical application of platelets.

Concerning the predisposition to stroke, the osmotic fragility of erythrocytes was also examined in selected male and female adults aged 40–59 from among 2000 inhabitants under our community health control program [22]. Erythrocytes from men with stronger genetic disposition to stroke were more fragile than those from age-matched men without obvious genetic disposition in their family history (Table 2). This difference in osmotic fragility was significant in males but not in females.

CONCLUSIONS

Biomembrane characteristics noted not only in erythrocytes or platelets, but also in synaptosomes in SHR and SHRSP may be related to the genetic pathogenesis of hypertensive diseases. Even if these findings were not of pathogenic importance, they may be used as genetic markers of hypertensive diseases and be useful for the early detection of predisposition to these diseases.

Table 2. Osmotic fragility of erythrocytes in men with genetic disposition to stroke*

Groups (No. of subjects)	Osmotic fragility (mM)	
	Hemolysis start-point	Hemolysis end-point
Males +(16)	58.7 ± 0.9**	36.4 ± 0.5**
−(9)	55.0 ± 0.9	33.5 ± 0.6
Females +(11)	59.8 ± 0.9	37.5 ± 0.7
−(19)	57.9 ± 0.8	36.1 ± 0.5

* Genetic disposition to stroke; + indicates individuals age 40–59, with at least one parent who had suffered from stroke; and − indicates individuals with both parents alive, over 70, who had no history of stroke.
** Significant differences from − group ($p < 0.05$).

142

ACKNOWLEDGMENTS

The authors express their cordial appreciation to Dr. Takeo Kimura, Technical Research Laboratory of Asahi Chemical Industry Co., Ltd, who helped the development of special electrodes and equipment for measuring ion permeability of erythrocytes. This study was supported by the Science and Technology Agency of the Japanese Government, Mitsubishi Foundation for Natural Science, Ministry of Education, and National Institutes of Health, U.S.A. (Grant HL 17754).

REFERENCES

1. Garay RP, Meyer P: A new test showing abnormal net Na^+ and K^+ fluxes in erythrocytes of essential hypertensive patients. Lancet i: 349–353, 1979
2. Gross F, Meyer P, Tosteson DC, Yamori Y (eds): Membrane in Hypertension. Table Ronde Roussel-Uclaf No. 42, Roussel Uclaf, Romanville, 1981
3. Hermsmeyer K: Cellular basis for increased seneitivity of vascular smooth muscle in spontaneously hypertensive rats. Circ Res Suppl 2, 38: 53–57, 1976
4. Hermsmeyer K: Electrogenesis of increased norepinephrine sensitivity of arterial vascular muscle in hypertension. Circ Res 38: 362–367, 1976
5. Jones AW: Altered ion transport in vascular smooth muscle from spontaneously hypertensive rats. Circ Res 33: 563–572, 1973
6. Jones AW: Altered ion transport in large and small arteries from spontaneously hypertensive rats and the influence of calcium. Circ Res Suppl 1, 34–35: 117–122, 1974
7. Mattiasson I, Mattiasson B, Hood B: The efflux rate of norepinephrine from platelets and its relation to blood pressure. Life Sci 24: 2265–2272, 1979
8. Nara Y, Yamori Y, Horie R, Kihara M, Ooshima A, Lovenberg W: Synaptosomal membrane characteristics in stroke-prone SHR (SHRSP). Jap Heart J 21: 558, 1980
9. Okamoto K (President): Proceedings of the 3rd international symposium on the SHR and related studies. Jap Heart J 20, suppl I, 1979
10. Okamoto K, Aoki K: Development of a strain of spontaneously hypertensive rats. Jap Circ J 27: 283–293, 1963
11. Okamoto K, Yamori Y, Nagaoka A: Establishment of the stroke-prone spontaneously hypertensive rat (SHR). Circ Res 34, 35, Suppl 1: 143–153, 1974
12. Postnov YUV, Orlov SN, Gulak PV, Shevchenko AS: Evidence of altered permeability of the erythrocyte membrane for sodium and potassium ions in spontaneously hypertensive rats. Clin Sci Mol Med 51: 196s–172s, 1976
13. Tanase H, Suzuki Y, Ohshima A, Yamori Y, Okamoto K: Genetic analysis of blood pressure in spontaneously hypertensive rats. Jap Circ J 34: 1197–1212, 1970
14. Yamori Y, Horie R, Akiguchi I, Nara Y, Ohtaka M, Fukase M: Pathogenic mechanisms and prevention of stroke in stroke-prone SHR. In: De Jong W, Provoost AP, Shapiro APA (eds), Progress in brain research. Elsevier, Amsterdam, 1977
15. Yamori Y, Horie R, Handa H, Ohtaka M, Nara Y, Fukase M: Pathogenic approach to the prophylaxis of stroke and atherogenesis in SHR. In: spontaneous hypertension. DHEW Publication No. (NIH) 77–1179, 1977
16. Yamori Y, Horie R, Sato M, Sasagawa S, Okamoto K: Experimental studies on the pathogenesis and prophylaxis of stroke in stroke-prone spontaneously hypertensive rats (SHR). (1) Quantitative estimation of cerebrovascular permeability. Jap Circ J 39: 611–615, 1975

17. Yamori Y, Lovenberg W, Freis E (eds): Prophylactic approach to hypertensive diseases. Raven Press, New York, 1979
18. Yamori Y, Nagaoka A, Okamoto K: Importance of genetic factors in hypertensive cerebrovascular lesions: An evidence obtained by successive selective breeding of stroke-prone and resistant SHR. Jap Circ J 38: 1095–1100, 1974
19. Yamori Y, Nara Y, Horie R, Ohtaka M: Ion permeability of erythrocyte membrane in SHR. Jap Heart J 18: 604–605, 1977
20. Yamori Y, Nara Y, Horie R, Ohtaka M: Biomembrane characteristics and chronic effect of tocopherol in models for hypertension and stroke. In: Hayaishi O (ed), Tocopherol, Oxygn and Biomembranes. Excepta Medica, Amsterdam, 1977
21. Yamori Y, Nara Y, Horie R, Ohtaka M, Ohta K, Mitani F: Biomembrane characteristics in stroke-prone spontaneously hypertensive rats (SHRSP). Jap Heart J 19: 597–598, 1978
22. Yamori Y, Nara Y, Horie R, Ooshima A: Abnormal membrane characteristics of erythrocytes in rat models and men with predisposition to stroke. Clin Exp Hypert 2: 1009–1021, 1980

V. THE ANTIHYPERTENSIVE HORMONES OF THE KIDNEY

11. HYPERTENSION INDUCED BY JG-LIKE CELLS GROWN IN TISSUE CULTURE

E.E. MUIRHEAD, J.A. PITCOCK, W.A. RIGHTSEL, P.S. BROWN, M.F. HALL, B. BROOKS

We have succeeded in developing a monolayer tissue culture of cells having the major characteristics of juxtaglomerular cells-termed JG-like cells. This was accomplished by following a suggestion made by Khayat, Lewis, and Smeby [5] of the Cleveland Clinic.

The renal cortex of kidneys from neonate rats was minced and subjected to tissue culture. By selecting culture bottles containing cells that formed whorls, eventually the JG-like cells were derived. By cloning and recycling as transplants *in vivo,* a nearly pure cell line was developed.

1. Characteristics of the cultured cells. The cultured cells have the following major features of JG cells, as determined by transmission electron microscopy (Figures 1, 2, 3): peripheral dense bodies and myofibrils, indicative of a smooth muscle origin; rough endoplasmic reticulum containing fluffy precipitate, suggestive of protein synthesis; and a large Golgi apparatus surrounded by granules. Some granules are dense and have an even texture surrounded by a membrane (often with shrinkage of the matrix away from the membrane), consistent with secretory granules; others have an uneven texture surrounded by a membrane, consistent with lysosomes.

2. Transplantation of JG-like cells. The cells were derived from kidneys of our syngeneic rat line (Wistar/GM). Thus, they could be retransplanted into recipients of the same line and have a relatively prolonged take.

Forty-five to 100 million cells were harvested, as previously described for renomedullary interstitial cells (RIC) [7], and injected as a small track subcutaneously. A good take was indicated by a nodule developing at this site which expanded, as demonstrated by palpation, over a day's time. This nodule remained for two to three weeks, then slowly disappeared.

3. Hypertension induced by JG-like cells (n = 15). Transplantation of the JG-like cells followed by uninephrectomy (under pentobarbital, 30 mg/kg i.p.) 24 hours later, was associated with the development of hypertension. The mean arterial pressure (MAP) increased over two to three weeks' time from 110–120 to 160–200 mm Hg (Figure 4). When both kidneys remained *in situ,* the hypertensive

Sambhi, M.P. (ed.) Fundamental fault in hypertension
© *1984, Martinus Nijhoff Publishers. Boston/The Hague/Dordrecht/Lancaster.*
ISBN 978-94-010-9006-3

148

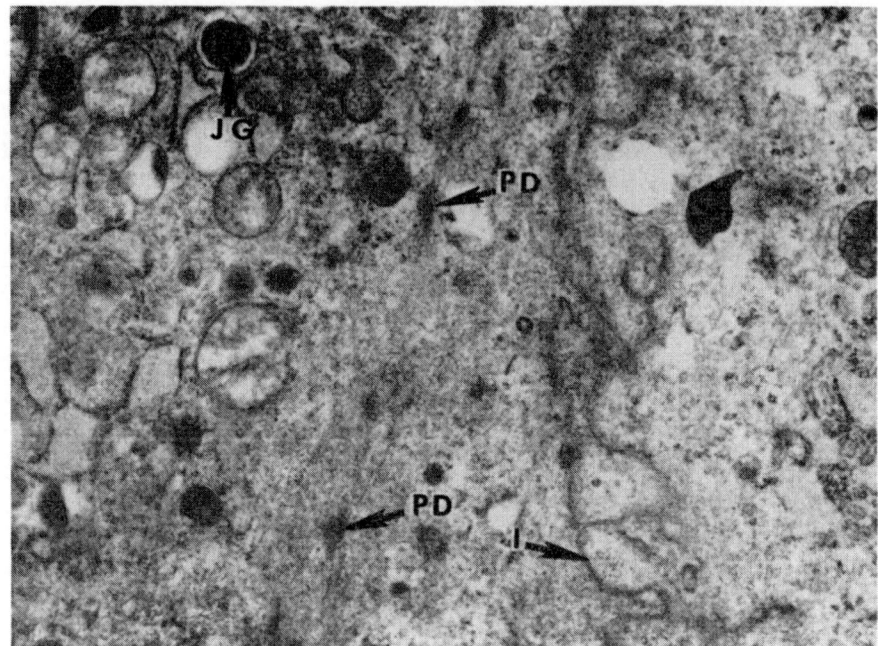

Figure 1. Cultured JG-like cells displaying peripheral dense bodies (*PD*), secretory granules (*JG*) and the cytoplasmic imbrication (*I*).

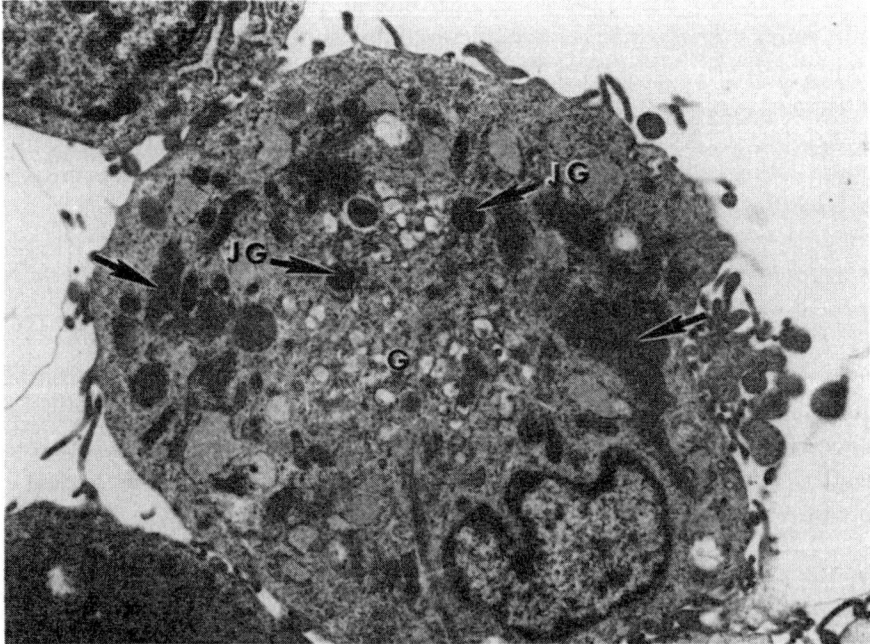

Figure 2. Cultured JG-like cell displaying a prominent Golgi apparatus (*G*) surrounded by secretory granules (*JG*). Note also rough endoplasmic reticulum containing precipitated fluffy material (plain arrows).

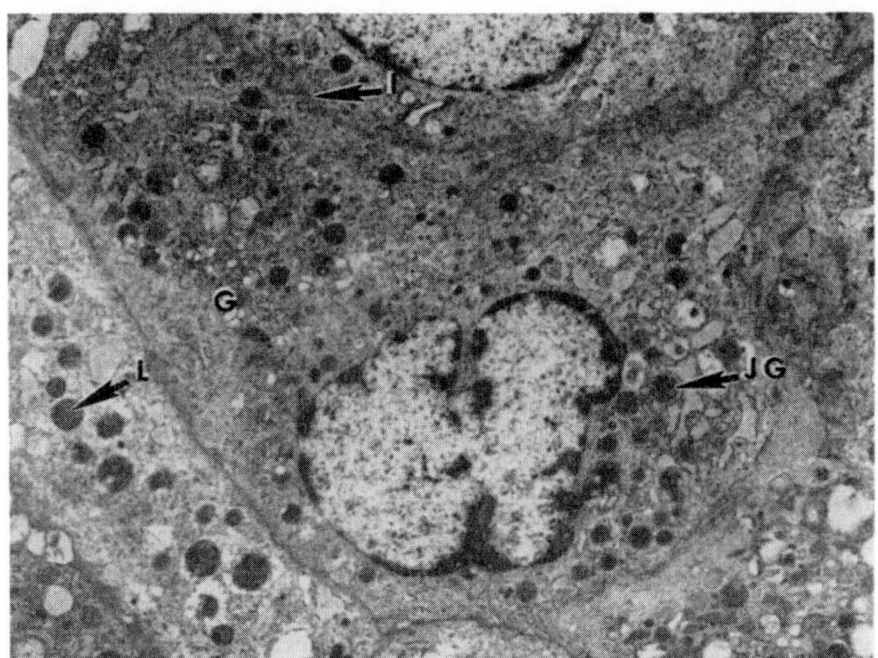

Figure 3. Cultured JG cell illustrating prominent granulation, including granules having the characteristics of secretory granules (*JG*) and granules resembling lysosomes (*L*). There is also a prominent Golgi apparatus (*G*) and imbrication between cells (*I*).

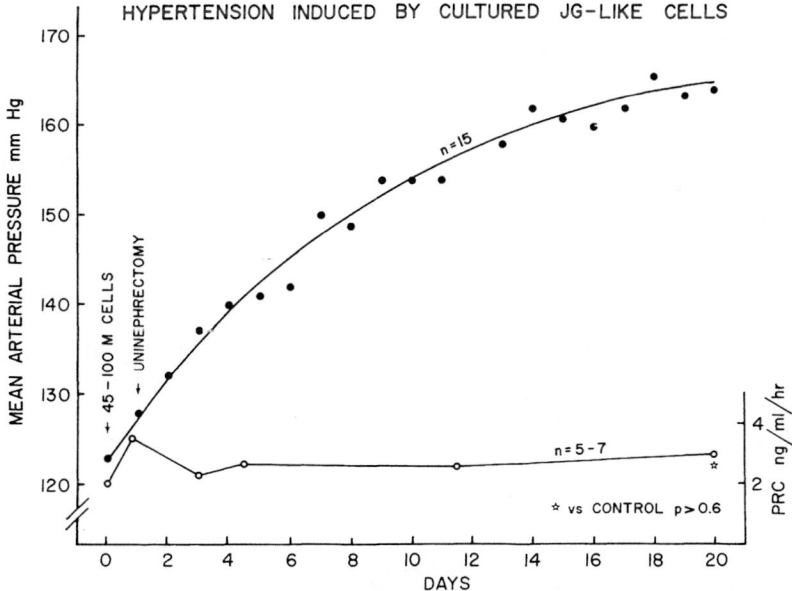

Figure 4. Evolution of the hypertension induced by cultured JG-like cells, depicted for 15 rats. The solid line is idealized for the points. The arterial pressure tends to level at about three weeks. Plasma renin concentration remained at control levels throughout.

state was less pronounced (MAP average 125 to 137 mm Hg), indicating some protection against the hypertension by renal tissue (Figure 5).

Controls (same rat line) consisted of uninephrectomized rats (n = 7), rats receiving a malignant cell line under the same conditions (n = 4), and rats receiving a transplant of cultured RIC followed by uninephrectomy 24 hours later (n = 8). None of these animals developed hypertension.

4. Some characteristics of this hypertensive model. (a) Plasma renin concentration, as measured by the micromethod of Carvalho et al. [2], remained at control level (~3 ng/ml/hr) throughout (Figure 4), i.e., during the developmental and the maintenance phases of the hypertensive state. There was no change in plasma renin substrate level. Thus, this was a normoreninemic state.
(b) Volume measurements: Blood, plasma, and extracellular fluid volumes, determined as described previously [8] were the same as those of paired controls (uninephrectomized animals followed for the same length of time as the hypertensive animals). Thus, this did not appear to be a volume-expanded state.
(c) Vascular disease: All animals displayed medial hypertrophy of small arteries and arterioles of the viscera. Some animals displayed fibrinoid necrosis and onion skin lesion of similar vessels, and polyarteritis nodosa of mesenteric arteries (Figures 6, 7, 8).

The combination of a non-expanded state (normal volume measurements) and severe arterial-arteriolar disease suggests to us the existence of a constricted arterial vascular tree (Johnson and Muirhead, 1979).

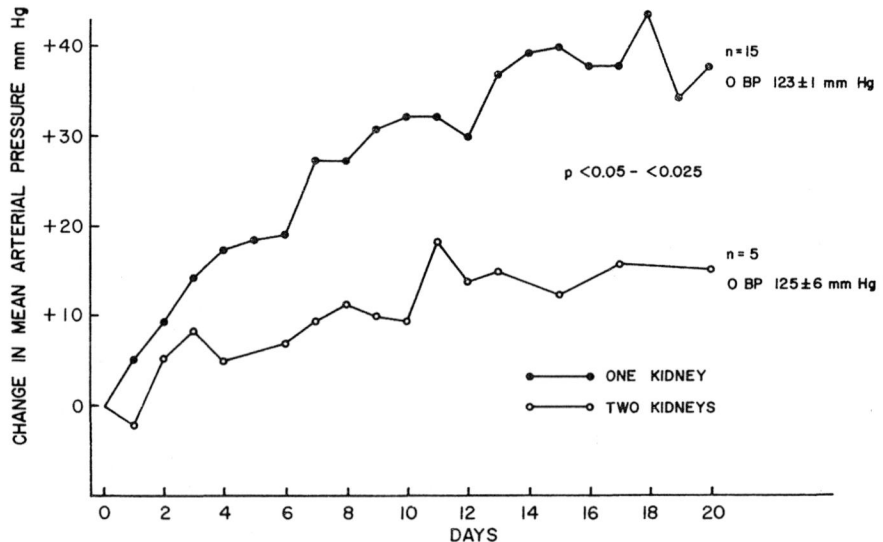

Figure 5. Protection against the hypertension induced by cultured JG-like cells when both kidneys remain intact (line with open circles).

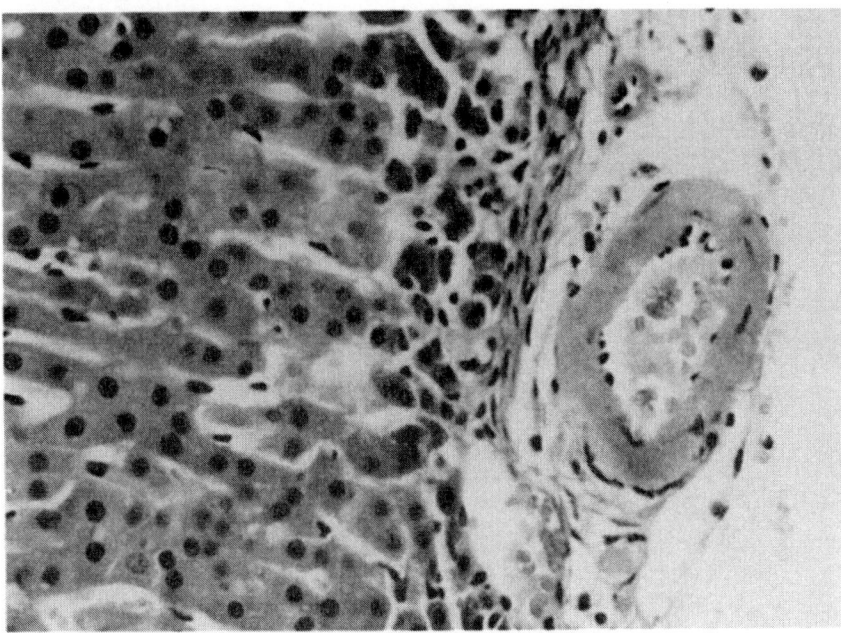

Figure 6. Necrotic small artery in the capsule of the adrenal, a consequence of hypertension induced by JG-like cells. Note that most of the nuclei of the media are absent, and the media is assuming a pseudo-hyalin appearance. This is what Byrom termed atypical necrosis.

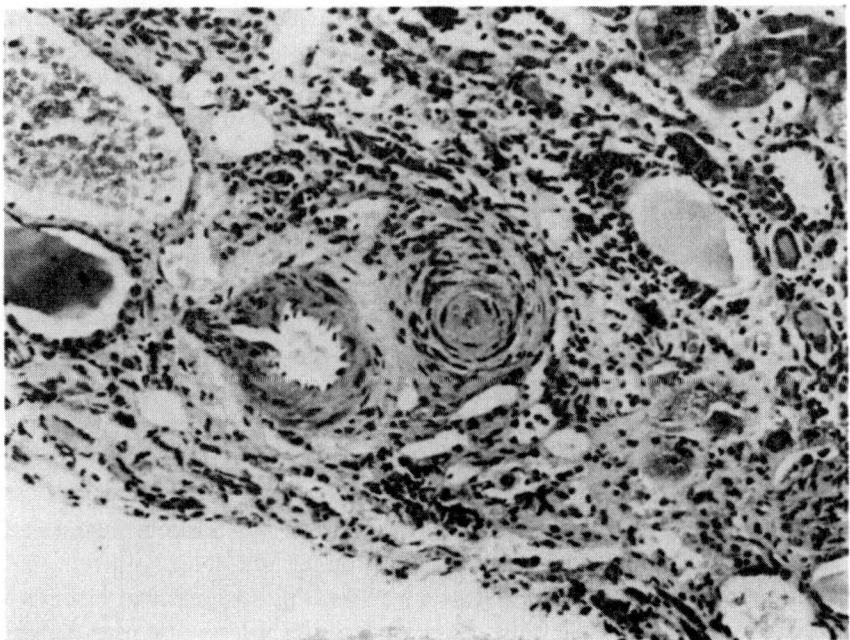

Figure 7. A markedly thickened small artery, shown in the center of the kidney. The lumen is virtually obliterated.

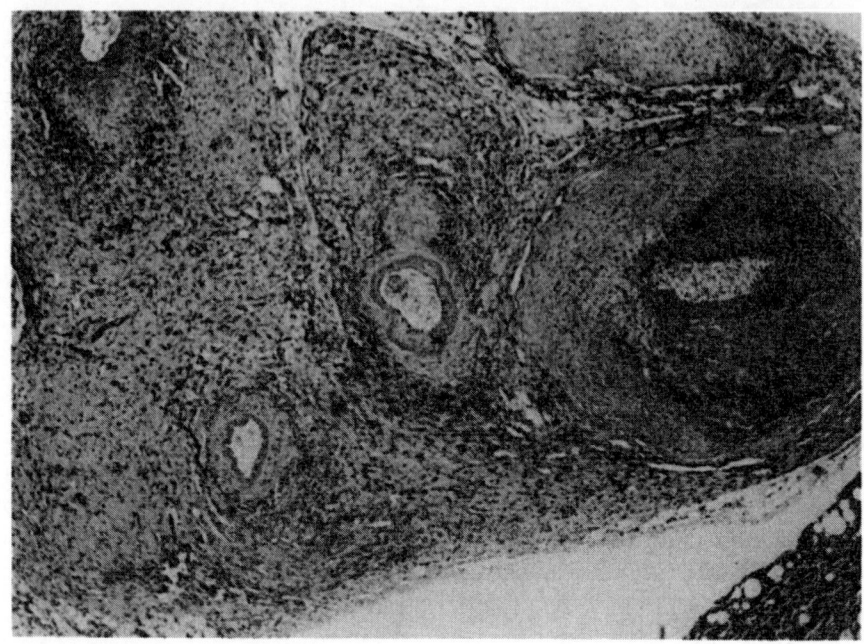

Figure 8. Polyarteritis nodosa of the mesenteric artery, as seen in the hypertension due to JG-like cells.

(d) Effect of captopril: The converting enzyme inhibitor captopril (SQ 14,225), when administered starting at the time of the transplantation (10 mg/kg/day p.o., n = 8), prevented the hypertension. In the face of a seeming normoreninemic state, these results present a puzzlement.

(e) Removal of the transplant of JG-like cells: Removal of the transplant at three days was attended by failure of the hypertensive state to evolve. Removal of the transplant at 6, 9, 11, and 12 days was followed by the MAP returning to near control levels, i.e., reversion of the hypertensive state. Removal of the transplant at 14–16 days did not alter the course of the hypertensive state. Thus, it appeared that the JG-like cells had to remain *in situ* for a period of time (about two weeks) for the hypertension to develop and enter the maintenance phase. This raises the question of what happened during this developmental period to establish the maintenance phase. The hypertension persisted after three weeks despite disappearance of the transplanted JG-like cells, at least from their subcutaneous location. Controls for the ablation of the transplant consisted of sham operated, similarly hypertensive animals. These had no change in MAP.

In these respects, the hypertension induced by the JG-like cells resembled the one-kidney, one-clip Goldblatt model, there being two phases, developmental and maintenance. It remains to be shown whether this resemblance extends to an angiotensin dependent phase (developmental) and a non-angiotensin dependent phase (maintenance). The results with captopril are consistent with this interpretation.

(f) Effect of transplant of RIC late in the course of the hypertension: Transplants of RIC, performed as described earlier [7], and introduced after one month of sustained hypertension, caused a significant lowering of the MAP over four days' time (average, −35 mm Hg from 182 ± 6.5 mm Hg, n = 7, p<0.01). It should be recalled that at this time the transplanted JG-like cells had disappeared, a small scar being left in their wake.

Effect of transplant of RIC at the same time as transplant of JG-like cells: When RIC were transplanted at the same time as the JG-like cells, but at a different site, the hypertension was not prevented. Thus, the RIC behaved differently during the developmental phase; i.e., they did not exert their anti-hypertensive action, as opposed to the maintenance phase, in which they exerted their antihypertensive action.

5. Morphologic and morphometric studies.
(a) Zona glomerulosa of the adrenal gland [10]: Comparison of the width of the zona glomerulosa of the hypertensive animals with that of the normotensive (uninephrectomized) controls indicated a significant increase in the width of this zone in the hypertensive animals.
(b) Juxtaglomerular index (JGI) [3]: The JGI of the hypertensive animals was significantly lower than that of the control (normotensive) animals.
(c) State of the RIC: The RIC of the remaining kidney were evaluated by a morphometric method previously described [9]. A comparison was made between the RIC in the kidney of the hypertensive animal during the established phase and those of the uninephrectomized controls (n = 8 each). There was a significant decrease in the number of RIC and the number of their osmiophilic granules (lipid-containing) in the kidneys of the hypertensive animals.
(d) The JG-like cell transplant: The transplant has been studied three to 16 days after its introduction. By three days, a compact nodule was formed. By one week, the structure was well vascularized, having capillaries traversing its substance.

The cells had the same characteristics as the cells in the culture bottle (Figures 9 and 10), including the peripheral dense bodies and myofibrils, rough endoplasmic reticulum containing fluffy material, and the Golgi apparatus surrounded by granules having the appearance of secretory granules and lysosomes. Of additional interest was the manner in which the cells had an imbricated arrangement of their surfaces, as described for JG cells in the kidney.

6. Attempts to extract renin from the cultured cells and the culture media.
On two occasions, we shipped to Dr. Jean Sealey an ample number of the JG-like cells and an ample volume of the media used to maintain the cells. She was not able to detect renin, prorenin, or angiotensin in this material. We also were not successful in detecting renin in said material. We have also homogenized the transplant that caused the hypertension and incubated this homogenate with rat renin substrate, and failed to detect the generation of angiotensin I. These findings remain enigmatic.

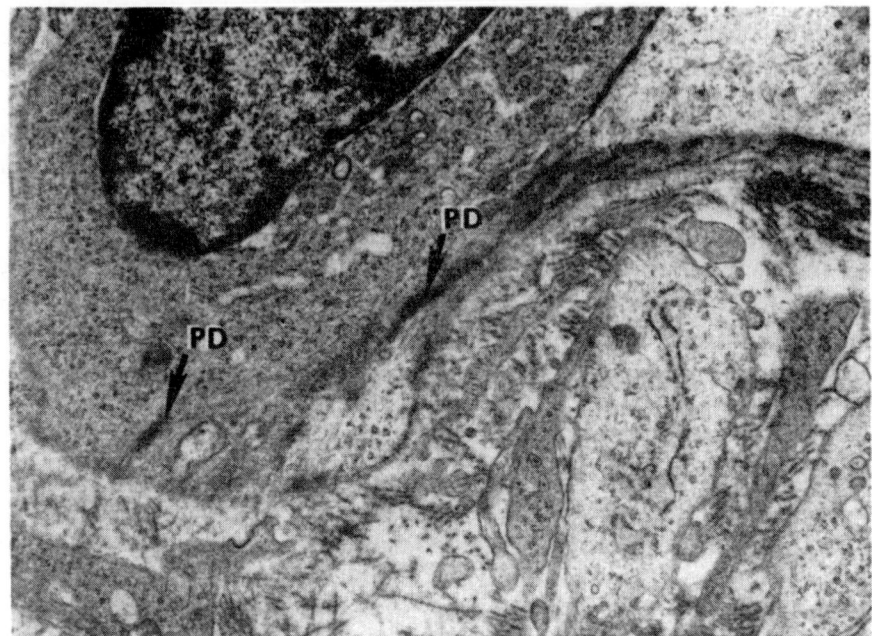

Figure 9. Examples from the transplant of the JG-like cell that induced hypertension. Note peripheral dense bodies (*PD*) with myofibrils between them; this is in keeping with the smooth muscle origin of the cells.

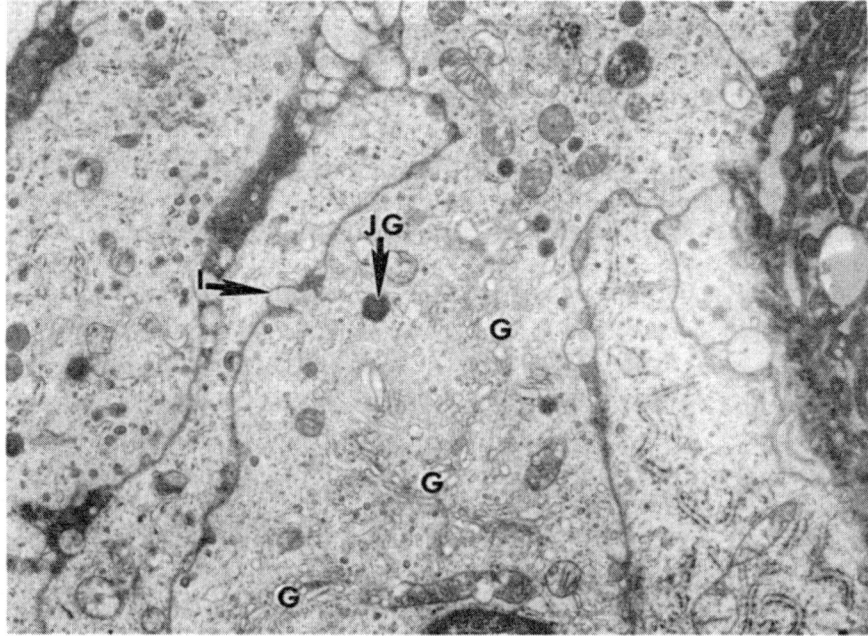

Figure 10. Cells also from the transplant of JG-like cells that induced hypertension. Notice the prominent Golgi (*G*), the secretory type granules (*JG*) of varying size surrounding the Golgi, and the imbrication of cytoplasm of cells (*I*).

7. Plasma angiotensin level. Since we met at Innisbrook, the puzzle concerning the constrictor agent appears to have been resolved. As the hypertension evolved, Dr. Ted Goodfriend analyzed serial plasma samples from six animals for circulating angiotensin. He reported extremely high plasma angiotensin levels in these animals, during the developmental phase of the hypertensive state (ave. control 391, during development 11,550 pc/ml). The plasma angiotensin level returned to baseline after 30 days in three animals followed for this period (Figure 11). Dr. Goodfriend's antibody does not discriminate between angiotensin II and angiotensin III. Studies aimed at this resolution are now in progress.

Widening of the zona glomerulosa of the adrenal gland is in keeping with the elevation of circulating angiotensin. We are evaluating the state of aldosterone. Lowering of the JGI could also be due to the high angiotensin level (negative feedback), but could also be related to the hypertensive state.

COMMENT

The hypertensive state resulting from the transplantation of JG-like cells, grown as a monolayer tissue culture, represents a new experimental model in the rat. In the absence of volume expansion, the severe vascular disease is likely due to increased peripheral vascular resistance. The constrictor agent appears to be angiotensin. How this agent is generated in the presence of a normal plasma renin concentration remains a puzzle.

The Goodfriend data demand a mechanism for angiotensin generation. It does

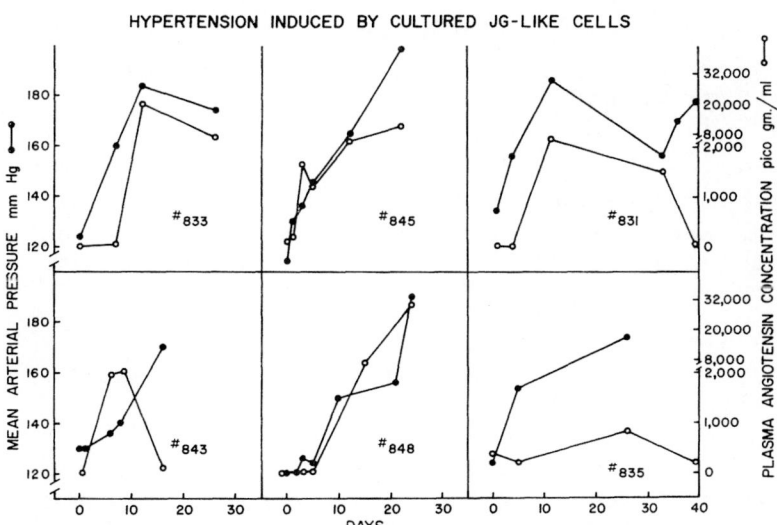

Figure 11. Preliminary data derived by Dr. Ted Goodfriend on the state of plasma angiotensin levels. As the blood pressure increased (solid circles), plasma angiotensin levels became extremely high (open circles). In time, the angiotensin levels returned toward baseline.

not appear to be due to the action of tonin [1], as it is our understanding that captopril does inhibit the actions of tonin (M. Antonaccio, personal communication). We continue to expect renin to be involved, but thus far lack proof of it.

The hypertensive state induced by the JG-like cells appears to have two phases-one dependent on the transplanted cells and their high generation of angiotensin (initiation phase) and one not so dependent (maintenance phase). The maintenance phase appears partly due to the prominent vascular disease of the viscera, including the kidney. This hypertensive state resembles that due to infusions of angiotensin II [6], as it should, in accordance with Goodfriend's angiotensin measurements.

SUMMARY

1. We have developed a near pure monolayer culture of JG-like cells from a syngeneic rat line (Wistar/GM).
2. These cells cause hypertension when transplanted into uninephrectomized syngeneic recipients.
3. The hypertensive state has the following characteristics:
a. Normal plasma renin concentration
b. High plasma angiotensin level
c. Protection by the entire renal mass
d. Severe necrotizing arterial disease
e. Thick zona glomerulosa
f. Normal body fluids
g. Decreased number of RIC and RIC lipid granules
h. Reversal when the transplant is removed after up to 12 days
i. Inhibition by captopril

In conclusion
1. A new hypertensive model of the rat is being described.
2. It is a normoreninemic, normovolemic hypertensive state induced by JG-like cells.
3. The constrictor agent appears to be angiotensin, the generation of which remains enigmatic.

REFERENCES

1. Boucher R, Demassieux S, Garcia R, Genest J: Tonin, angiotensin II system. A review. Circ Res (Supp. II) 41: 26–29, 1977
2. Carvalho JS, Shapiro R, Hopper P, Page LB: Methods for serial study of renin-angiotensin system in the unanesthetized rat. Am J Physiol 228: 369–375, 1975

3. Hartroft PM, Hartroft WS: Studies on renal juxtaglomerular cells. I. Variations produced by sodium chloride and desoxycorticosterone acetate. J Exper Med 97: 415–428, 1953
4. Johnson JG, Muirhead EE: Vascular complications of the hypertensive state. Dialogues in Hypertension 1: 38–51, 1979
5. Khayat A, Lewis LJ, Smeby RR: Renin release from cultured cells. Fed Proc 37(3): 290 (abs.), 1978
6. Koletsky S, Rivera-Vel JM, Pritchard WH: Production of hypertension and vascular disease by angiotensin. Arch Path 82: 99–106, 1966
7. Muirhead EE, Germain GS, Armstrong FB, Brooks B, Leach BE, Byers LW, Pitcock JA, Brown P: Endocrine-type antihypertensive function of renomedullary interstitial cells. Kidney Intern 8: S-271–282, 1975
8. Muirhead EE, Leach BE, Davis JO, Armstrong FB, Pitcock JA, Brosius WL Jr: Pathophysiology of angiotensinsalt hypertension. J Lab & Clin Med 85: 735–745, 1975
9. Pitcock JA, Brown P, Brooks B, Clapp WL, Muirhead EE: Renomedullary deficiency in partial nephrectomy-salt hypertension. Hypertension, 2: 281–290, 1980
10. Pitcock JA, Hartroft PM: The juxtaglomerular cells in man and their relationship to the level of plasma sodium and to the zona glomerulosa of the adrenal cortex. Am J Path 34: 863–883, 1958

12. THE GLANDULAR KALLIKREIN-KININ SYSTEM IN HYPERTENSION

OSCAR A. CARRETERO, ALFONSO G. SCICLI

ABSTRACT

Kallikreins are enzymes that release kinins, potent vasodilator peptides from plasma substrates called kininogens. In the microdissected nephron, prekallikrein and kallikrein are localized in the granular part of the distal and cortical collecting tubules (connecting tubules). Urinary kinins are formed in this part of the nephron and in the papilla and pelvis of the kidney. The intrarenal concentration of kinins may be affected by factors other than kallikrein, such as: kininogen, kininases, presence of kallikrein inhibitors, concentration of electrolytes, and hydrogen ions. There are important interrelationships between the kallikrein-kinin, renin-angiotensin-aldosterone, and prostaglandin systems. Kallikrein or other serine protease(s) inhibited by aprotinin appear to play a role within the kidney, controlling renal vascular resistance, salt and water excretion, and renin release. However, the final role of this system still remains to be elucidated. In patients or animals with primary or secondary hypertension, urinary kallikrein excretion is frequently decreased. In mineralocorticoid induced hypertension kallikrein excretion is normal or increased. It has not been proven that the decrease in kallikrein excretion indicates a decrease in the intrarenal formation of kinins and that this decrease participates in the pathogenesis of hypertension. There is evidence that some of the acute pharmacological effects of the converting enzyme inhibitors (CEI) are due to an increase in kinin concentration which directly, or through the release of prostaglandins, could affect local and peripheral vascular resistance and sodium and water excretion. The role of kinins in the chronic antihypertensive of CEI, if any, has not yet been determined.

THE KALLIKREIN-KININ SYSTEM

Vasoconstrictor and vasodilator peptides are important components of the many complex mechanisms that control tissue perfusion and blood pressure. It is recognized that hypertension may result either from an excess of vasopressor substances or from a deficiency of vasodepressor substances.

Kinins are a group of potent vasodilator oligo-peptides that contain bradykinin

Sambhi, M.P. (ed.) Fundamental fault in hypertension
© 1984, Martinus Nijhoff Publishers. Boston/The Hague/Dordrecht/Lancaster.
ISBN 978-94-010-9006-3

or bradykinin analogs in their structure. Figure 1 shows the structure of some of the known kinins. Bradykinin, bradykinin-containing peptides, kinin-releasing enzymes, and/or peptides that inhibit kinin-destroying enzymes have been isolated from jellyfish toxin, wasp and snake venom, the skin and bladder of the frog, as well as from tissues and exocrine secretions of mammals [1–4].

The early appearance of bradykinin, the conservation of its structure through evolution, and its wide distribution in the animal kingdom suggest that the presence of kinins in mammals is not an inconsequential 'accident' of evolution. It is easy to envision the role of kinins or of a kinin-generating system as vasodilators in venoms, highly specialized fluids intended to harm the victim. The snake venom not only has enzymes that release kinins, but it also contains peptides that inhibit the destruction of kinins [1, 3]. The evolutionary advantage, at least for the snake, of increasing blood flow to the area of the bite is obvious since the venom can then pass rapidly from that area into the systemic circulation. Although the role of kinins in other biological fluids has not yet been determined, it is interesting to note that kinin-generating enzymes in amphibians and mammals occur mainly in tissues with an active transport in water and electrolytes.

In mammals, kinins are released from inactive precursors, the kininogens, by a group of serine proteases named kininogenases. Although many enzymes have kininogenase activity, such as trypsin, uropepsin, and plasmin, the two main kininogenases are plasma and glandular kallikreins. The two main forms of kininogens or kallikrein substrates, low (LMWK) and high (HMWK) molecular weight kininogen are found in plasma [5]. Plasma kallikrein, also known as Fletcher factor, releases bradykinin only from HMWK, also known as Fitzgerald factor. Plasma kallikrein is found in the zymogen form (prekallikrein) and, together with HMWK and the Hageman factor, is involved in coagulation, fibrinolysis, and possibly in the activation of the complement system [6]. It is not known whether the plasma kallikrein-HMWK system, through the release of bradykinin, is involved in blood flow and blood pressure regulation. Plasma kallikrein has a molecular weight of ≃100,000 daltons and differs from glandular

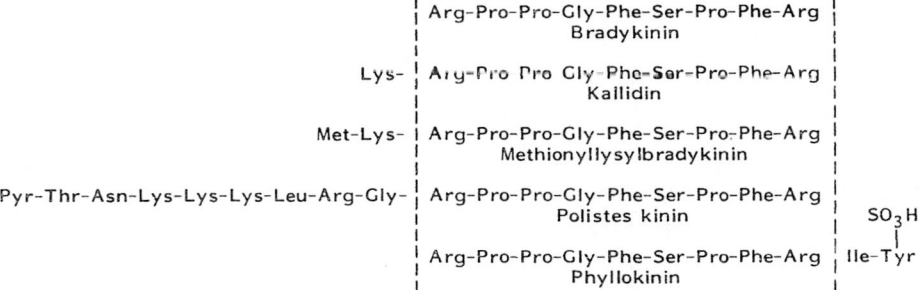

Figure 1. Structure of some of the known kinins. Bradykinin, kallidin, and methionyllysylbradykinin have been isolated from mammals, while polisteskinin and phyllokinin have been isolated from the venom of wasps and the skin of amphibians, respectively. Bradykinin is also found in the skin of many amphibians. Modified from Pisano [2].

kallikrein in its biochemical, immunological, and functional characteristics. The role of plasma kallikrein in coagulation and fibrinolysis will not be discussed here. For further information, the reader is referred to a recent review on the subject [6].

Glandular kallikreins are found in the kidney, pancreas, intestine, salivary and sweat glands, and in the exocrine secretion of these organs. We and others have found that there is also immunoreactive glandular kallikrein in plasma [7, 8, 9]. This immunoreactive kallikrein appears to be mainly in the inactive form [10]. However, recently it has been reported that some of the plasma glandular kallikrein is in the active form [11]. Further, there is evidence that kinins may be generated by glandular kallikrein or kininogenases other than plasma kallikrein [12, 13]. In man [14] and rabbit, 50% or more of the urinary kallikrein is in the inactive form, while in the rat, most of it is in the active form. Glandular kallikreins release kinins *in vitro* from both low and high molecular weight kininogen. However, the natural substrate for this enzyme is probably low molecular weight kininogen, since a patient with a congenital deficiency of plasma high molecular weight kininogen (Fitzgerald trait) has normal amounts of kinins in blood [12] and urine (unpublished data). Glandular kallikreins release kallidin (lysylbradykinin), which is partially converted to bradykinin by an aminopeptidase present in plasma and urine [15]. Rat urinary kallikrein may be an exception since it has recently been reported that it releases bradykinin [16]. Methionyl-lysyl-bradykinin is formed by uropepsine, when the urine is collected at acidic pH [14, 17]. Kinins are rapidly inactivated by enzymes called kininases, which are found in blood and other tissues. The two main kininases have been named kininase I and II. Kininase I is an arginine carboxypeptidase and kininase II, also known as angiotensin I converting enzyme, is a peptidyl dipeptidase [18]. Figure 2 shows the mechanism of kinin generation and destruction. In this review, emphasis will be placed on the renal kallikrein-kinin system and its possible role in the regulation of renal function since the kidney plays an important role in the long-term regulation of blood pressure and in the pathogenesis of hypertension.

LOCALIZATION OF THE KALLIKREIN-KININ SYSTEM IN THE NEPHRON

Over 90% of the kallikrein in the kidney is found in the cortex, decreasing from the outer to the inner cortex, with very little kallikrein in the medulla and papilla. Isolated glomeruli have a small amount of kallikrein activity compared to the kallikrein concentration in the total cortex [19]. We recently studied the localization of both active and inactive kallikrein in the microdissected rabbit nephron and found that both forms of the enzyme were localized in the granular portion of the distal and cortical collecting tubules [20]. This segment of the nephron contains more than 85% of the active and inactive kallikrein found in the total microdissected nephron. Only very small amounts of active and inactive kal-

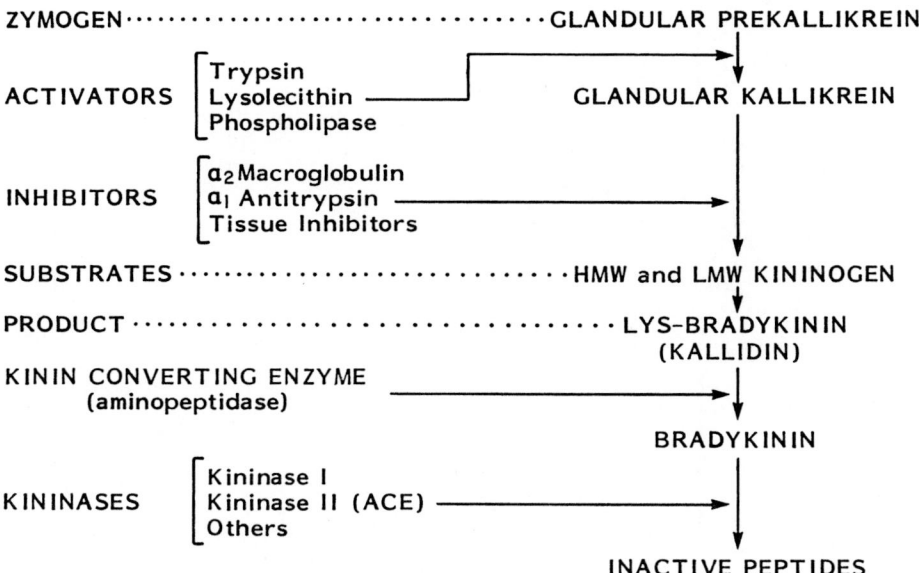

Figure 2. Mechanisms of kinin generation and destruction. ACE = angiotensin-I convering enzyme; HMW = high molecular weight; LMW = low molecular weight.

likrein were found in other segments, including the bright portion of the distal segment which has the macula densa (Figure 3).

The granular portions of the distal convoluted and cortical collecting tubules form a single nephron segment called the connecting tubule, which has two types of cells; the connecting tubule cells, and the intercalated cells. Since the connecting tubule cells and kallikrein localize only in the granular part of the distal and collecting segment, and the intercalated cells are thoroughly distributed from the granular distal tubule to the medullary collecting tubule, it is reasonable to assume that kallikrein is synthesized in the connecting cells. The discrete localization of kallikrein suggests a specific role of renal kallikrein in association with these nephron segments.

Kinins present in the urine are released in the kidney itself since when bradykinin is infused into the renal artery, less than 0.2% appears in the urine and more than 90% is inactivated in the vascular compartment of the kidney by kininases [21, 22]. There are two main types of kininases: kininase I and II. Kininase II has been studied more extensively than kininase I, partly because kininase II, in addition to hydrolyzing kinins, converts angiotensin I to angiotensin II (angiotensin I converting enzyme). The brush border of the proximal tubule is rich in kininase II, which prevents filtered kinins from reaching the distal nephron [23]. Carone et al. [24] have shown that when labeled bradykinin was injected into the proximal tubule it was almost completely destroyed. However, when this peptide was injected into the distal tubule, it appeared almost intact in

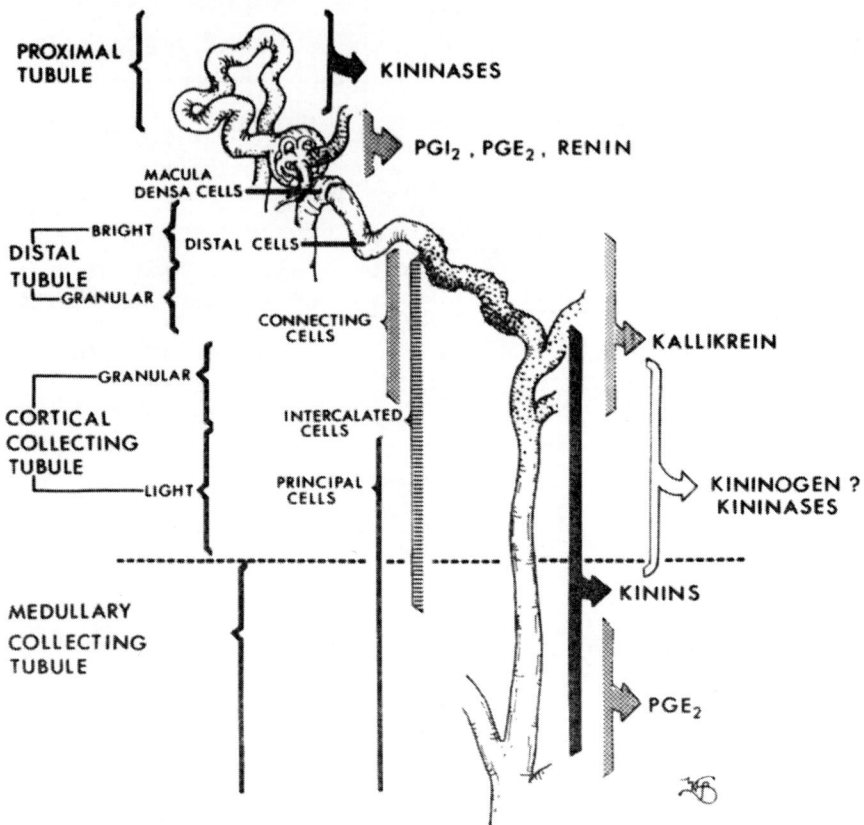

Figure 3. Localization of the kallikrein-kinin system, renin and prostaglandins in the nephron (right brackets), anatomical subdivisions of the nephron (outer left brackets) and type of cells found in the distal nephron (inner left brackets). PGE_2 = prostaglandin E_2, PGI_2 = prostacyclin.

the urine. The evidence, plus the fact that renal kallikrein is secreted into the urine at the level of the distal tubule, seems to indicate that urinary kinins may be formed in the distal part of the nephron. We have confirmed this possibility by using the stop-flow technique and found that kinins are formed in the distal part of the nephron, with the highest concentration located in the final segment of the nephron or even in the renal papilla and pelvis [25]. No evidence of kinin formation was found in the fraction representing the proximal nephron.

The origin of the kininogen (substrate) needed for the formation of kinins in the lumen of the nephron is not known. The plasma is very rich in kininogen and a small amount of plasma kininogen reaching the distal nephron could account for the kinins found in the urine. In human urine, there is a significant amount of immunoreactive kininogen, however kininogen is found in small amounts when measured by its capability to generate kinins [14]. It could be that most of the kininogen has already been consumed by the urinary kallikrein. It has been reported that urinary kinins are absent in a subject with a congenital deficiency of plasma low and high molecular weight kininogen [26]. On the other hand, in a patient without plasma high molecular weight kininogen but with near normal low molecular weight kininogen (Fitzgerald trait), we found that the urine contained normal amounts of kinins (unpublished observation). This indicates that kinins in urine are formed from low molecular weight kininogen and that they are not formed by plasma kallikrein, since this enzyme releases kinins only from high molecular weight kininogen.

Recently, Proud et al. [27] using antibody to low molecular weight kininogen and immunohistochemical techniques, have localized kininogen in cells of distal and collecting tubules. In rabbit renal tissue, we have been unable to demonstrate the presence of kininogen (K. Omata, A.G. Scicli, and O.A. Carretero, unpublished results). The presence of an inhibitor of glandular kallikrein has also been demonstrated in the rat kidney tubules [28]. It is feasible that this inhibitor could play a role in the regulation of intrarenal formation of kinins.

Factors that control the intrarenal formation of kinins are not well defined. We have found no correlation between kallikrein and kinin excretion in urine collected directly from the ureter of the rat [29]. Further, we found that acidification of the urine by sodium sulfate infusion, decreased kinin excretion while it increased kallikrein excretion. It is possible that the lower pH within the distal nephron decreases the kininogenase activity of renal kallikrein since the optimum pH of kallikrein is 8.5. Alkalinization of normally acidic urine of the rat by infusion of sodium bicarbonate increases kinin excretion especially when the animals receive a converting enzyme inhibitor [30]. It is possible that renal kininase activity increased since their optimum pH is above 7.0; and therefore alkalinization of the urine could result in an increase in both formation and destruction of kinins.

It has recently been reported that the concentration of electrolytes also affects the rate of kinin formation [31, 32]. Thus, the intrarenal concentration of kinins may depend on their rates of formation and destruction (Figure 2). In turn, these rates may depend on the intrarenal concentration of kallikrein, kininogen, kininases, kallikrein inhibitors, electrolytes and hydrogen ions.

RELATIONSHIP AMONG THE KALLIKREIN-KININ, RENIN-ANGIOTENSIN-ALDOSTERONE, PROSTAGLANDIN AND VASOPRESSIN SYSTEMS

Plasma and glandular kallikrein *in vitro* convert inactive renin to active renin, and it has been suggested that renal and plasma kallikrein activate renin *in vivo* [33]. Suzuki [34] reported that urinary kallikrein stimulates renin release from superfused isolated kidney slices. Neither bradykinin in high doses nor trypsin were able to release renin under these experimental conditions, indicating that kallikrein acts directly on the renal tissue to release renin. However, recently, investigators from the same group, have been unable to confirm that kallikrein stimulates renin release in the kidney slices preparation [35]. Using isolated superfused glomeruli we have been able to show that both kallikrein and bradykinin stimulate renin release [36]. The effect of bradykinin in a molar basis was more potent than that of isoproterenol. *In vivo,* bradykinin infused into the renal artery of dogs stimulates the release of renin [37].

Abe et al. [38] reported that aprotinin infused in the renal artery of dogs inhibits the renin release stimulated by a converting enzyme inhibitor. This study may suggest that the release of renin was stimulated either by renal kallikrein directly, or by kinins released by this enzyme since aprotinin has frequently been used to inhibit kallikrein. However, aprotinin inhibits dog glandular kallikrein poorly or not at all [39]. Furthermore, since aprotinin is a polyvalent inhibitor of serine proteases, its effect on renin release in the dog may be mediated by inhibition of other enzymes. Inhibition of renin release by aprotinin has also been reported in humans and rats [40, 41]. These findings indicate that kallikrein or other serine proteases may participate in the control of renin release.

The angiotensin I converting enzyme (kininase II) further links the kallikrein-kinin and renin-angiotensin systems. Converting enzyme is found in high concentrations on the endothelial cell surface of the vascular bed of the lung and has the concurrent functions of converting angiotensin I to II and destroying kinins. There is evidence that over 90% of the kinins administered in the venous site of the systemic circulation are destroyed by one passage through the lung, thus most of the kinins formed in tissues which might enter the vascular compartment would be destroyed before they reach the peripheral circulation. This suggests that the biological effects of kinins take place within the confines of the organ in which they are released.

Mineralocorticoid administration increases urinary kallikrein excretion and renal tissue kallikrein concentration, while spironolactone, an aldosterone antagonist, decreases it [42–45]. In dogs, this increase in urinary kallikrein excretion by the administration of deoxycorticosterone acetate (DOCA) was found only after the dogs escaped from the sodium-retaining effects of DOCA [44]. Thus, at the present time it is not clear whether aldosterone stimulates renal kallikrein secretion directly or through an alteration of water and electrolyte metabolism. Angiotensin has also been reported to stimulate renal kallikrein excretion [46].

Kinins infused into the renal artery stimulate the synthesis of prostaglandins, probably prostaglandin E_2 (PGE_2) in the collecting duct and renal medulla, and prostacyclin (PGI_2) in the arterioles [47, 48]. This effect of kinins is produced by an increased release of arachidonic acid as a consequence of the activation of phospholipase A_2. Furthermore, part of the renal vasodilator and natriuretic effect of kinins is mediated through the release of prostaglandins and can be inhibited by prostaglandin synthesis inhibitors such as indomethacin and meclofenamate. However, these findings are not universal and some investigators have been unable to demonstrate that the renal vasodilator effects of kinins are mediated by prostaglandins [48]. On the other hand, prostaglandins have been reported to stimulate, while prostaglandin synthesis inhibitors suppress, renal kallikrein release [46, 48].

The interactions between the kallikrein-kinin system, the renin-angiotensin-aldosterone, and the prostaglandin systems are depicted in Figure 4. These interactions may play an important physiological role. It could be speculated that increased activity in the renin-angiotensin system would produce both a peripheral and renal vasoconstriction that could impair renal blood flow. However, angiotensin II and aldosterone stimulate the release of renal kallikrein and prostaglandin, which could produce local vasodilation and maintain renal blood flow even in the presence of high concentrations of angiotensin II.

Antidiuretic hormone (ADH) stimulates the release of kallikrein and the intrarenal formation of kinins [49, 50]. Further, kinins antagonize the effect of ADH in the toad bladder and in the kidney [51, 52]. Thus, it is possible that kinins antagonize or modulate the effects of ADH in the kidney either directly or through the release of prostaglandins.

In conclusion, there are numerous complex interactions between the kallikrein-kinin, renin-angiotensin-aldosterone, ADH, and prostaglandin systems. Many are not completely understood and some of them may be of no physiological importance.

PHYSIOLOGICAL ROLE OF THE RENAL KALLIKREIN-KININ SYSTEM

Although some of the actions of renal kallikrein, such as the activation of inactive renin, may be due to its direct catalytic effect, most of its effect seems to be mediated by kinin release. The infusion of kinins into the renal artery results in an increased blood-flow diuresis and natriuresis without changing the glomerular filtration rate. Like most vasodilator drugs, kinins produce a greater increase in blood flow in the inner cortex than in the outer. Unlike other vasodilators, kinins

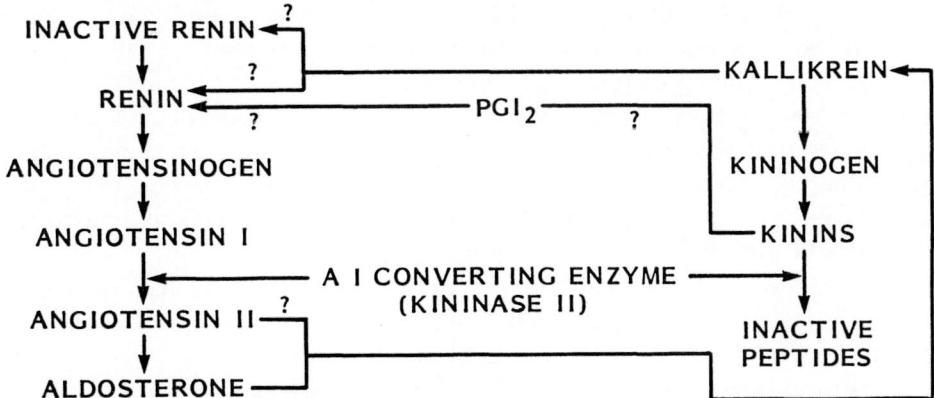

Figure 4. Interactions between the kallikrein-kinin, renin-angiotensin-aldosterone and prostaglandin systems. A–I = angiotensin-I; PGI_2 = prostacyclin.

do not decrease proximal sodium and water reabsorption in outer cortical nephrons available for micropuncture [53]. Accordingly, the natriuretic effect of kinins is either due to inhibition of sodium reabsorption in the distal part of the nephron or to changes in deep nephron reabsorption. Kinins may affect sodium reabsorption as the result of a direct effect on the transport of sodium in the nephron, a vasodilator effect with changes in the interstitial fluid pressure, changes in the osmotic gradient of the renal medulla, or a combination of all these effects. Changes in the osmotic gradient of the renal medulla could explain the decrease in urinary osmolality and vasopressin-resistant diuresis caused by kinins [54].

Kinins administered into the renal artery probably do not mimic the effects produced by kinins formed intrarenally by endogenous kallikrein, since their sites of action or concentration could be different. Kauker [55] has shown that kinins administered directly into the late proximal tubule increase sodium excretion, suggesting that kinins in the lumen of the nephron have natriuretic effects.

The role of endogenously generated kinins in the regulation of renal blood flow and water and electrolyte excretion has been studied by using angiotensin converting enzyme inhibitors (CEI). These inhibitors increase the concentration of endogenous kinins by inhibiting kininase II. After CEI administration, renal blood flow increases in the juxtamedullary cortex with a simultaneous increase in the fractional excretion of sodium [56]. However, the use of CEI does not allow for differentiation between the potentiation of kinin activity and the inhibition of the conversion of angiotensin I to angiotensin II. Administration of aprotinin, an inhibitor of kallikrein and other serine proteases, to volume-expanded rats decreased GFR, renal blood flow, urinary volume, sodium, potassium, and PGE_2 excretion [57]. Furthermore, administration of antibodies against kinins to saline-infused rats resulted in a decrease in sodium excretion [58]. These findings suggest that intrarenally released kinins cause natriuresis, diuresis, and release of prostaglandins.

Recently, Johnston et al. [59, 60] have shown that aprotinin increases renal vascular resistance under conditions of dietary sodium restriction or with reduced renal perfusion pressure. While aprotinin may not be acting specifically against kallikrein, their results support a role for a serine protease(s) in the regulation of renal blood flow. Using the isolated perfused kidney, it has been demonstrated that kallikrein is secreted not only into the nephron, but also into the interstitial and vascular space of the kidney [61]. However, we have recently found that the difference in arteriovenous concentration of immunoreactive glandular kallikrein is negative, suggesting that the kidney not only releases, but also depurates immunoreactive glandular kallikrein from plasma [62]. Locally formed kinins could participate in the regulation of renal blood flow distribution. It has recently been reported that when kinins are applied to the serosa of the intestine, the transport of chloride is stimulated from the serosal to the mucosa [63, 64]. Whether this effect also occurs in the nephron is not known, but it suggests that kinins may be important in the regulation of electrolytes.

THE RENAL KALLIKREIN-KININ SYSTEM IN HUMAN AND EXPERIMENTAL
HYPERTENSION

The theoretical possibility that hypertension results from either an excess of
vasopressor substances or from a deficiency of vasodepressor substances has
stimulated research on the role of the renal kallikrein-kinin system in the pathogenesis of various types of human and experimental hypertension. Furthermore,
the kidney, which is considered one of the most important determinants in the
long-range control of blood pressure, has both vasopressor (renin-angiotensin
system) and vasodepressor (kallikrein-kinin-prostaglandin system) components.
These vasoactive substances could also participate in the regulatory capacity of
the kidney to excrete sodium and water.

There are many reports which indicate that urinary kallikrein excretion is
decreased in patients with essential hypertension [65–71]. However, it has been
reported that if variables such as renal function and race are taken into consideration, urinary kallikrein excretion is comparable in hypertensive and control
subjects [72, 73, 74]. However, we and others [75–78] have reported that kallikrein excretion is decreased in patients with essential hypertension and normal
renal function when compared to normotensive controls matched for age, race,
and sex. The reasons for the discrepancy among these studies are not known,
however, it is interesting to note that many hypertensive patients have normal
kallikrein excretion whereas others have conspicuously low amounts of kallikrein
[75].

In an epidemiological study in which urinary kallikrein concentration (esterase
activity) was measured in a large population of normal children and their moth-
ers, there was a significant familial clustering of urinary kallikrein excretion [78,
79]. Urinary kallikrein concentration was significantly lower in black children
than in white children. It was altered by season (lower in summer) and by time of
day (highest in morning). Families with the lowest mean kallikrein concentrations tended to have higher blood pressure than families with the highest kallikrein concentrations, suggesting concomitant and genetic influence on both
blood pressure and kallikrein excretion. In this regard, it is interesting to note that
urinary kallikrein excretion is decreased in three different models of genetically
hypertensive rats developed by selective inbreeding on the basis of their blood
pressure [80–83]. Perhaps one of the genetic loci which controls blood pressure is
linked to one which controls renal kallikrein. At the present time, it is not clear
whether these are concomitant phenomena functionally unrelated to each other,
or whether the decrease in kallikrein excretion is a pathogenetic factor in the
development of hypertension. Another possibility is that the kallikrein excretion
is decreased secondary to the increase in blood pressure; however, decreased
urinary kallikrein is seen in normotensive children of patients with essential
hypertension and also in rats of the New Zealand genetically hypertensive strain
and in the Dahl salt-sensitive rat prior to the development of hypertension [78–
83].

Urinary kallikrein excretion is decreased in rats bred to be susceptible to the hypertensive effect of salt (Dahl's salt-sensitive rats) [83]. It may be that a decrease in kallikrein-kinin system activity may alter sodium and water excretion in susceptible rats and thereby promote hypertension during high sodium intake. It is even possible that similar defects occur in some cases of patients with essential hypertension and very low urinary kallikrein excretion. Furthermore, it has recently been reported that patients with essential hypertension and low kallikrein excretion responded to the oral administration of glandular kallikrein with a greater decrease in blood pressure than patients with normal kallikrein excretion [84, 85]. However, these studies need to be repeated. Kallikrein excretion and renal tissue kallikrein are also decreased in renovascular hypertension [74, 82, 86], whereas they are increased in those types of hypertension resulting from an excess of mineralocorticoids such as primary aldosteronism and deoxycorticosterone-salt experimental hypertension [42, 69, 73, 82]. According to a recent report, kallikrein excretion also increased in mice with genetic hypertension [87].

In conclusion, urinary kallikrein excretion is frequently decreased in patients and animals with primary or secondary hypertension, with the exception of mineralocorticoid-induced hypertension in which kallikrein excretion is normal or increased. It has not yet been proven that the decrease in kallikrein excretion indicates a decrease in the intrarenal formation of kinins and that this decrease participates in the pathogenesis of hypertension.

ROLE OF KININS IN THE PHARMACOLOGICAL EFFECTS OF CONVERTING ENZYME INHIBITORS

The antihypertensive effect of converting enzyme inhibitors (CEI) may be due to a blockade of the formation of the vasoconstrictor peptide angiotensin II, or to the inhibition of destruction of the potent vasodilator peptides, kinins. Evidence indicates that the blockade of angiotensin II formation is an important mechanism in the antihypertensive effects of CEI. Captopril, an orally active CEI, is an effective antihypertensive, not only in high-renin hypertension, but also in clinical and experimental models of hypertension in which the renin-angiotensin system has not been pathogenetically implicated [88]. Thus, the effects of CEI may be mediated either by an increase in the concentration of kinins or by a yet undetermined mechanism. Reports on the concentration of kinins in blood or plasma after the administration of CEI differ as to whether it is increased, unchanged, or decreased [88–92]. These conflicting results may be a consequence of methodological problems in the determination of kinins in blood or plasma. Kinins in the urine have been reported consistently increased after the administration of CEI, which indicates an increase in their concentration in the renal tissue [91, 93, 94]. This increase in kinins may participate in the antihypertensive effect of CEI by altering renovascular resistance and by increasing sodium and water excretion. It has been shown that teprotide (SQ 20, 881), another CEI induces increases in both uteroplacental blood flow and plasma PGE_2 in pregnant, nephrectomized rabbits [95, 96]. Since these increases can be blocked by kinin antibodies, part of the effect of CEI on the blood flow may be mediated by an increase in kinins directly and/or through the release of prostaglandins.

It has also been reported that aprotinin, an unspecific inhibitor of kallikrein and other proteases, blocks the acute antihypertensive effect of captopril in patients with low- and normal-renin essential hypertension [97]. Further, in spontaneously hypertensive rats (SHR) and in two-kidney, one-clip renovascular hypertensive rats, the acute antihypertensive effects of this CEI is almost completely blocked by high titer antibodies against kinins [98]. These antibodies do not alter the vasodepressor effect of the CEI in sodium-depleted normotensive rats. There are also reports that PGE_2 and its metabolites are increased in patients with essential hypertension after the administration of captopril [99]. In addition, the antihypertensive effect of captopril is partially blocked by indomethacin, a prostaglandin synthesis inhibitor [100].

In conclusion, these data suggest that some of the acute pharmacological effects of the CEI are due to an increase in kinin concentration, which directly, or through the release of prostaglandins, could affect local and peripheral vascular resistance and sodium and water excretion. For further detail on the role of kinins in the pharmacological effect of CEI, see Carretero et al. [98]. The role of kinins in the chronic antihypertensive effect of CEI has not yet been determined.

ACKNOWLEDGMENTS

Supported in part by National Institutes of Health Grants HL 15839, HL 24650, and HL 28982. A.G. Scicli is a recipient of a RCDA, HL 00682.

REFERENCES

1. Rocha E, Silva M, Beraldo WT, Rosenfeld G: Bradykinin a hypotensive and smooth muscle stimulating factor released from plasma globulin by snake venoms and by trypsin. J Physiol 109: 488, 1949
2. Pisano JJ: Kinins of non-mammalian origin. In: Handbook of Experimental Pharmacology. Erdos EG (ed), New York: Springer, New York, 1970, Vol 25, pp. 589–595
3. Ferreira SH, Greene LJ, Alabaster VA, Bakhle YS, Vane JR: Activity of various fractions of bradykinin potentiating factor against angiotensin I converting enzyme. Nature 225: 379, 1970
4. Hartman KR, Calton GJ, Burnett JW: The utilization of the bradykinin radioimmunoassay for the study of a kinin-like factor in jellyfish toxin. Comp Biochem Physiol 66: 163, 1980

170

5. Jacobsen S: Substrates for plasma kinin-forming enzymes in human, dog and rabbit plasma. Br J Pharmacol 26: 403, 1966
6. Colman RW: Patho-physiology of the kallikrein system. An Clin Lab Sci 10: 220, 1980
7. Rabito SF, Scicli AG, Carretero OA: Immunoreactive glandular kallikrein in plasma. In: Enzymatic release of vasoactive peptides. Vogel GF (ed), Raven Press, New York, 1980, pp. 245–258
8. Nustad K, Ørstavik TB, Gautvik KM: Radioimmunological measurements of rat submandibular gland kallikrein (RSK) in tissues and serum. Microvasc Res 15: 115, 1978
9. Fink E, Scifert J, Guttel C: Development of a direct radioimmunoassay for pig pancreatic kallikrein and its application in physiological studies. Fresenius Z Anal Chem 290: 183, 1978
10. Lawton WS, Proud D, Warner ME, Pierce JV, Keiser HR, Pisano JJ: Characterization and origin of immunoreactive glandular kallikrein in rat plasma. Biochem Pharmacol 30: 1731–1737, 1981
11. Geiger R, Clausnitzer B, Fink E, Fritz H: Isolation of an enzymatically active glandular kallikrein from human plasma by immunoaffinity chromatography. Hoppe-Zyler's Z Physiol Chem 361: 1795–1803, 1980
12. Scicli AG, Mindroiu T, Carretero OA: Blood kinins, their concentration in normal subjects and in patients with congenital deficiency in plasma prekallikrein and kininogen. A new method for its determination. J Lab Clin Med 100(1): 81–93, 1983
13. Scicli AG, Rabito SF, Ørstavik TB, Carretero OA: Blood kinins during changes in renal and submandibular gland kallikrein. Proc Intern Conf Kallikrein, Kinins, Kininogens, Kininases, Kinin 1981, Munich
14. Pisano JJ, Corthorn J, Yates K, Pierce JV: The kallikrein-kinin system in the kidney. Contrib Nephrol 12: 116–125, 1978
15. Brandi CM, Prado ES, Prado MJBA, Prado JL: Kinin-converting aminopeptidase from human urine: partial purification and properties. Int J Biochem 7: 335–341, 1976
16. Alhenc-Gelas F, Marchetti J, Allegrini J, Corvol P, Menard J: Measurement of urinary kallikrein activity. Species differences in kinin production. Biophys Biochem Acta 677: 477–488, 1981
17. Hial V, Keiser HR, Pisano JJ: Origin and content of methionyl-lysyl-bradykinin, lysyl-bradykinin and bradykinin in human urine. Biochem Pharmacol 25: 2499–2503, 1976
18. Erdös EG: Conversion of angiotensin I to angiotensin II. Am J Med 60: 749–759, 1976
19. Scicli AG, Carretero OA, Oza NB, Schork A: Distribution of kidney kininogenase. Proc Soc Exp Biol Med 151: 47–60, 1976
20. Omata K, Carretero OA, Scicli AG, Jackson BA: Localization of active and inactive kallikrein in isolated tubular segments of the rabbit nephron. Kidney Int 22: 602–607, 1982
21. Abe K: Urinary excretion of kinin in man with special reference to its origin. Tohoku J Exp Med 87: 175–184, 1965
22. Nasjletti A, Colina-Churio J, McGiff JC: Disappearance of bradykinin in the renal circulation of dogs: effects of kininase inhibition. Circ Res 37: 59–65, 1975
23. Nishimura K, Erdös EG: Membrane bound kininase and kallikrein: enzymatic release of vasoactive peptides. Gross F, Vogel G, Raven Press, New York, 1980, pp. 225–234
24. Carone FA, Pullman TN, Oparil S, Nakamura S: Micropuncture evidence of rapid hydrolysis of bradykinin by rat proximal tubule. Am J Physiol 230: 1420–1424, 1976

25. Scicli AG, Gandolfi R, Carretero OA: Site of formation of kinins in the dog nephron. Am J Physiol 234 (Renal Fluid Electrolyte Physiol 3): F35, 1978
26. Hial V, Keiser HR, Pisano JJ: Methionyl-lysyl-bradykinin (MLBK) in human urine and the absence of kinins in subjects with congenital deficiency of kininogen. Fed Proc 35: 692, 1976
27. Proud D, Perkins M, Pierce JV, Yates KN, Highet PF, Herring PL, Mangkorn-kanok/Mark M, Bahu, R, Carone F, Pisano JJ: Characterization and localization of human renal kininogen. J Biol Chem 256: 10634–10639, 1981
28. Geiger R, Mann K: A kallikrein-specific inhibitor in rat kidney tubules. Hoppe-Seylers Z Physiol Chem 357: 553–558, 1976
29. Scicli AG, Diaz M, Carretero OA: Effects of pH and amiloride in the intrarenal formation of kinins. Am J Physiol 245: F198–F203, 1983
30. Brukman J, Carretero O, Churchill P, Scicli A: Effect of urinary alkalinization of intrarenal formation of kinins. Physiologist 26(4): A130, 1983
31. Lieberthal W, Oza NB, Bernard DB, Levinsky NG: The effect of cations on the activity of human urinary kallikrein. J Biol Chem 257(18): 10827–10830, 1982
32. Chao J, Tanaka S, Margolius HS: Inhibitory effects of sodium and other monovalent cations on purified versus membrane-bound kallikrein. J Biol Chem 258(10): 6461–6465, 1983
33. Sealey JE, Atlas SA, Laragh JH: Linking the kallikrein and renin system via activation of inactive renin. Am J Med 65: 994–1000, 1978
34. Suzuki S, Franco-Saenz R, Tan SY, Mulrow PJ: Direct action of rat urinary kallikrein on rat kidney to release renin. J Clin Invest 66: 757–762, 1980
35. Doi Y, Hinko A, Franco-Saenz R, Mulrow PJ: Reexamination of the effect of urinary kallikrein on renin release: Evidence that kallikrein does not release renin but protects renin from destruction. Endocrinology 113(1): 114–118, 1983
36. Beierwaltes WH, Arora ML, Carretero OA: Stimulation of renin by kallikrein and kinin in isolated glomeruli. The Physiologist 25(40): 318, 1982
37. Flamenbaum W, Gagnon J, Ramwell P: Bradykinin induced renal hemodynamic alterations: renin and prostaglandin relationships. Am J Physiol 237: F433–F440, 1979
38. Abe Y, Miura K, Imanishi M, Yukimura T, Komori T, Okahara T, Yamamoto K: Effects of an orally active converting enzyme inhibitor (YS-980) on renal function in dogs. J Pharmacol Exp Ther 214(1): 166–170, 1980
39. Moriwaki C, Miyazaki K, Matsuda Y, Moriya H, Fujimoto Y, Veki H: Dog renal kallikrein: purification and some properties. J Biochem (Tokyo) 80: 1277–1285, 1976
40. Overlack A, Stumpe KO, Heck I, Ressel C, Kunhert M, Kruck F: Identification of angiotensin II and kinin-dependent mechanisms in essential hypertension. In: Hypertension: Mechanisms and Management. Phillipp T, Distlber A (ed) Springer-Verlag, Berlin Heidelberg, 1980, pp 183–191
41. Seto S, Kher V, Scicli AG, Carretero OA: Effect of aprotinin, a serine protease inhibitor on renin release. The Physiologist 25(4): 318, 1982
42. Margolius HS, Horowitz D, Geller RG, Alexander RW, Gill JR, Pisano JJ, Keiser HR: Urinary kallikrein excretion in normal man. Relationships to sodium intake and sodium-retaining steroids. Circ Res 35: 812–819, 1974
43. Nasjletti A, McGiff JC, Colina-Chourio J: Interrelations of the renal kallikrein-kinin system and renal prostaglandins in the conscious rats: influence of mineralocorticoids. Circ Res 43: 799–807, 1978
44. Marin-Grez M, Oza NB, Carretero OA: The involvement of urinary kallikrein in the renal escape from the sodium retaining effects of mineralocorticoids. Henry Ford Hosp Med J 21: 85–90, 1973
45. Margolius HS, Chao J, Kaizu T: The effects of aldosterone and spironolactone on

renal kallikrein. Clin Sci Mol Med 51 (Suppl 3): 279S–282S, 1976
46. Mills IH: Kallikrein, kininogen and kinins in control of blood pressure. Nephron 23: 61–71, 1979
47. Terragno NA, Lonigro AJ, Malik KU, McGiff JC: The relationship of the renal vasodilator action of bradykinin to the release of prostaglandin E-like substances. Experentia 28: 437–439, 1972
48. Nasjletti A, Malik KU: Relationships between the kallikrein-kinin and prostaglandin system. Life Sci 25: 99–110, 1979
49. Fejes-Toth G, Zahajszky T, Filep J: Effect of vasopressin on renal kallikrein excretion. Am J Physiol 239: F388–392, 1980
50. Robertson GL, Conder ML: Regulation of urinary kinin excretion (abstr). Circ Res 28: 536, 1980
51. Furtado MRF: Inhibition of the permeability response to vasopressin and oxytocin in the toad bladder: effects of bradykinin, kallidin, eledoisin, and physalaemin. J Membrane Biol 4: 165–178, 1971
52. Carvounis CP, Carvounis G, Arbeit LA: Role of endogenous kallikrein-kinin system in modulating vasopressin stimulated water flow and urea permeability in the toad bladder. J Clin Invest 67: 1792–1796, 1981
53. Stein JH, Congbalay RC, Karsh DL, Osgood RW, Ferris TF: The effect of bradykinin on proximal tubular sodium reabsorption in the dog: evidence for functional nephron heterogeneity. J Clin Invest 51: 1709–1721, 1972
54. Willis LR: Effect of bradykinin on the renal medullary osmotic gradient in water diuresis. Eur J Pharmacol 45: 173–183, 1977
55. Kauker ML: Bradykinin action of the efflux of luminal Na in the rat nephron. J Pharmacol Exp Ther 214: 119–123, 1980
56. Bailie MD, Barbour JA: Effect of inhibition of peptidase activity on distribution of intrarenal blood flow. Am J Physiol 228: 850–853, 1975
57. Kramer HJ, Moch T, vonSicherer L, Dusing R: Effects of aprotinin of renal function and urinary prostaglandin excretion in conscious rats after acute salt loading. Clin Sci 56: 547–553, 1979
58. Marin-Grez M: The influence of antibodies against bradykinin on isotonic saline diuresis in the rat. Pflüegers Arch 350: 231–239, 1974
59. Johnston PA, Bernard DB, Perrin NS, Arbeit L, Lieberthal W, Levinsky NG: Control of rat renal vascular resistance during alterations in sodium balance. Circ Res 48: 728–733, 1981
60. Johnston PA, Perrin NS, Bernard DB, Levinsky NG: Control of rat renal vascular resistance at reduced perfusion pressure. Circ Res 48: 734–739, 1981
61. Roblero J, Croxatto H, Garcia R, Corthorn J, DeViot E: Kallikrein-like activity in perfusates and urine of isolated rat kidneys. Am J Physiol 231: 1383–1389, 1976
62. Rabito SF, Scicli AG, Kher V, Carretero OA: Immunoreactive glandular kallikrein in rat plasma: a radioimmunoassay for its determination. Am J Physiol 242: H602–H610, 1982
63. Cuthbert AW, Margolius HS: Kinins stimulate net chloride secretion by the rat colon. Br J Pharmac 75: 587–598, 1982
64. Manning DC, Snyder SH, Kachur JF, Miller RJ, Field M: Bradykinin receptor-mediated chloride secretion in intestinal function. Nature 299: 256–259, 1982
65. Elliot AH, Nuzum FR: The urinary excretion of a depressor substance (kallikrein by Frey and Kraut) in arterial hypertension. Endocrinol 18: 462–474, 1934
66. Abe K, Seino M, Otsuka Y, Yoshinga K: Urinary kallikrein excretion and sodium metabolism in human hypertension. In: Chemistry and biology of the kallikrein-kinin system in health and disease. Pisano JJ, Austen KF (eds), U.S. Government Printing Office, Washington, 1976, Fogarty Center Proceedings No. 27

67. Margolius HS, Geller R, Pisano JJ, Sjoerdsma A: Altered urinary kallikrein excretion in human hypertension. Lancet II: 1063–1065, 1971
68. Werle E, Korsten H: Der Kallikreingehalt des Harns, des Speichels und des Blutes bei Gesunden und Kranken. Z Ges Exp Med 103: 153, 1938
69. Seino M, Abe K, Otsuka Y, Saito T, Irokawa N, Yasujima M, Chiba S, Yoshinga K: Urinary kallikrein excretion and sodium metabolism in hypertensive patients. Tohoku J Exp Med 116: 359–367, 1975
70. Greco AV, Porcelli G, Croxatto HR: Kallikrein excretion in diverse types of hypertension. In: Chemistry and biology of the kallikrein-kinin system in health and disease. Pisano JJ, Austen KF (eds),U.S. Government Printing Office, Washington, 1977, Fogarty International Center Proc. No. 27, pp 439–440
71. Mersey J, Williams G, Emanuel R, Dluhy R, Wong P, Moore T: Plasma bradykinin levels and urinary kallikrein excretion in normal renin essential hypertension. J Clin Endocrinol Metab 48: 642–647, 1979
72. Lawton WS, Fritz AE: Urinary kallikrein in normal renin essential hypertension. Circ 56: 856–859, 1977
73. Holland OB, Chud JM, Braunstein H: Urinary kallikrein excretion in essential and mineralocorticoid hypertension. J Clin Invest 65: 347, 1980
74. Shkhuatsabaya I, Nekrasova A, Chernova N, Khukarev V: Kinin system of the kidneys in pathogenesis of hypertensive disease. Ter Arkh 45: 71, 1973
75. Carretero OA, Scicli AG: The renal kallikrein-kinin system in human and experimental hypertension. Klin Wochenschr 56, Suppl. I: 113–125, 1978
76. Horwitz D, Margolius HS, Kerser HR: Effects of dietary potassium and race on urinary excretion of kallikrein and aldosterone in man. J Clin End Metab 47: 296–299, 1978
77. Levy SB, Liley JJ, Frignon RP, Stone RA: Urinary kallikrein and plasma renin activity as determinants of renal blood flow. J Clin Invest 60: 129–138, 1977
78. Zinner SH, Margolius HS, Rosner B, Kass EH: Familial aggregation of urinary kallikrein concentrations in childhood. Am J Epidemiol 104: 124–132, 1976
79. Zinner SH, Margolius HS, Rosner B, Kass EH: Stability of blood pressure rank and urinary kallikrein concentration in childhood: an eight year follow-up. Circ 58: 905–915, 1978
80. Carretero OA, Polomski C, Hampton A, Scicli AG: Urinary kallikrein, plasma renin, and aldosterone in New Zealand genetically hypertensive (GH) rats. Clin Exp Pharmacol Physiol 3, Suppl.: 55–59, 1976
81. Carretero OA, Scicli AG, Piwonska A, Koch J: Urinary kallikrein in rats bred for susceptibility and resistance to the hypertensive effect of salt in New Zealand genetically hypertensive rats. Mayo Clin Proc 52: 465–467, 1977
82. Keiser HR, Geller RG, Margolius HS, Pisano JJ: Urinary kallikrein in hypertensive animal models. Fed Proc 35: 199–202, 1976
83. Carretero OA, Amin VM, Ocholik T, Scicli AG, Koch J: Urinary kallikrein in rats bred for their susceptibility and resistance to the hypertensive effect of salt. A new radioimmunoassay for its direct determination. Circ Res 42: 727–731, 1978
84. Overlack A, Stumpe KO, Zywzok W, Ressel C, Kruck F: Defect in kallikrein-kinin system in essential hypertension and reduction of blood pressure by orally given kallikrein. In: Kinins II: Biochemistry pathophysiology, and clinical aspects, Fujii S, Moriya H, Suzuki T (eds), Plenum, 1979, New York, Vol. B, pp 539–547
85. Overlack A, Stumpe KO, Kolloch R, Reeseland C, Krueck F: Antihypertensive effect of orally administered glandular kallikrein in essential hypertension. Hypertension 3 Suppl. I: 18–21, 1981
86. Carretero OA, Oza NB, Scicli AG, Schork A: Renal tissue kallikrein, plasma renin, and plasma aldosterone in renal hypertension. Acta Physiol Lat-Am 24: 448, 1974

87. Sustarsic DL, McPartland RP, Rapp JP, Schlager G, Yan SY: Urinary kallikrein and urinary prostaglandin E_2 in genetically hypertensive mice. Proc Soc Exp Biol Med 163: 193–199, 1980

88. DeBryn J, Man in't Veld A, Wenting G et al.: Converting enzyme inhibitor affects blood pressure equally in renovascular hypertension, essential hypertension and the anephric state. Clin Sci 59, 83s, 1980

89. Swartz SL, Williams GH, Hollenberg NK et al.: Converting enzyme inhibition in essential hypertension: the hypotensive response does not reflect only reduced angiotensin II formation. Hypertension 1: 106, 1979

90. Swartz SL, Williams GH, Hollenberg NK et al.: Captopril-induced changes in prostaglandin production. J Clin Invest 65: 1257, 1980

91. Vinci JM, Horwitz D, Zusman RM et al.: The effect of converting enzyme inhibition with SQ-20,881 on plasma and urinary kinins, prostaglandin E, and angiotensin II in hypertensive man. Hypertension 1: 416, 1979

92. Hulthen UL, Hokfelt B: The effect of converting enzyme inhibitor SQ-20,881 on kinins, renin-angiotensin-aldosterone and catecholamines in relation to blood pressure in hypertensive patients. Acta Med Scand 204: 497, 1978

93. McCaa RE: Studies in vivo with angiotensin I converting enzyme (kininase II) inhibitors. Fed Proc 38: 2783, 1979

94. Scicli AG, Rabito S, Albertini R, Carretero, OA: Lack of feedback between urinary kinins and kallikrein in the anesthetized and saline expanded dog. Physiologist 21(4): 106, 1978

95. Seino M, Albertini R, Scicli AG, Carretero OA: Isorenin, kinins, and prostaglandins in the regulation of blood pressure and uteroplacental blood flow during pregnancy. Am J Physiol 242: H142, 1982

96. Albertini R, Seino M, Scicli AG, Carretero OA: Uteroplacental renin in regulation of blood pressure in the pregnant rabbit. Am J Physiol 239: H266, 1980

97. Overlack A, Stumpe KO, Sealey JE: Altered blood pressure (BP) and renin (PRA) responses to converting-enzyme (CE) inhibition after aprotinin (AP) induced kallikrein-kinin-system (KKS)-blockade. Clin Sci 59: 129s, 1980

98. Carretero OA, Scicli AG, Maitra SR: Role of kinins in the pharmacological effects of converting enzyme inhibitors. In: Angiotensin converting enzyme inhibitors: mechanisms of action, Horovitz ZP (ed), Urban and Schwarzenberg, Munich, 1981, p 105

99. Swartz SL, Williams GH, Hollenberg NK et al.: Captopril-induced changes in prostaglandin production. J Clin Invest 45: 1257, 1980

100. Abe K, Ito T, Sato M et al.: The role of prostaglandin in antihypertensive mechanism of captopril in low renin hypertension. Clin Sci 59: 141s, 1980

VI. THE ROLE OF THE CENTRAL NERVOUS SYSTEM: MEDIATION OR INITIATION?

13. THE MECHANISM OF HYPERTENSION – A PERSONAL VIEW

AUSTIN E. DOYLE

With the exception of a few well-defined varieties of secondary hypertension, the processes that initiate the development of high blood pressure usually occur too early in the disease to allow definition. For this reason, most observations on human hypertension relate to the established phase of the disease, and most have of necessity been directed to elucidating the mechanisms that lead to maintenanc of the hypertension. These sustaining processes are comparatively well defined, but may not necessarily be the same as the factors that initiate hypertension.

It is nevertheless useful to attempt to define the possible factors that operate to maintain high blood pressure in the chronic hypertensive, and then to consider which of these may be relevant initiating mechanisms.

THE AUTONOMIC NERVOUS SYSTEM

The autonomic nervous system is of considerable importance in the control of the circulation, particularly in man because of his habit of walking upright. Most of the autonomic mechanisms concerned in the control of the circulation seem better designed to monitor potential falls in blood pressure and to reverse them, rather than to moderate factors leading to rises in blood pressure. Thus, autonomic dysfunction, such as may occur as a result of many disease processes or the use of some anti-hypertensive drugs, leads to an inability to maintain normal blood pressure in the erect posture. For the most part, blood pressure in such instances can be maintained at adequate levels in the recumbent sodium-replete normal individual, which suggests that the autonomic nervous system in normal man is mainly concerned with buffering and preventing falls in blood pressure in response to such stimuli as the erect posture, sodium depletion, or hemorrhage.

There is no doubt that in hypertensive patients the autonomic nervous system continues to exert a major influence in preventing falls of blood pressure in response to such stimuli, as evidenced by the very large falls of blood pressure that can be obtained in the erect posture in hypertensive patients when autonomic reflexes are interfered with by drugs. In hypertension, postural falls of blood pressure are uncommon in the absence of drug treatment, and the blood pressure is maintained at an elevated level equally well in the recumbent and the erect

Sambhi, M.P. (ed.) Fundamental fault in hypertension
© *1984, Martinus Nijhoff Publishers. Boston/The Hague/Dordrecht/Lancaster.*
ISBN 978-94-010-9006-3

178

positions. This phenomenon implies that the blood pressure is being regulated to a new high level with the active connivance of the autonomic nervous system. It is of interest that this appears to be the case not only in patients with essential hypertension but in many patients in whom the hypertension is obviously second-ary to some other cause, such as primary aldosteronism. This raises the possibility that, regardless of the initiating cause of the hypertension, the function of the autonomic nervous system is to regulate blood pressure to a preset level.

The evaluation of the function of the sympathetic nervous system in man is of necessity difficult, and indirect methods must be used. These include responses to drugs that interfere with the autonomic nervous system, and the measurement of the neurotransmitter, norepinephrine. Soon after the introduction of the gang-lion blocking drugs for the treatment of hypertension, it became apparent that these caused very large falls in blood pressure in hypertensive patients. Doyle and Smirk [6] in 1955 reported the effects of large doses of the ganglion blocking drug, pentolinium, given intravenously in hypertensive patients and in normotensive controls (Figure 1). Very large doses of these drugs produced only small falls of blood pressure in recumbent normotensive controls, whereas the same doses given to hypertensive patients produced much larger falls of blood pressure. The responses to ganglion blockage in individual hypertensives varied considerably. A few hypertensive patients had falls of blood pressure no larger than those in normotensives, whereas other hypertensive patients had much greater falls of blood pressure, of sufficient magnitude to reduce the resting systolic and diastolic blood pressures to normal levels. This variation in the response to functional

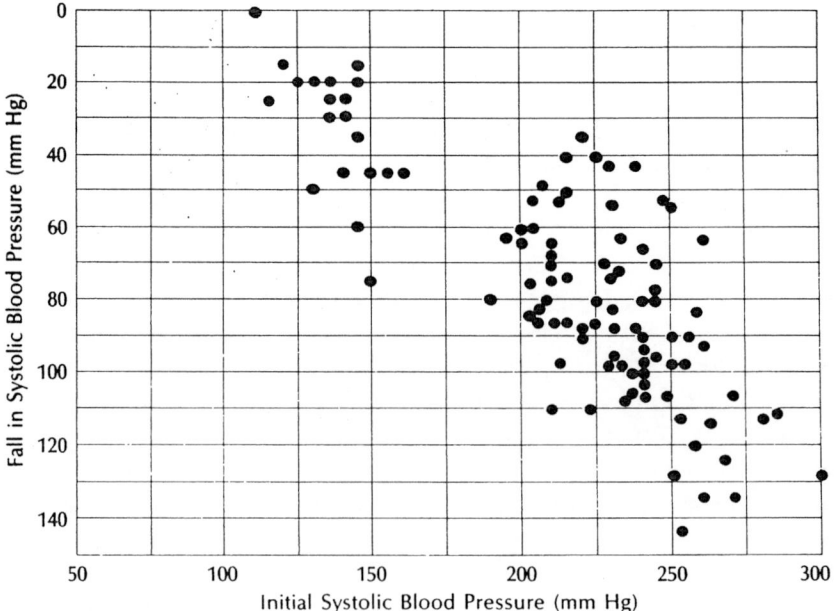

Figure 1. From Doyle, A.E. [2], with permission.

autonomic denervation strongly suggests that in many hypertensive patients the involvement of the autonomic nervous system in maintaining the high level of blood pressure far exceeds that which would be required for pressure regulation, and indicates that the major sustaining component in many hypertensives is the activity of the autonomic nervous system.

It was also clear from these early studies that the magnitude of the autonomic component is not fixed. In any given individual it obviously increases with assumption of the erect posture; in separate experiments the autonomic component could be shown to decrease with small infusions of pressor substances such as angiotensin or norepinephrine. These small infusions, although ineffective in inducing large rises in blood pressure in hypertensive patients, greatly reduced the fall in blood pressure induced by ganglion blockade (Figure 2). These observations suggest that blood pressure was being regulated to a comparatively fixed point by a combination of autonomic and non-autonomic factors, and that any increase in the non-autonomic component was readily buffered by a reduction in the autonomic component. Because in many hypertensive patients the autonomic component seemed to be very large, factors tending to raise blood pressure could be readily resisted by reduction of the autonomic component, thus obviating the need for the baroreflex response in heart rate, which is well known to be less marked in hypertensive subjects than in normals, in whom there is presumably a smaller resting component of autonomic activity.

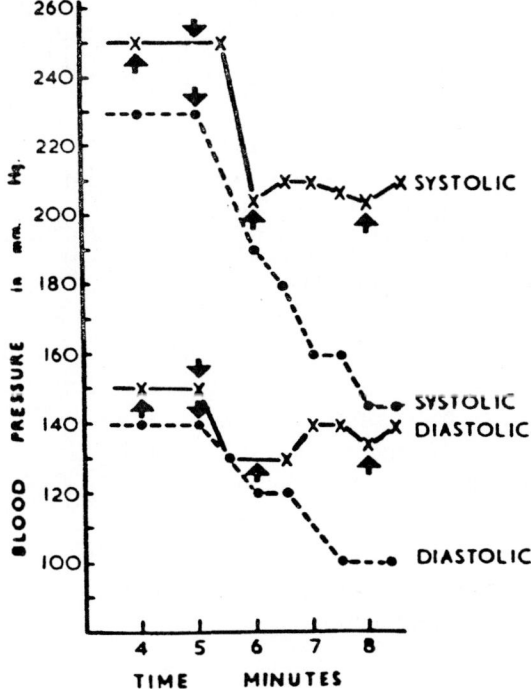

Figure 2. Doyle, A.E. & Smirk E. [5], with permission.

The second line of evidence relating to the activity of the autonomic nervous system has been derived from studies related to the circulating levels of the neurotransmitter, norepinephrine. It has to be emphasized that information concerning autonomic activity provided by the measurement of circulating norepinephrine is at best indirect and may be misleading. The neurotransmitter is released into the synaptic cleft by a process of exocytosis; much of the released transmitter is either taken up again into the nerve ending for re-use, or else is inactivated by enzyme systems such as catecholomethyltransferase or monoamine oxidase, so that only a small proportion of the released neurotransmitter finds its way into the circulation. Several groups, de Quattro and Chan [17], de Champlain et al. [1] and Louis et al. [12] have reported that in some, but by no means all, patients with essential hypertension, plasma levels of norepinephrine are higher than those found in normotensive individuals. Some doubt about the validity of these observations has been cast by other groups who have found no statistically significant differences between the norepinephrine levels in normotensives and hypertensives [18, 20]. The situation is further complicated by the fact that plasma norepinephrine levels seem to become elevated with advancing age. Because circulating norepinephrine levels at best can only be expected to provide a crude index of autonomic activity, and because the methodology is complex and difficult, these differences are probably not surprising. Furthermore, the circumstances relating to the sampling of blood for norepinephrine levels are obviously of great importance, as such factors as assumption of the erect posture, anxiety, lack of familiarity with the procedure, and the state of sodium balance may greatly influence plasma norepinephrine levels. These have often not been carefully controlled.

There is also considerable controversy as to the extent to which plasma norepinephrine levels correlate with the blood pressure at the time of measurement. Many studies have reported no relationship between the level of blood pressure and the level of plasma norepinephrine. However, Louis et al. [11, 12] using basal levels of blood pressure and basal levels or norepinephrine in hypertensive patients studied three days after hospitalization, did find a relationship between diastolic blood pressure and plasma levels of norepinephrine (Figure 3). Perhaps of more significance is the close relationship found between the hypotensive responses to pentolinium, a ganglion blocking drug, and the falls in plasma norepinephrine induced by this agent (Figure 4). Patients who had larger falls in blood pressure in response to a small intravenous dose of pentolinium also had greater falls in plasma norepinephrine in response to this drug. The importance of this finding is that it suggests that the large anti-hypertensive responses to drugs that interfere with autonomic activity occur because such patients have excess autonomically induced vasoconstriction.

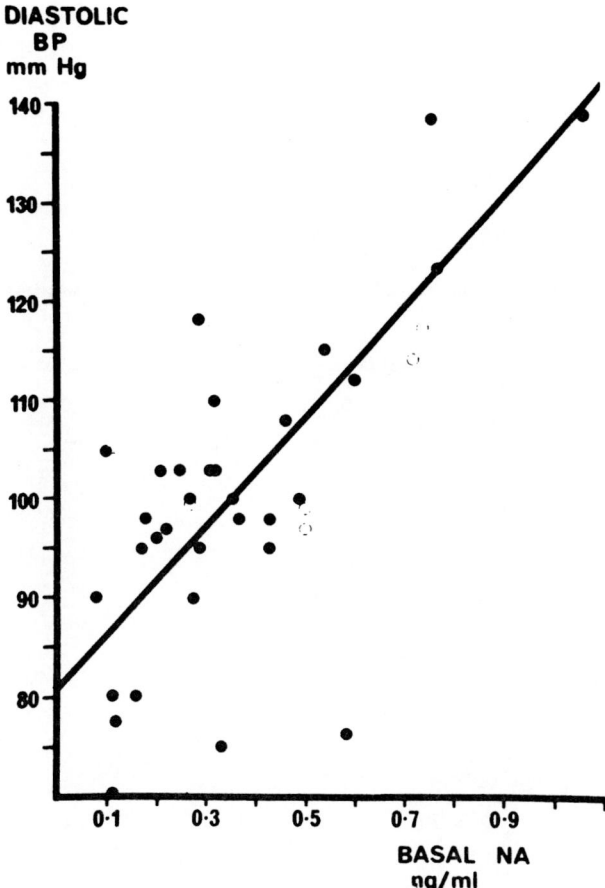

Figure 3. Louis, W.J. et al. [12], with permission.

VASCULAR REACTIVITY

It has been known for many years that in established human hypertension the resistance vessels have greater responses to a given constrictor stimulus than in normotension. These findings have been made in the hand using adrenaline [6], in the nail bed with epinephrine and norepinephrine [9], in the finger following sympathetic blockade by indirect heat or ganglion blocking drug [14, 15], and in muscle using norepinephrine [16]. All these workers have reported increased reactivity in hypertension. Doyle, Fraser, and Marshall [4], used intra-arterial infusion of norepinephrine, angiotensin, and 5-hydroxy tryptamine in dose-response studies and reported that a given constrictor response to norepinephrine could be induced in hypertensive patients with approximately one-half of the dose required in normotensives. The same workers also found a close relationship between the vascular responses of individual patients to norepinephrine and 5-hydroxy tryptamine (Figure 5), but the responses to angiotensin in hypertensive

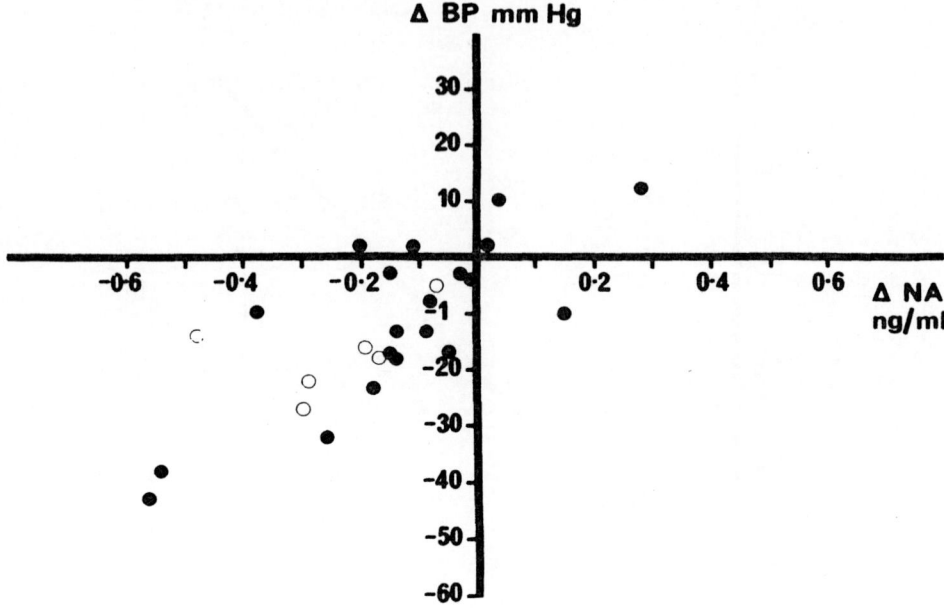

Figure 4. Louis, W.J. et al. [12], with permission.

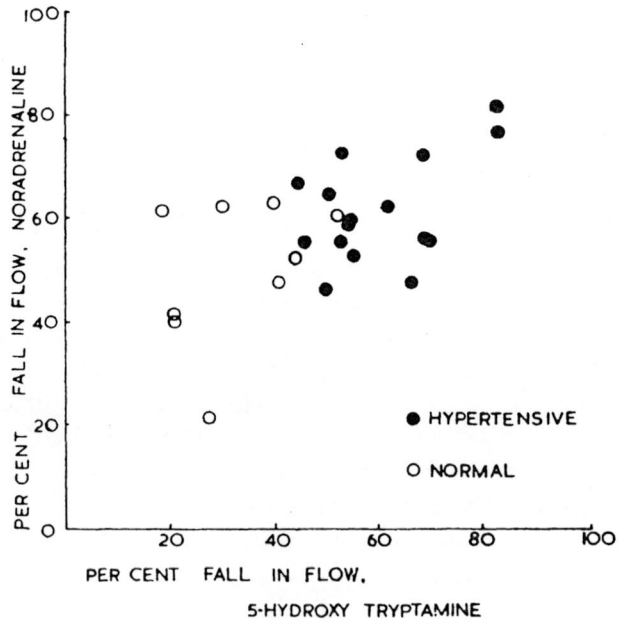

Figure 5. Doyle, A.E. et al. [4], with permission.

patients were less exaggerated. This latter finding suggests that the increase in vascular reactivity may not be due entirely to structural hypertrophy of vascular smooth muscle, although this is no doubt an important factor [8]. It is possible that there may be a specific lack of responsiveness to angiotensin. However, McGregor and Smirk [13], and later Haeusler and Finch [10], found that the mesenteric vascular bed of the New Zealand strain of hypertensive rats had a specific increase in sensitivity to 5-hydroxy tryptamine but not to norepinephrine. This raises the possibility that increased vascular reactivity in hypertension may contain an element of supersensitivity as well as being due in part to muscle hypertrophy.

Increased vascular reactivity could be an important sustaining mechanism in hypertension as an amplification system in conjunction with either the autonomic nervous system or with other pressor systems. This would greatly facilitate the regulation of blood pressure to a preset elevated level. It would partly account for the exaggerated falls of blood pressure that follow autonomic blockade in hypertensives. It also has to be taken into account when evaluating depressor responses to agents that interfere with the renin angiotensin system.

THE RENIN ANGIOTENSIN SYSTEM

The renin angiotensin system, like the autonomic nervous system, may play a significant role in the regulation of blood pressure, particularly in relation to sodium depletion and in the erect posture. Although high plasma renin or angiotensin levels are often regarded as evidence of primary involvement of this system in hypertension, they may be merely another example of a secondary sustaining mechanism in maintaining hypertension at a preset level.

For example, the two-kidney (2k) Goldblatt hypertensive rat is often cited as a renin-dependent model. In this model, blood pressure rises (Figure 6), and so in many instances does plasma renin activity (Figure 7). The rise in blood pressure is often accompanied by sodium depletion. If a radioactive sodium equilibration technique [7] is used, plasma renin activity (PRA) remains high, but exchangeable sodium levels rise as well [3]. In the two-kidney rat model, Captopril induces a prompt fall in blood pressure (Figure 8), the magnitude of which does not correlate well with the pre-existing PRA (Figure 9). This could be taken as evidence of angiotensin dependency, and as presumptive evidence of the role of angiotensin as an initiating mechanism. However, removal of the opposite kidney in hypertensive 2K rats, thus converting them to the 1K model, is accompanied by a fall in PRA (Figure 10) and a loss of response to Captopril (Figure 11), without any significant change in blood pressure (Figure 12).

It appears therefore that the presence of the contralateral kidney leads in some way to an increased output of renin from the clipped kidney as a homeostatic response to maintain blood pressure at elevated levels. An important question is,

184

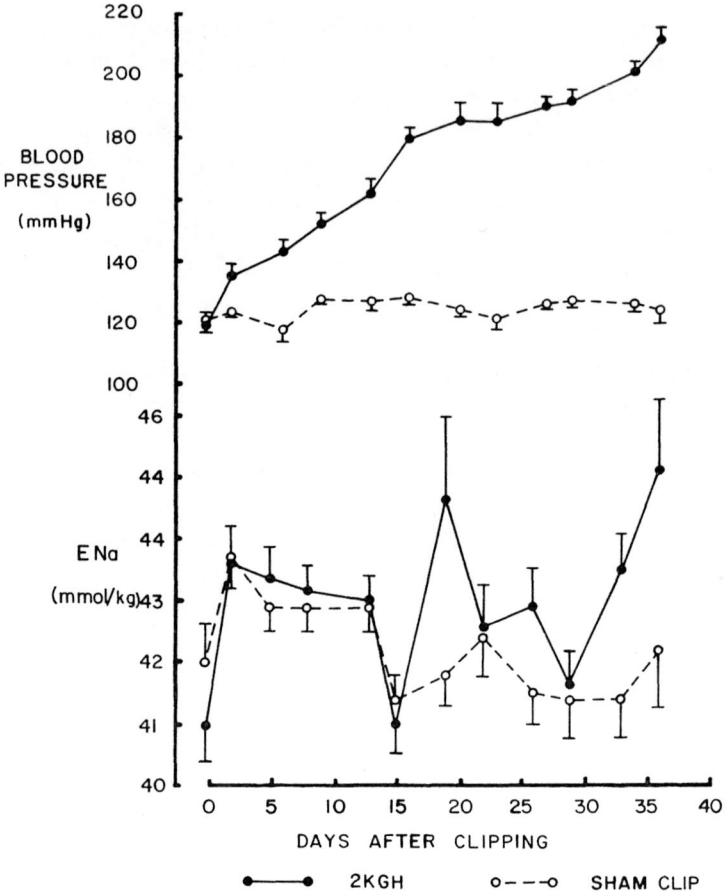

Figure 6. The changes in blood pressure and exchangeable sodium (ENa) in clipped 2 KGH rats
(●——●) and sham clipped rats (○– – –○).

why is this necessary? It does not appear to be due to overall depletion of body
sodium, since it still occurs in animals drinking sodium chloride solution, whose
total exchangeable sodium is normal or elevated. Presumably, the application of
a clip to one kidney provides some signal that induces a rise in blood pressure. The
fact that resetting of the baroreceptors occurs very early in experimental one-
kidney renal hypertension [19] suggests that even in this model the autonomic
nervous system may be involved.

To summarize, the balance of evidence suggests that high blood pressure is
sustained by activity of the autonomic nervous system and increased vascular
responses acting together. These mechanisms are supplemented when necessary
by others, such as the renin angiotensin system. Sustained hypertension is dominated by the need to maintain the capacity of the circulation to respond in as
normal a manner as possible to changes in internal or external environment. In
some respects the situation may be analogous to that in chronic obstructive lung

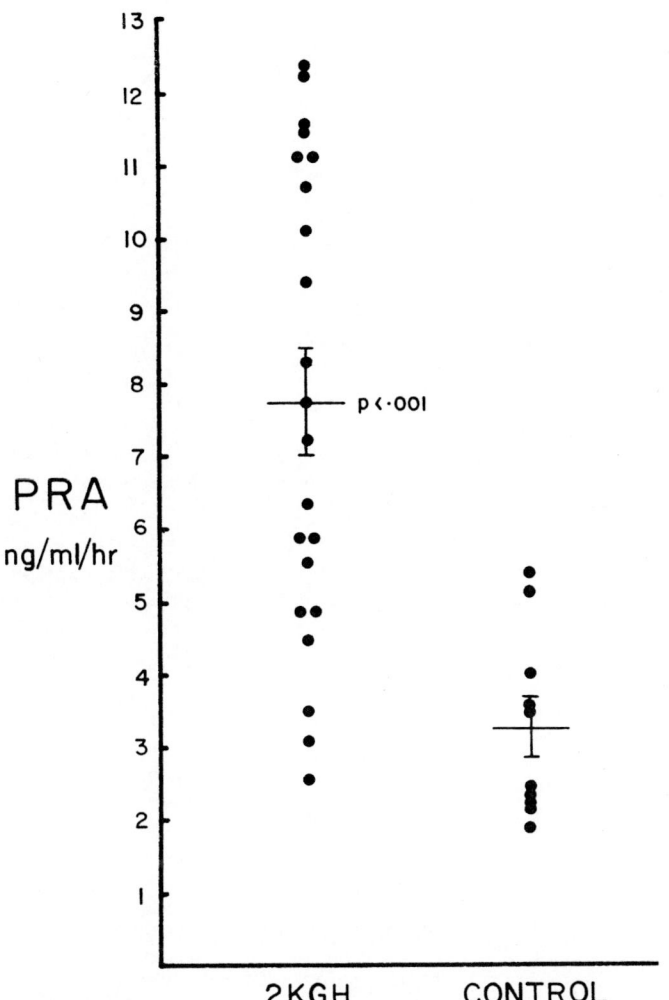

Figure 7. Plasma renin activity (PRA) in 2-kidney hypertensive rats and sham-operated controls, 36 days after the procedure.

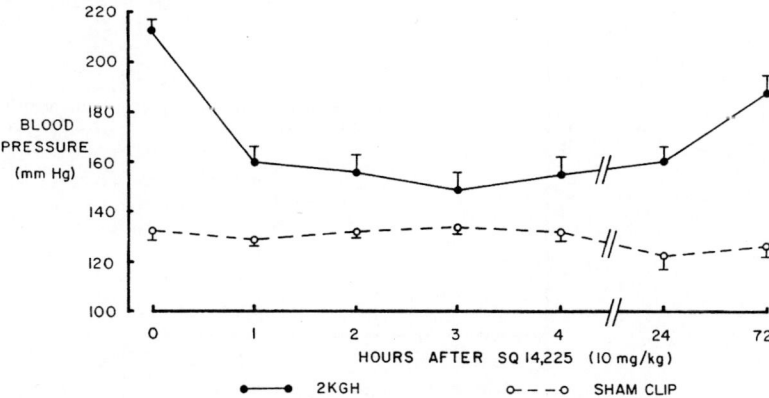

Figure 8. Changes in blood pressure following the oral administration of 10 mgm/kg of Captopril to 2-kidney hypertensive rats and control sham-operated animals.

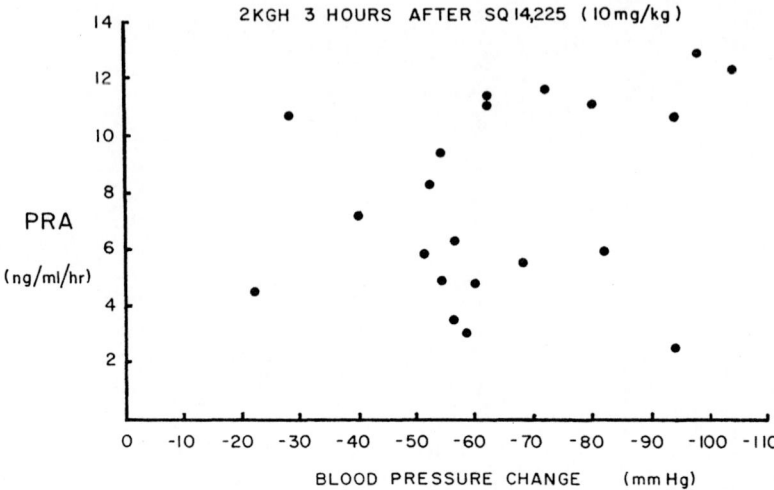

Figure 9. The absence of relationship between plasma renin activity (PRA) before Captopril and the change in blood pressure 3 hr after an oral dose of 10 mgm/kg of Captopril.

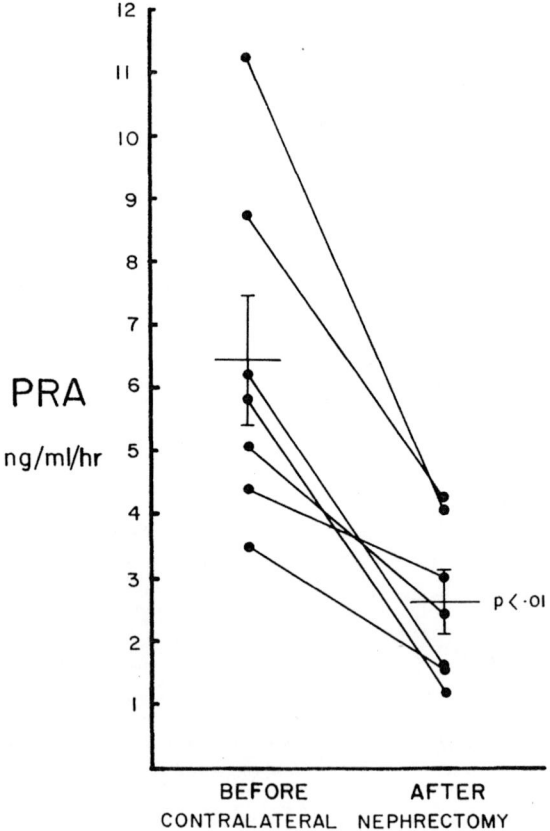

Figure 10. The effect of contralateral nephrectomy on plasma renin activity (PRA) in 2-kidney hypertensive rats.

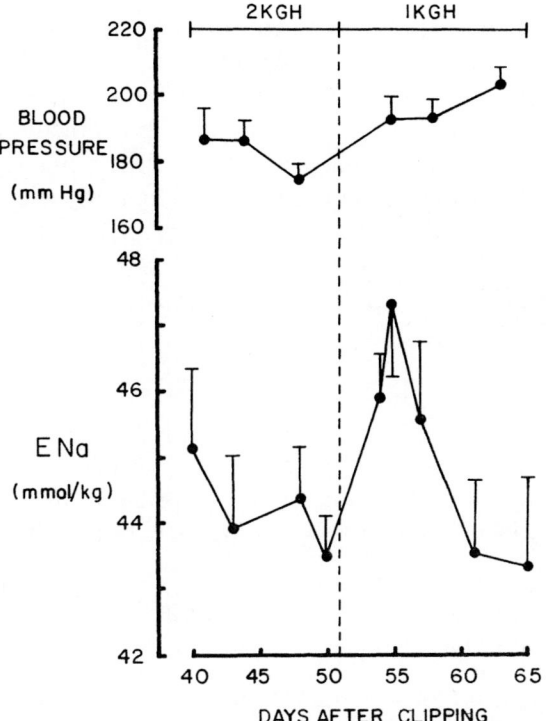

Figure 11. The effect on blood pressure of an oral dose of 10 mgm/kg of Captopril, before (●——●) and after (○– – –○) removal of the untouched kidney, in 2-kidney hypertensive rats.

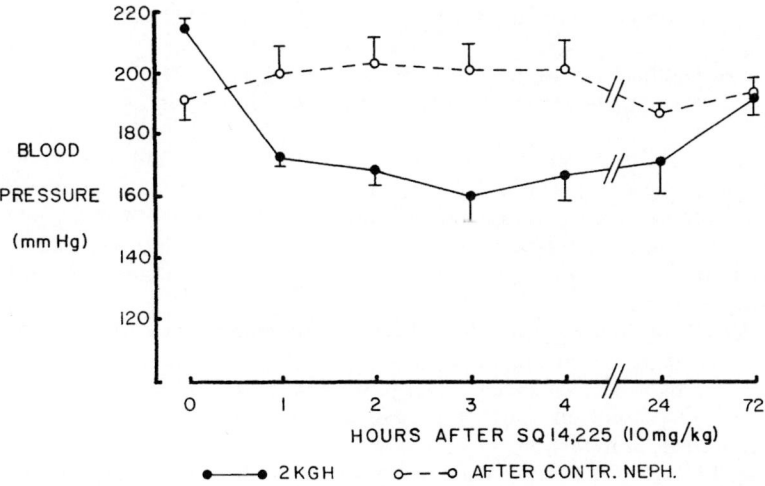

Figure 12. The effect of removal of the untouched kidney (dashed vertical line) on blood pressure and exhangeable sodium (ENa) in the 2-kidney hypertensive rat.

188

disease, in which the need to regulate respiratory responses leads to an acceptance by the organism of high levels of arterial P_{CO_2}.

It seems very likely that a wide variety of pathophysiological events, such as sodium retention, renal ischemia, primary autonomic overactivity, or loss of a depressor mechanism, may initiate the process. Once the initial stages of hypertension have occurred, regulation of blood pressure to normotensive levels must become progressively more difficult to achieve and in certain instances one may speculate that, even if the primary cause has disappeared, the hypertensive process is sustained by the secondary involvement of the autonomic nervous system.

REFERENCES

1. de Champlain J, Farley L, Cousineau D, Van Ameringen MR: Circulating catecholamine levels in human and experimental hypertension. Circulation Res 38: 109, 1976
2. Doyle AE: Sympathetic nervous activity and hypertension. In: Hypertension mechanisms, diagnosis and management. Davis JO, Laragh JH, Selwin A (eds), Hospital Practice Publishing Co. Inc., New York, 1977
3. Doyle AE, Duffy S, MacDonald GJ: Exhangeable sodium in experimental hypertension in rats. Clin Sci and Mol Med 51: 1335, 1976
4. Doyle AE, Fraser JRE, Marshall RJ: Reactivity of forearm vessels to vasoconstrictor substances in hypertensive and normotensive subjects. Clin Sci 18: 441, 1959
5. Doyle AE, Smirk FH: The neurogenic component in hypertension. Circulation 12: 543, 1955
6. Duff RA: Adrenaline sensitivity of peripheral blood vessels in hypertension. Brit Heart J 19: 45, 1957
7. Dusting GJ, Harris GS, Rand MJ: A specific increase in cardiovascular reactivity related to sodium retention in DOCA-salt treated rats. Clin Sci and Mol Med 45: 571, 1973
8. Folkow B, Hallback M, Lundgren G, Weiss L: Background of increased flow resistance and vascular reactivity in spontaneously hypertensive rats. Acta Physiol Scand 80: 93, 1970
9. Greisman SE: The reaction of the capillary bed of the nailfold to the continuous intravenous infusion of levo-norepinephrine in patients with normal blood pressure and with essential hypertension. J Clin Invest 33: 975, 1954
10. Haeusler G, Finch L: Vascular resistance and reactivity to various vasoconstrictor agents in hypertensive rats. In: Spontaneous hypertension. Okamoto K (ed), Igaku Shoin, Tokyo, 1972
11. Louis WJ, Doyle AE, Anavekar SN: Plasma norepinephrine levels in essential hypertension. New Eng J Med 288: 599, 1973
12. Louis WJ, Doyle AE, Anavekar SW, Johnston CI: Sympathetic and reflex mechanisms. In: Hypertension, current problems. Distler A, Wolff HP (eds). George Thieme Verlag, Stuttgart, 1974
13. McGregor DD, Smirk FH: Vascular responses to 5 hydroxytryptamine in genetic and renal hypertensive rats. Am J Physiol 219: 687, 1970
14. Mendlowitz M, Gitlow SE, Wolf RL, Naftchi NE: Mechanisms in essential hypertension. Am J Cardiol 9: 100, 1962

15. Mendlowitz M, Naftchi N, Wolf RL, Gitlow SE: Reactivity of the digital blood vessels to angiotensin II in normal and hypertensive subjects. Am Heart J 62: 221, 1961
16. Moulton R, Spencer AG, Willoughby DA: Noradrenaline sensitivity in hypertension measured with a radioactive sodium technique. Brit Heart J 20: 224, 1958
17. de Quattro V, Chan S: Raised plasma catecholamine levels in some patients with primary hypertension. Lancet 1: 806, 1972
18. Sever PS, Birch M, Osikowska B, Tunbridge RDG: Plasma noradrenaline in essential hypertension. Lancet 1: 1078, 1977
19. Sleight P, Robinson JL In: Modern aspects in the treatment of arterial hypertension. Zanchetti A, Enrico M (eds). Boehringer Ingelheim, Firenze, 1973
20. Ziegler MG, Lake CR, Kopin IJ: Plasma noradrenaline increases with age. Nature 261: 333, 1976

14. ARTERIAL BAROREFLEXES IN HUMAN BEINGS

GIUSEPPE MANCIA, ALBERTO ZANCHETTI

Arterial baroreflexes have been extensively studied in experimental animals and a large body of information has been collected. It has been shown that *1.* baroreceptors in both the carotid sinuses and the aortic arch exert an important circulatory control; *2.* this control is partly different for these two reflexogenic areas and is not exerted uniformly on the various cardiovascular effectors; *3.* it is deranged, sometimes to a marked degree, in a number of pathological conditions [13].

Little of this information has been directly verified in man, however, the reason being primarily the lack of suitable methods of study. Few satisfactory techniques are available in this field. The one most extensively used consists of altering the activity of the arterial baroreceptors by injection of vasopressor and vaso-depressor drugs [17, 33]; this allows exploration of the baroreceptor control of heart rate (as well as of other cardiac functions), but obviously does not offer any information on the reflex control of blood pressure, and more generally of peripheral circulation. Another techniques makes use of the Valsalva maneuver. Although in this instance measurements have been made of either the cardiac or vasomotor reflex responses [16], there is no doubt that a major drawback is the complexity of the stimulus being applied to the various reflexogenic areas, which prevents the contribution of the arterial baroreflexes to be selectively sorted out. Another technique consists of reducing central blood volume and arterial blood pressure by application of negative pressure to the lower half of the body [34, 41]. This allows measurement of reflex changes in some vascular beds (those of the upper side of the body) as well as in the heart, and also exploration of possible differences between reflex control exerted by receptors in the high and low pressure areas. Still, only one side of the reflexes (i.e., reduction in receptor activity) can be investigated; moreover, under these circumstances no blood pressure responses can be assessed.

A fourth technique for studying reflex control of circulation in human subjects is the variable pressure neck chamber [8], a plastic collar with double rubber valves that adhere below to the shoulders and above to the chin, the ear lobes, and the occiput of the subject. Pneumatic pressure inside the chamber can be altered in a positive or a negative direction, with corresponding reduction and increase in transmural pressure across the carotid arteries, and therefore with

Sambhi, M.P. (ed.) Fundamental fault in hypertension
© *1984, Martinus Nijhoff Publishers. Boston/The Hague/Dordrecht/Lancaster.*
ISBN 978-94-010-9006-3

corresponding reduction and increase in the activity of the carotid sinus baro-receptors. This technique allows the study of reflex control from a baroreceptor area of paramount importance, and the estimation of a large number of reflex effects that include arterial blood pressure. In addition, the reflex function can be evaluated over a range of baroreceptor activities from below to above the existing level.

In the past few years we have applied the variable pressure neck chamber technique in normotensive subjects and in subjects with arterial hypertension while measuring blood pressure and other reflex responses. As a result, data have been collected on the characteristics of the carotid baroreceptor reflex in normal conditions and in conditions in which blood pressure is chronically elevated. A description of these data is provided in the following pages, along with other data gathered with the use of other techniques, in combination with the neck chamber or alone, to add to our information on reflex circulatory control in human beings.

THE VARIABLE PRESSURE NECK CHAMBER TECHNIQUE

Before applying the variable pressure neck chamber in systematic studies, a number of theoretical uncertainties about the technique were investigated [19]. For example, we observed that application of positive chamber pressure up to 60 mmHg did not cause a reduction in cerebral blood flow, thus ruling out the possibility that cerebral ischemia was involved in the genesis of the cardiovascular responses to be measured. We also gained evidence against a participation of the carotid chemoreceptors in the reflex changes that could be observed. Most importantly, we were able to determine the amount of positive and negative neck chamber pressures that are transmitted through the neck tissues to the region of the carotid sinuses. This point was investigated by applying a series of different positive and negative pressures within the neck chamber, while simultaneously measuring pressure from a tissue catheter placed close to the walls of a carotid sinus. The results in 10 subjects (6 normotensives and 4 hypertensives) studied in this way are shown in Figure 1 [19]. There was a very strict linear relationship between charges in positive and negative neck chamber pressure and changes in neck tissue pressure (in each subject, r was greater than 0.989, $p < 0.001$). Trans-mission, though prompt, was incomplete, however, since on average 86% of the positive neck chamber pressure, and only 64% of the negative one were transmit-ted to the tissue catheter. It can be seen from the confidence limits shown in Figure 1 that individual regression coefficients were close to the means. These can therefore be meaningfully used as correction factors for the applied pneumatic pressures, so as to achieve a more accurate estimation of the stimuli applied to the carotid baroreceptors under the various circumstances of the study.

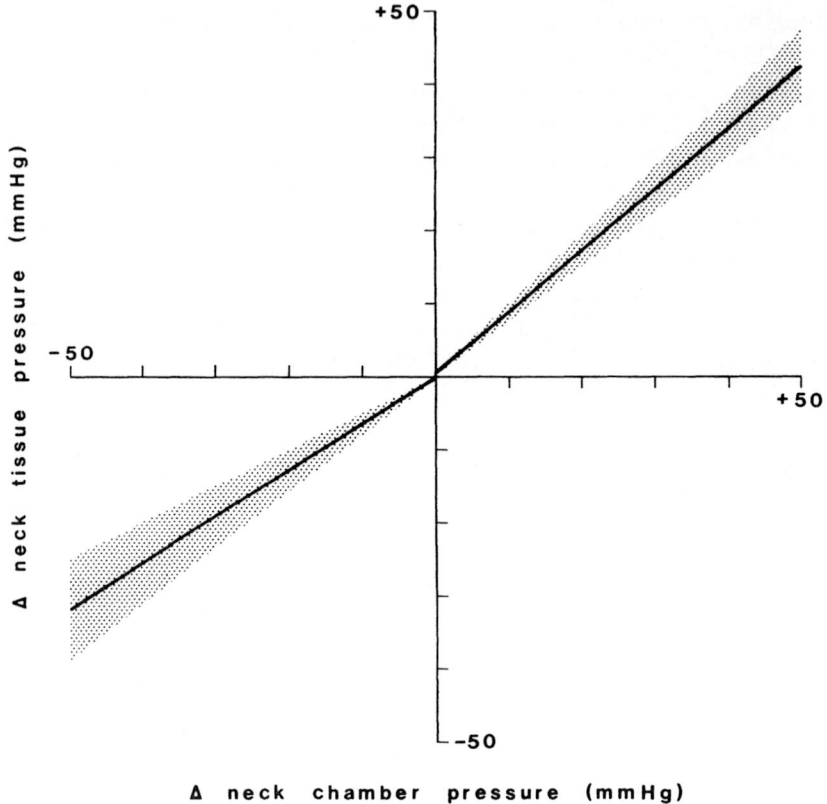

Figure 1. Relationship of change in neck chamber pressure to change in tissue pressure adjacent to a carotid sinus. Separate mean regression lines and 90% confidence limits are shown for positive and negative applied pressures. Each of the lines and its limits was constructed from the individual calculated regressions of 10 subjects (5 to 10 observations for each regression in each subject). From Mancia et al. [19], by permission.

CAROTID BARORECEPTOR REFLEX IN NORMOTENSIVE SUBJECTS

Reflex effects of carotid baroreceptors on blood pressure and heart rate were investigated in 11 normotensive subjects whose mean age was 36 ± 4 years [23]. In each subject a series of 4 to 6 negative and 4 to 6 positive neck chamber pressures were applied within the range of ± 50 mmHg. Each stimulus was maintained for 2 min, its reflex effects being evaluated both shortly after stimulus application and in its last phase (for their characteristics, these responses were called 'early or transient' and 'late or steady-state', respectively). In almost every circumstance the magnitude of the applied stimulus and the resulting response displayed a linear relationship, which allowed us to take the regression coefficient as the measure of the reflex function.

The results of our study on normotensive subjects is summarized in Figure 2, which shows the relationship between changes in tissue pressure outside the carotid sinuses and the resulting changes in mean arterial pressure and heart rate (expressed as R-R interval). The data are presented as means ± standard errors of the regression coefficients obtained in the individual subjects, the dashed lines representing the early responses and the solid lines the steady-state responses.

Three findings are worthy of mention. One, heart rate responses were not invariably sustained through the duration of the stimulus; in particular, the bradycardia accompanying the negative neck chamber pressure, though evident in the early phase, almost disappeared in the late one. Two, blood pressure changes were invariably sustained through the duration of the stimulus, as indicated by the fact that the steady-state responses were either greater or similar to the early ones. Three, the responses obtained with positive neck pressures were greater than those with negative ones, a finding that was particularly significant during the steady state. This last result is in line with that obtained by other investigators [37]; we have discussed elsewhere two hypotheses that can explain it [28]. One would be that carotid baroreceptors discharge at basal blood pressure near their maximal level, thus making the decrease in baroreceptor firing induced by a decrease in carotid transmural pressure greater than the increase in baroreceptor firing induced by an increase in carotid transmural pressure. This must not be regarded as unlikely, as the carotid sinuses have thin and highly compliant walls that can be easily distended by the pulse pressure wave to provide a strong stimulus for the local stretch receptors. A second hypothesis is that what has been speculated for the carotid baroreceptors (near maximal stimulus provided by the existing blood pressure value) does in fact hold for the aortic (or cardio-aortic) baroreceptors. In this case, the depressor response

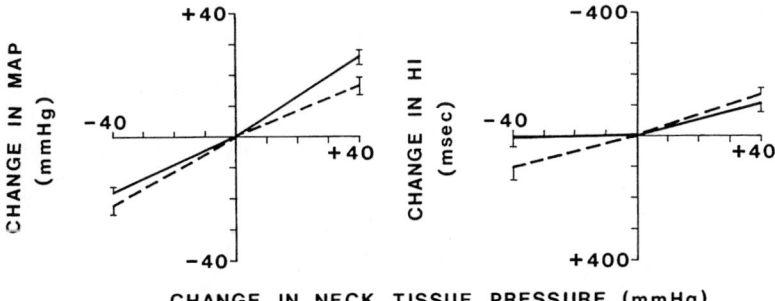

CHANGE IN NECK TISSUE PRESSURE (mmHg)

Figure 2. Changes in mean arterial pressure (MAP) and R-R interval (HI) induced by changes in tissue pressure outside the carotid sinuses (neck tissue pressure). Data are shown as means ± SE of individual regression coefficients in 11 subjects. The dashed line represents the early response (average of the values between the 5th and the 15th sec. following the change in neck tissue pressure); the solid line shows the steady-state response (the average value that occurred in the last 30 sec. of the change in neck tissue pressure). Changes in neck tissue pressure were calculated from changes in neck chamber pressure, using correction figures for pressure transmission through neck tissue (see text). From Mancia, Ferrari, Gregorini, Valentini, Ludbrook and Zanchetti: Circ Res 41:170, 1978. By permission.

194

induced by an increase in carotid baroreceptor activity would be more effectively buffered than the pressor response induced by the decrease in carotid baroreceptor activity, thus accounting for the asymmetry we observed. This is less likely for a number of reasons: that the aortic walls are much less compliant than the carotid sinuses, that no asymmetry of this sort has ever been shown in animals (if anything, the aortic baroreceptors have been shown to be close to threshold at normal blood pressure values), and that no pressor response ensues in normotensive humans, when the ongoing cardioaortic baroreceptor influence is suddenly eliminated by vagal anesthesia [9].

It seems therefore likely that the asymmetry observed by our group and by Thron et al. [37] refers to a peculiar role of the carotid baroreflex, which in human beings with normal blood pressure levels may well have a greater ability to counteract a decrease rather than an increase in carotid transmural pressure, thus acting as a more effective antihypotensive than an antihypertensive mechanism.

CAROTID BARORECEPTOR REFLEX IN SUBJECTS WITH ARTERIAL
HYPERTENSION

The carotid baroreceptor reflex was studied in a population of 35 subjects with essential hypertension (mean age, 45 ± 5 years). The study was conducted in the same way as for the normotensives, and the results are shown in Figure 3. As in Figure 2, means ± standard errors of individual regression coefficients are shown, the dashed and solid lines representing the early and steady-state responses, respectively.

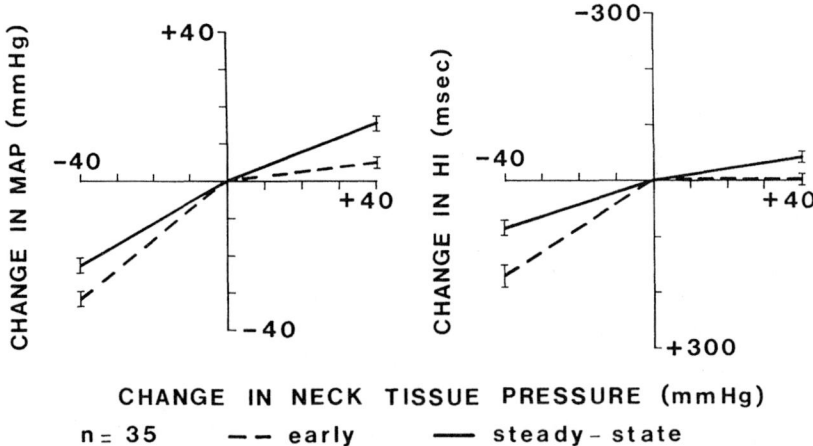

Figure 3. Changes in mean arterial pressure (MAP) and R-R interval (HI) by changes in tissue pressure outside the carotid sinuses (neck tissue pressure). Data are shown as means ± SE of individual regression coefficients in 35 subjects with essential hypertension. All symbols and details as in Fig. 2. see text for further explanation. From Mancia et al. [26], by permission.

In this case, three major conclusions were reached. One, the carotid baro-receptor reflex continues to have a homeostatic role in essential hypertension, as both reduction and increase in carotid baroreceptor activity cause reflex responses linearly related to the stimuli. Two, in hypertensive subjects there is also a significant asymmetry of the reflex, but the asymmetry is opposite to that observed in normotensives and consists of greater responses in increase rather than to decrease in carotid sinus transmural pressure; this means that in essential hypertension there is a reset of the baroreceptor reflex which favors its antihypertensive function.

Three, differences not only in shape but also in magnitude of the reflex functions exist between normotensives and patients with essential hypertension. By comparison of the two sets of data with the unpaired t test, the responses to reduction in carotid transmural pressure appear to be smaller in hypertensives than in normotensives, while the responses to increase in carotid transmural pressure appear to be greater. This point is further developed in Figures 4 and 5,

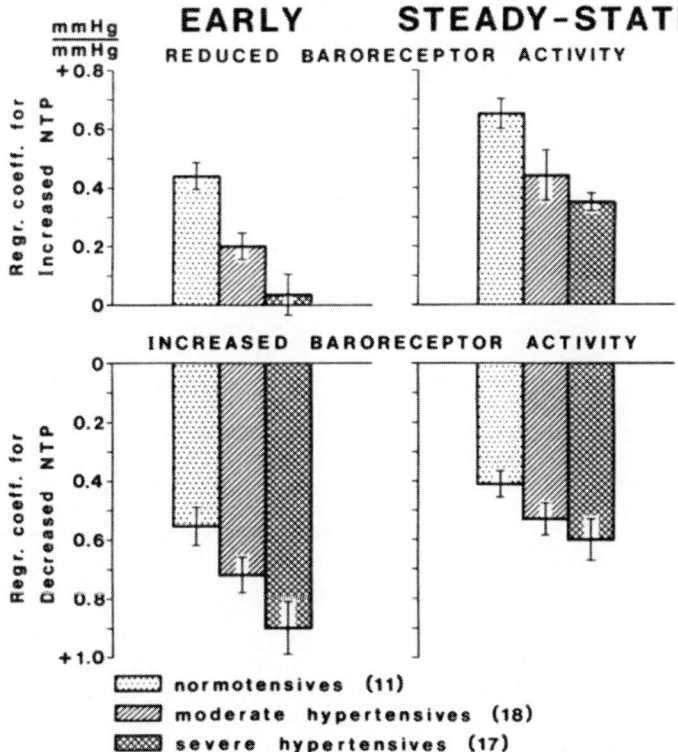

Figure 4. Carotid baroreceptor influence on blood pressure in 11 normotensive, 18 moderately hypertensive, and 17 more severely hypertensive subjects. The data are shown as the averages ($\pm$ SE) of individual regression coefficients (regr. coeff.) relating changes in mean arterial pressure (mmHg) to changes in tissue pressure outside the carotid sinuses (NTP, mmHg) *Top*: Data for increased NTP, i.e., reduced baroreceptor activity. *Bottom*: Data for decreased NTP, i.e., increased baroreceptor activity. Both early (left panels) and late or steady-state responses (right panels) are shown. From Mancia et al. [26], by permission.

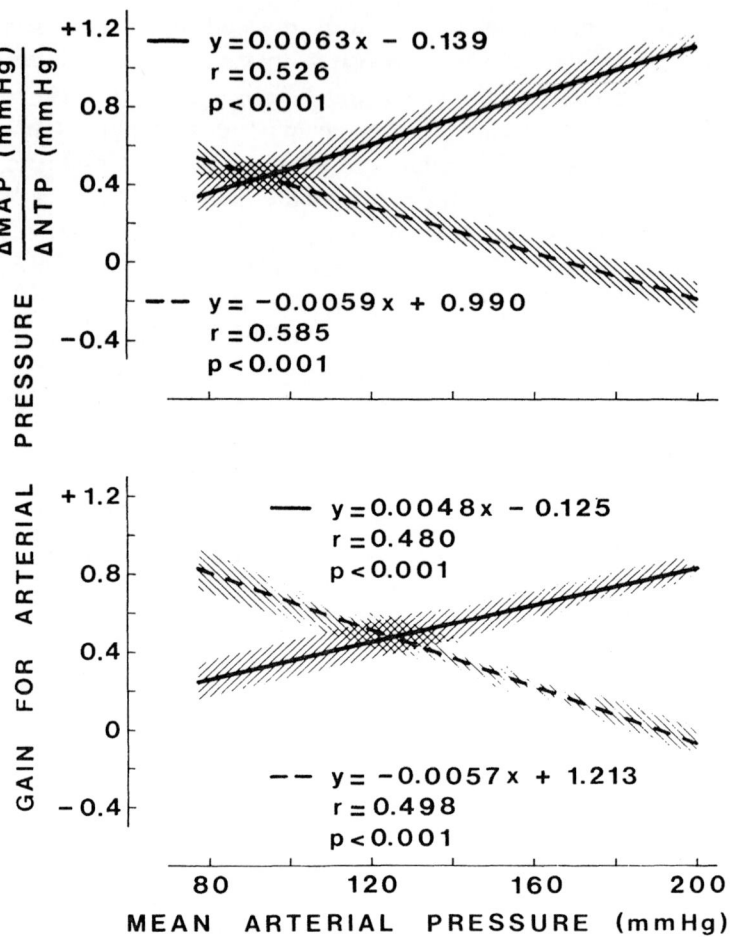

Figure 5. Relation between regression coefficients for mean arterial pressure (gain) and basal mean arterial pressure in 11 normotensive and 35 hypertensive subjects. The gain is expressed as changes in mean (arterial) pressure (MAP) induced by changes in tissue pressure outside the carotid sinuses (NTP). *Top*: early response; *bottom*: late or steady-state response s lines: Gains for reflex responses to increased baroreceptor activity; dashed lines: gains for reflex responses to reduced baroreceptor activity. The hatched areas represent the standard errors of the regressions. The equations of the regressions are also shown (*p* = probability; *r* = correlation coefficient). From Mancia et al. [28], by permission.

which show individual regression coefficients (expressing the magnitude of the reflex responses) as a function of the individual basal mean arterial pressure for three separate groups of subjects defined as normotensive, moderate, and severe hypertensive (Figure 4) and for the entire population of normotensive and hypertensive subjects taken together (Figure 5). It is clear that these two variables were linearly related. That is, the depressor response to increase in carotid transmural pressure became progressively greater as mean arterial pressure moved from the lowest to the highest values, while the pressor response to reduction in carotid transmural pressure showed an exactly opposite pattern.

Again, the hypotheses that can be made to explain these findings have been discussed in detail elsewhere [26]. One hypothesis is clarified by expressing the data as in Figure 6 and by applying the schema of Figure 7. In brief, it can be suggested that the progressively reversing asymmetry shown by the carotid baroreflex on going from normotensive to mild and more severe hypertensive subjects is due to the fact that under these circumstances the basal blood pressure level becomes a progressively less effective stimulus for the carotid baroreceptors. In normotensive subjects the basal blood pressure level may be capable of inducing a near maximal carotid baroreceptor activation (see above), thereby allowing large decreases but only small further increases in the receptor activity to occur with the use of the neck chamber. In hypertensive subjects, however, the stimulus provided by the basal blood pressure may become progressively less effective, and finally it may just move above the baroreceptor threshold, creating conditions under which smaller decreases but not larger increases in the receptor activity can be produced by the neck chamber. This is tantamount to suggesting that the carotid baroreflex undergoes a resetting in essential hypertension, and that the resetting is so marked that it does not limit itself to maintaining the set-

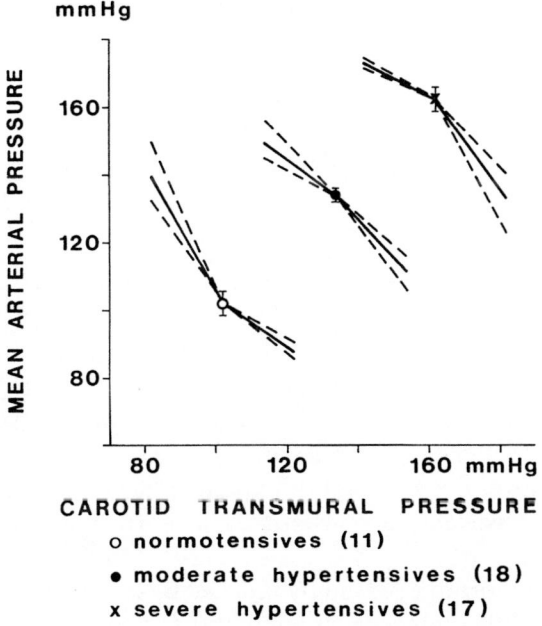

Figure 6. Carotid baroreceptor influence on blood pressure in the same 3 groups of subjects as in Figure 4.The open circle, the closed circle, and the cross represent the average (± S.E.) mean arterial pressure during the control period in each group, respectively. The solid lines represent the average of individual regression coefficients relating mean arterial pressure to increased or decreased carotid transmural pressure with respect to control values, the dashed lines indicating the standard errors of the regressions. The data are shown for the late or steady-state effects of the neck chamber, the carotid transmural pressure being calculated as the difference between the mean arterial pressure and the tissue pressure outside the carotid sinuses. From Mancia et al. [26], by permission.

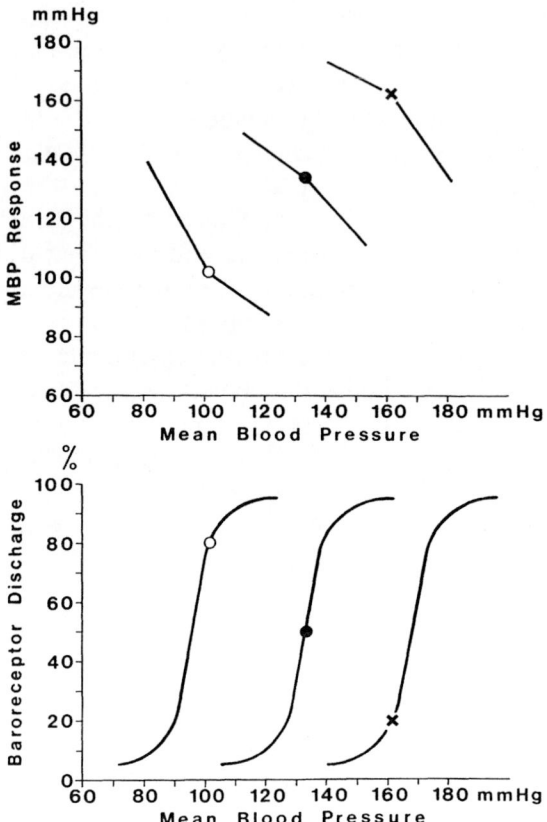

Figure 7. Schematic drawing of the stimulus response curves relating arterial blood pressure and carotid baroreceptor firing. The set-point of the reflex (i.e., the point corresponding to the stimulus provided by the existing blood pressure) may be located near baroreceptor saturation in normotensive subjects (left curve) and migrate progressively towards the baroreceptor threshold in moderate and in severe hypertension.

point of the reflex along the stimulus-response curve, but it actually moves it in a direction opposite to that predictable on the basis of the increasing pressure stimulus. A resetting of the baroreflex in hypertension has been repeatedly shown in animal hypertensive models [31, 35], and it may well be that the larger duration of human hypertension makes it even more significant than it was originally supposed.

The change in the baroreflex sensitivity induced by essential hypertension is a controversial issue. While there is no doubt that the sensitivity of the baroreceptor control of heart rate is reduced in this disease [3, 17] (and our data would suggest that this is so because of an impairment of aortic baroreflexes, see below), there are data that suggest that carotid sinus reflex control of blood pressure may be preserved to a greater degree [25, 26, 39, 12, 2]. The reasons for this may be complex, and more than one factor at different sites of the reflex arch may be responsible.

At any rate, our data have a number of clinical implications. For example, the greater response to increase in carotid transmural pressure we found in hypertensives suggests a better protection of these subjects against further sudden rises in pressure above the already high existing levels. On the other hand, the blunted response to reduction in carotid transmural pressure should leave hypertensive subjects less resistant to the effects of hemorrhage, and perhaps explains why they are more prone to orthostatic hypotension[6]. It is possible, however, that this decrease in the reflex function favors antihypertensive therapy, in that attempts at pharmacological reductions of blood pressure should in theory be facilitated by attenuation of a negative feed back system controlling this variable. A further facilitation of the effects of antihypertensive drugs may result from the baroreflex resetting that seems to be produced by several antihypertensive agents (see below).

Three other topics we have investigated in subjects with arterial hypertension will be briefly mentioned. One refers to reflex changes in cardiac output and total peripheral resistance induced by increase and decrease in the activity of the carotid baroreceptors. This point was examined in 27 subjects with essential hypertension in whom cardiac output (thermodilution technique) was measured before and during the steady-state phase of the blood pressure response to changes in neck chamber pressure over $\pm$ 40 mmHg [28]. The results (Table 1) indicate that the depressor responses to increases in carotid transmural pressure can be accounted for both by reduction in cardiac output and by decrease in total peripheral resistance. On the other hand, the pressor responses to reductions in carotid transmural pressure are not associated with any increase in cardiac output, and therefore appear to be caused entirely by an increase in total peripheral resistance. These findings reveal a major difference with the patterns of response observed by other investigators in normotensives, as in these subjects an increase in cardiac output was found to be the major cause for the reflex pressor response. It may be that subjects with established hypertension have less ability to increase cardiac output in the presence of an increasing afterload above the already elevated existing level.

Table 1. Hemodynamic responses to changes in neck chamber pressure in 27 subjects with essential hypertension*

	Control	Decrease in NTP	Control	Increase in NTP
Mean arterial pressure (mmHg)	139.3 ± 3.8	121.9 ± 4.2	137.1 ± 3.9	153.1 ± 4.0
Cardiac output (L/min)	6.20 ± 0.23	5.77 ± 0.24	6.12 ± 0.25	6.11 ± 0.29
Total peripheral resistance (Units)	23.3 ± 1.0	22.1 ± 1.0	22.8 ± 1.1	26.6 ± 1.3

* Data are shown as means ± SE. Cardiac output was measured during the steady-state phase of the blood pressure responses to the decrease and increase in neck tissue pressure (NTP), which amounted to −35.8 ± 0.8 and 32.6 ± 1.0 mmHg.

A second topic is related to the possibility that carotid baroreceptors reflexly influence secretion of renin from the kidneys. It has long been established that renin secretion can be powerfully modified by neural factors [7], and recent evidence has involved various reflexes in renin control [4, 36, 21, 40]. In this respect, however, information refers to animal experiments with almost no direct evidence in man.

In our study [24], 11 supine patients with essential hypertension were fitted with the neck chamber while they were undergoing catheterization of the aorta and a renal vein for clinical reasons. Positive and negative neck chamber pressures (all above ± 40 mmHg) were applied for 5 min., and plasma renin activity was measured by radioimmunoassay from blood samples withdrawn via the catheters before and during the 5th minute of pressure application. Basal values of plasma renin activity from the aorta and a renal vein were 0.30 ± 0.06 and 0.40 ± 0.10 ng/ml/h. These values became 0.34 ± 0.10 and 0.44 ± 0.15 ng/ml/h during application of negative, and 0.32 ± 0.08 and 0.47 ± 0.10 during application of positive neck chamber pressure. Only the last difference (plasma renin activity in the renal vein before and during positive neck pressure) was statistically significant at $p<0.05$, though this difference was indeed very small. In 5 of the 11 subjects the results obtained with application of positive neck pressures were compared to those obtained with 5 min. of head-up tilting (Figure 8). This was done because tilting reduces central blood volume as well as arterial blood pressure at the carotid sinus level, and thus deactivates a much larger population of receptors than the positive neck chamber application. With tilting, plasma renin activity from the renal vein increased significantly and markedly, though the calculated reduction in carotid transmural pressure was no greater than that induced by the neck chamber. Similar findings were obtained in another study in which hypertensive subjects with a high renin secretion were investigated [20]. We concluded from these data that the carotid baroreceptors do not exert a relevant control of renin release in essential hypertension. A reflex control of renin is present in this condition, but is likely due to receptors in the low pressure area.

The third topic refers to possible differences in the carotid baroreceptor reflex function in different forms of hypertension, a study currently under investigation. Data on carotid baroreceptor control of blood pressure in renovascular vs. essential hypertension seem to indicate that, whenever the age and the basal blood pressure values of the subjects are matched, there is no major difference in the baroreflexes of these two pathological conditions.

CAROTID BARORECEPTOR REFLEX DURING ANTIHYPERTENSIVE THERAPY

The problem of whether baroreceptor control of blood pressure is altered during treatment with antihypertensive drugs is of both practical and theoretical interest. Practical interest derives from the well-known fact that interference with the

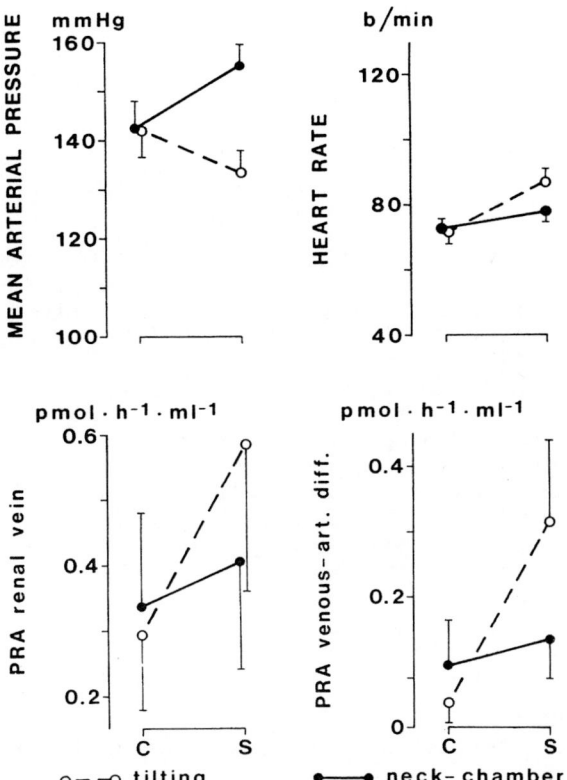

Figure 8. Effects of head-up tilting (dashed lines) and application of positive pressures in the neck chamber (solid lines) on plasma renin in 5 patients with essential hypertension. Results are shown as means ± SE. *C*: values during control; *S*: values during 5 minutes of tilting or positive neck pressure; *PRA*: plasma renin activity; *v + a*: difference in PRA between a renal vein and the aorta. From Mancia et al. [24], by permission.

baroreflex function induces a pronounced lability of arterial blood pressure in animals [5, 10, 18]. Theoretical interest is related to the hypothesis (also derived mainly from animal experiments) that currently used drugs such as clonidine and alpha-methyldopa exert their hypotensive effect by reducing the activity of the sympathetic vasoconstrictor nerves [14, 38], and that in the case of clonidine this is in part due to potentiation of the baroreflexes [14, 15].

We have tested the carotid baroreceptor reflex function in 16 patients with essential hypertension before and after intravenous administration of clonidine at doses of 150 μg (8 patients) and 300 μg (8 patients) [27]. As mentioned above, the magnitude of the reflex response was established by the regression coefficient of the changes in mean arterial pressure or heart rate (expressed as R-R interval) and the changes in neck tissue pressure. The difference in the reflex responses induced by the drug was assessed in individual subjects by covariant analysis, and in the group by paired t-test. The results of the study with the lesser dose of clonidine are shown in Table 2. In brief, no significant difference was found in the

Table 2. Cardiovascular responses to changes in neck tissue pressure (NTP) before and after administration of clonidine (150 μg i.v.) in 8 subjects with essential hypertension

		Decreased NTP			Increased NTP	
		Control	Early	Steady-state	Early	Steady-state
Mean arterial pressure	B	145 ± 4	0.59 ± 0.04	0.48 ± 0.08	0.17 ± 0.08	0.57 ± 0.14
	A	123 ± 4	0.59 ± 0.06	0.50 ± 0.06	0.07 ± 0.09	0.51 ± 0.12
	P	<0.005	ns	ns	ns	ns
R-R interval	B	800 ± 64	−4.06 ± 0.85	−2.63 ± 0.56	−0.43 ± 0.68	−1.61 ± 0.56
	A	833 ± 56	−4.00 ± 1.20	−1.68 ± 0.67	−0.07 ± 0.81	−2.55 ± 0.70
	P	ns	ns	ns	ns	ns

Data are shown as means ± SE. Control refers to values (mmHg and msec) in the 30 sec. prior to the changes in neck tissue pressure. Responses to changes in neck tissue pressure are shown as regression coefficients of the changes in mean arterial pressure or R-R interval to the changes in neck tissue pressure. Regression coefficients are positive for arterial pressure because a reduction in neck tissue pressure was associated with a reduction in mean arterial pressure and vice versa; and negative for R-R interval because a reduction in neck tissue pressure was associated with a lenghtening of this interval (i.e., bradycardia) and vice versa. *B*: before and *A*: after clonidine.

reflex responses to either increase or decrease in carotid transmural pressure before and after administration of clonidine. Thus it seems unlikely that potentiation of the baroreflexes is a mechanism for the hypotension clinically induced by clonidine. As far as other drugs are concerned, we found a profound reduction of the carotid baroreceptor reflex response during administration of the ganglion blocking agent trimetaphan, but little change in the reflex during chronic therapy with alpha-methyldopa and prazosin [29, 30]. Thus, several drugs reputed to lower blood pressure by interfering with the autonomic nervous system do not affect baroreceptor reflex, at least as far as its gain is concerned. It must be mentioned, however, that preservation of similar baroreflex responses at lower blood pressure levels may indicate a resetting of the baroreflex, and that this may represent an effect of these drugs that would contribute to the persistence of their antihypertensive action.

REFLEXES FROM AREAS OTHER THAN THE CAROTID SINUSES

Despite the unequivocal demonstration in animals of a powerful reflex control from the aortic arch [32] and from the heart and lungs [22] in man data on baroreflexes from areas other than the carotid sinuses are somewhat conflicting. Several investigators have reported vascular responses attributable to receptors in the low pressure area [34]. Other investigators have denied this possibility, however [9].

We had thought that information on the topic of the extracarotid baroreceptor reflexes in man might derive from comparing, in the same subjects, the reflex changes in heart rate induced by the two techniques: the variable pressure neck chamber, which alters primarily the activity of the carotid baroreceptors, and the intravenous injection of pressor and depressor drugs that induce changes in the stimulus to baroreceptors located at any possible arterial site. We performed this study in 8 normotensive subjects and in 8 subjects with essential hypertension (mean ages, 40 ± 3 and 38 ± 5 years respectively). For comparison, the stimuli were calculated as changes in transmural pressure: for the drugs these were represented by the changes in mean arterial pressure, while for the neck chamber they were the changes in tissue pressure outside the carotid sinuses minus the resulting reflex alterations in mean arterial pressure. The responses induced by the drugs were calculated 10–15 sec. after the injection, when the reflex changes in heart rate were maximal and relatively stable. These responses were compared with the early or the steady-state responses induced by the neck chamber.

The results are shown in Figures 9 and 10, which represent means $\pm$ standard errors of individual regression coefficients of the relationship between stimuli and reflex responses. As in previous examples, changes in heart rate are shown as changes in R-R interval.

Two major points are evident. One, in normotensive subjects the reflex changes in heart rate induced by the drugs were about three times as great as

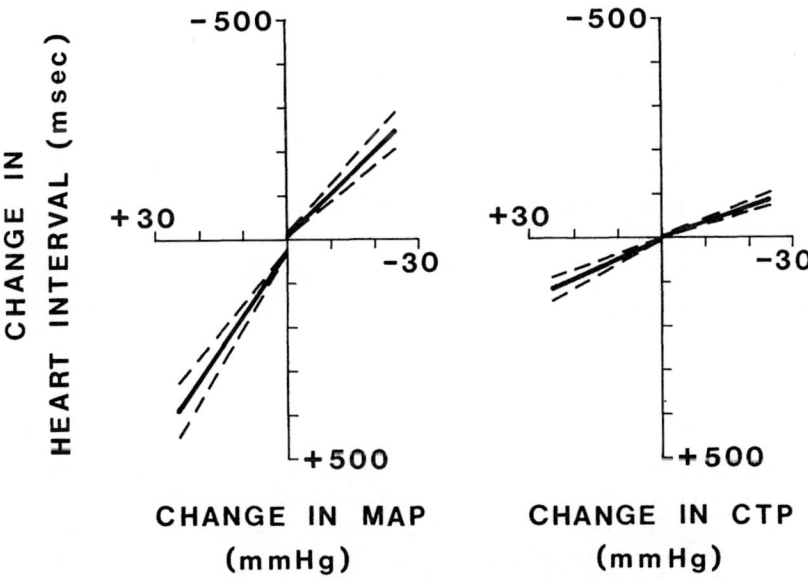

Figure 9. Changes in R-R interval (heart interval) with drug-induced changes in mean arterial pressure (MAP) (*left*) and with neck chamber-induced changes in carotid sinus transmural pressure (CPT) (*right*); means (solid lines) $\pm$ SE (dashed lines) of individual regression coefficients taken from 8 normotensive subjects in whom both techniques were used. For the neck chamber, the early heart interval responses were considered, the changes in carotid sinus transmural pressure being those at the time at which the responses were developed. Control mean arterial pressure and heart interval were 101 ± 5 mmHg and 864 ± 61 msec for the drug studies, and 791 ± 59 msec for the neck chamber studies. From Mancia et al. [23], by permission.

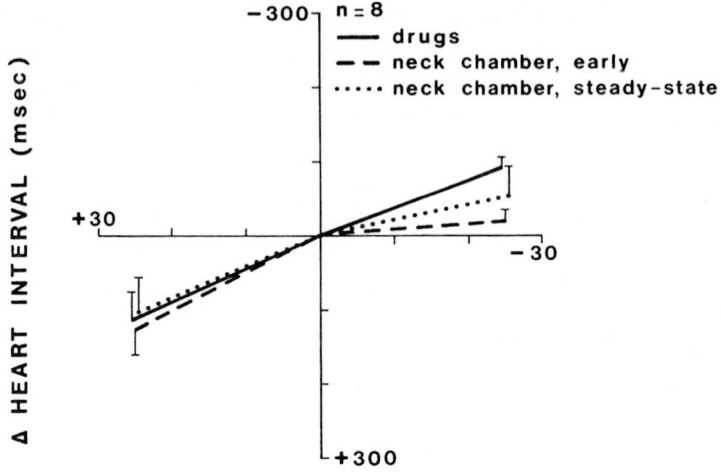

Δ ARTERIAL TRANSMURAL PRESSURE (mmHg)

Figure 10. Changes in R-R interval (heart interval) with changes in arterial transmural pressure induced by drugs or by the neck chamber. Means ± SE of individual regression coefficient taken from 8 subjects with essential hypertension in whom both techniques were used. For the neck chamber, both the early and the steady-state heart interval responses were considered, the changes in arterial transmural pressure being those at the actual time the response was measured. Control mean arterial pressure and heart interval were 138 ± 4.5 mmHg and 707 ± 28 msec for the drug studies, and 138 ± 5 and 706 ± 32 msec for the neck chamber studies. For further details see text. From Mancia et al. [26], by permission.

those induced by the neck chamber. In hypertensive, the reflex changes in heart rate induced by the drugs were about three times smaller than in normotensives, thus becoming similar to those induced by the neck chamber, which did not show appreciable modifications. This suggests that reflexes originating from extra-carotid baroreceptor areas are important in heart rate control in normotensive man, and that this function is markedly diminished in hypertensives [26].

REFERENCES

1. Angell-James JJE: Characteristics of single aortic and right subclavian baroreceptor fibre activity in rabbits with chronic renal hypertension. Circ Res 32: 149, 1973
2. Bevegard S, Castenfors J, Danielson M: Carotid baroreceptor function in hypertensive patients. Scand J Lab Invest 37: 495, 1977
3. Bristow SD, Honour AS, Pickering GW, Sleight P, Smyth HS: Diminished baroreceptor sensitivity in high blood pressure. Circulation 39: 48, 1969
4. Bunag D, Page IH, McCubbin JW: Neural stimulation of renin release. Circ Res 19: 851, 1966
5. Cowley AW, Liard JF, Guyton AG: Role of baroreceptor reflex in daily control of arterial pressure and other variables in dogs. Circ Res 32: 564, 1973
6. Cuche JL, Kuchel O, Barbeau A, Boucher R, Langlois Y, Genest J: Autonomic nervous system and benign essential hypertension. Circ Res 35: 290, 1974

7. Davis JO, Freeman RH: Mechanisms regulating renin release. Physiol Rev 56: 1, 1976
8. Ernsting J, Parry DJ: Some observations on the effect of stimulating the carotid arterial stretch receptors in the carotid artery of man. J Physiol 137, 45 pp, London
9. Guz A, Noble MIM, Trenchard D, Cochrane HJ, Makey AR: Studies on the vagus nerve in man: their role in respiratory and circulatory control. Clin Sci 27: 293, 1964
10. Heymans C, Neil E: Reflexogenic areas of the cardiovascular system. J. and A. Churchill Ltd London, 1958
11. Higgins CB, Vatner SF, Eckberg DE, Braunwald E: Alterations in the baroreceptor reflex in conscious dogs with heart failure. J Clin Invest 51: 715, 1972
12. Kezdi P: Sino-aortic regulatory system. Arch Int Med 91: 26, 1953
13. Kirchheim HP: Systemic arterial baroreceptor reflexes. Physiol Rev 56: 100, 1976
14. Kobinger W: Catapres as a tool for evaluation of cardiovascular regulating system in CNS. In: The Nervous System in Arterial Hypertension. Julius S, Esler M (eds), CC Thomas Publ, 1976, p 430
15. Korner PI, Oliver JR, Sleight P, Chalmers JP, Robinson JS: Effects of clonidine on the baroreceptor-heart rate reflex and on single baroreceptor fibre discharge. Europ J Pharmacol 28: 189, 1974
16. Korner PI, Tonkin AM, Uther JB: Reflex and mechanical circulatory effects of graded Valsalva maneuvers in normal man. J Appl Physiol 40: 434, 1976
17. Korner PI, West MJ, Shaw J, Uther JB: 'Steady-state' properties of the baroreceptor-heart rate reflex in essential hypertension in man. Clin Exp Pharmacol Physiol 1: 65, 1974
18. Kumazawa T, Baccelli G, Guazzi M, Mancia G, Zanchetti A: Hemodynamic patterns during desynchronized sleep n intact cats and in cats with sino-aortic deafferentation. Circ Res 24: 923, 1969
19. Ludbrook J, Mancia G, Ferrari A, Zanchetti A: The variable pressure neck chamber method for studying the carotid baroreflex in man. Clin Sci Mol Med 53: 165, 1977
20. Mancia G: Reflex control of renin release. In: Hayase S, Murao S (eds), International congress series no. 470, Proc VIII world congr of cardiology, Tokyo, Excerpta Medica, Amsterdam, 1978, p 450
21. Mancia G, Romero JC, Shepherd JT: Continuous inhibition of renin release by vagally innervated receptors in cardiopulmonary region in dogs. Circ Res 36: 529, 1975
22. Mancia G, Lorenz RL, Shepherd JT: Reflex control of circulation by heart and lungs. Internat Rev of Science, Cardiovascular Physiol II, Vol 9: 111, 1976
23. Mancia G, Ferrari A, Gregorini L, Valentini R, Ludbrook J, Zanchetti A: Circulatory reflexes from carotid and extracarotid baroreceptor areas in man. Circ Res 41: 309, 1977
24. Mancia G, Leonetti G, Terzoli L, Zanchetti A: Reflex control of renin release in essential hypertension. Clin Sci Molec Med 54: 217, 1977
25. Mancia G, Ferrari A, Gregorini L, Ludbrook J, Zanchetti A: Baroreceptor control of heart rate in man. In: Brown A, Malkani A, Schwartz PJ, Zanchetti A (eds), Nervous control of cardiac arrhythmias. Raven Press, New York, 1978, p 323
26. Mancia G, Ludbrook J, Ferrari A, Gregorini L, Zanchetti A: Baroreceptor reflexes in essential hypertension. Circ Res 43: 170, 1978
27. Mancia G, Ferrari A, Gregorini L, Zanchetti A: Clonidine and carotid baroreflex in essential hypertension. Hypertension 1: 362, 1979
28. Mancia G, Ferrari A, Gregorini L, Parati G, Ferrari MC, Pomidossi G, Zanchetti A: Control of blood pressure by carotid sinus baroreceptors in human beings. Am J Cardiol 44: 895, 1979
29. Mancia G, Ferrari A, Gregorini L, Terzoli L, Leonetti G, Zanchetti A: Methyldopa

and neural control of circulation in essential hypertension. Am J Cardiol 45: 1237, 1980

30. Mancia G, Ferrari A, Gregorini L, Ferrari MC, Bainchini C, Terzoli L, Leonetti G, Zanchetti A: Effects of prazosin on autonomic control of circulation in essential hypertension. Hypertension, 2: 700, 1980
31. McCubbin JW, Green JH, Page IH: Baroreceptor function in chronic renal hypertension. Circ Res 4: 205, 1956
32. Pelletier CL, Shepherd JT: Circulatory reflexes from mechanoreceptors in the cardio-aortic area. Circ Res 33: 131, 1973
33. Pickering TG, Gribbin B, Sleight P: Comparison of reflex heart rate responses to rising and falling arterial pressure in man. Cardiovasc Res 6: 277, 1972
34. Roddie IC, Shepherd JT: Receptors in the high-pressure and low-pressure vascular system. Their role in the reflex control of human circulation. Lancet 1: 493, 1958
35. Salgado HC, Krieger EM: Resetting of the baroreceptor in hypotension in rats. Clin Sci Mol Med 51: 351s, 1976
36. Stella A, Zanchetti A: Effects of renal denervation on renin release in response to tilting and furosemide. Am J Physiol 232: H500, 1977
37. Thron HL, Brechmann W, Wagner J, Keller K: Quantitative Untersuchungen uber die Bedentung der Gefassdehnungsreceptoren in Rahmen der Kreislaufhomoiestase beim Wachen Menschen. Pflüg Arch 293: 68, 1967
38. Van Zwieten PA: Centrally mediated action of alphapethyldopa. In: Onesti G, Fernandes M, Kim KE (eds), Regulation of blood pressure by the central nervous system. Grune-Stratton, 1976, p 293
39. Wagner S, Wackerbauer S, Hilger HH: Arterielles Blutdruck und Herzfrequenzerhalten bei Hypertonikern unter Anderung des Transmuralen Druckes im Karotismus-Bereich. Z Kreislauf 57: 703, 1968
40. Zehr JE, Hasbargen JA, Kurtz KD: Reflex suppressing of renin secrevion during distension of cardiopulmonary receptors in dogs. Circ Res 38: 232, 1976
41. Zoller RP, Mark AL, Abboud EM, Schmid PG, Heistad DD: The role of low-pressure baroreceptors in reflex vasoconstrictor responses in man. J Clin Invest 51: 2967, 1972

15. POSSIBLE MECHANISM OF PROTECTION FROM RENAL HYPER-TENSION BY ANTEROVENTRAL THIRD VENTRICLE (AV3V) LESIONS: ROLE OF RENAL AFFERENT NERVES

L.T. Mahoney, J.R. Haywood, R. Correy, N.P. Patel, A.K. Johnson, M.J. Brody

SUMMARY

Regional hemodynamic responses produced by renal afferent nerve stimulation (RANS) in rats are described. There responses were qualitatively similar to those produced by direct stimulation of the anteroventral third ventricle (AV3V).

A lesion of the AV3V, previously shown to prevent renal and mineralocorticoid hypertension, abolished the responses to RANS.

Deafferentation of the kidney by autotransplantation (AT) delayed the appearance of one-kidney (1-K) Grollman hypertension for two months. In contrast, AT did not affect the course of blood pressure elevation produced by deoxycorticosterone and salt (DOC-S).

These data suggest that renal afferent nerves, interacting with the region of the AV3V, may have a major role in the onset of 1-K Grollman hypertension, but do not appear to be involved in the pathogenesis of DOC-S hypertension.

INTRODUCTION

In the rat, the centrally mediated pressor activity of angiotensin is localized in the ventricular system in the preoptic hypothalamic region. The integrity of the anteroventral third ventricle (AV3V) region is essential for the development of renal [5], steroid-salt hypertension [9], and other forms of hypertension (for details, see Brody and Johnson [4]).

As the renin-angiotensin system is suppressed in deocycorticosterone and salt (DOC-S) hypertension [10], and probably plays no significant role in maintaining one-kidney (1-K) hypertension [6], other mechanisms, perhaps neural in origin, must be playing an essential role. Renal neural contributions to renal hypertension are probably not related to efferent sympathetic mechanisms [7]. The potential role of renal afferent sympathetic nerves in these models of hypertension has not been investigated, however.

The purposes of this study were (1) to test directly the functional nature of the afferent connections by recording regional hemodynamic effects produced by electrical stimulation of the renal afferent nerves; (2) to determine whether these

Sambhi, M.P. (ed.) Fundamental fault in hypertension
© *1984, Martinus Nijhoff Publishers. Boston/The Hague/Dordrecht/Lancaster.*
ISBN 978-94-010-9006-3

reflexes involve central neural connections to the area of the AV3V; and (3) to determine whether deafferentation of sensory connections between the kidney and the central nervous system by autotransplantation (AT) would protect rats from the development of 1-K and DOC-S hypertension.

METHODS

Using techniques described earlier, lesioning electrodes were places sterotaxically in the AV3V region of Sprague-Dawley rats [8]. Following a minimum recovery period of 24 hours, the animals were anesthetized with dialurethane. Using a modification of the pulsed Doppler flowmeter described by Hartley and Cole [11], miniature flow probes were places on the right renal artery, distal aorta, and superior mesenteric artery to record vascular resistance changes in those beds [12]. The left renal nerve was isolated and cut, the central end was placed on a bipolar stimulating electrode, and frequency response curves for arterial pressure and regional vascular resistance changes were recorded. Another group of rats was given hexamethonium to determine whether these changes were neurogenic in origin. The effect of bilateral adrenalectomy was also evaluated.

To determine directly whether the responses involved the region of the AV3V, frequency response curves were generated before and 30 min after either an electrolytic lesion of the AV3V or a sham lesion (either an asymmetric lesion that left one-half of the periventricular area intact or a lesion more anterior and superior in location). A third group of control rats was evaluated before and after a similar 30-minute waiting period with no lesion performed.

A related group of experiments consisted of total renal denervation performed by AT of the left kidney. The renal artery and vein were removed from their site of connection to the aorta and inferior vena cava, respectively, and re-anastomosed to their present vessel more caudally. The ureter was left intact. The right kidney was removed. Rats with intact renal nerves also underwent right nephrectomy and served as controls. Baseline arterial blood pressure (AP) and fluid intakes (FI) were obtained for all rats prior to figure-of-eight wrapping of the left kidney. AP and FI were monitored for 12 weeks. At the conclusion of the study period, the rats were infused with saralasin, an angiotensin antagonist, and their AP monitored.

In a separate study, a group of uninephrectomized AT and control rats was given weekly injections of deoxycorticosterone pivalate with 1% saline drinking water. AP and FI were monitored for an eight-week period.

RESULTS

The regional hemodynamic effects produced by renal afferent nerve stimulation (RANS) were recorded. The greatest peak resistance changes were seen in the vessels of the hindquarters, which exhibited vasodilatation, and in the superior mesenteric artery, where vasoconstriction was seen. The mean arterial pressure fell slightly, while the contralateral renal resistance increased slightly. All effects increased in a frequency-dependent fashion. These responses were abolished by hexamethonium, while bilateral adrenalectomy had no effect; therefore, these reflex responses appeared to be mediated exclusively via efferent sympathetic nerves.

Our hypothesis that renal afferent nerve function might be linked to the anterior hypothalamus was strenghtened by the observation of similarity of hemodynamic responses between RANS and data obtained by Fink et al. [9] during electrical stimulation of the AV3V. Furthermore, a lesion in this area essentially abolished the blood pressure and vascular resistance changes produced by RANS. In contrast, there was no difference in the responses obtained before and after sham lesioning, nor in intact animals tested before and after a similar 30-minute waiting period.

In a related study, the protective role of renal denervation by AT was demonstrated in the 1-K rat. The FI rose significantly in both the AT and control groups, and remained elevated. There was no difference in urine volume or electrolytes between groups in either baseline values or data obtained after wrapping during the 12-week study period. Intact rats became hypertensive within a week and their AP remained elevated throughout the study. AT rats remained normotensive for 8 to 10 weeks, when their AP began to rise. After 12 weeks, AT rats reached a hypertensive level not significantly different from controls. Electron microscopy confirmed that efferent sympathetic reinnervation had not occurred. The renin-angiotensin system played no apparent role in the subsequent AP increase in AT rats, as the infusion of saralasin had no effect on baseline AP. The efficacy of the saralasin dose was demonstrated by a significant attenuation of the AP increase following infusion of angiotensin II.

Another group of AT rats, given DOC pivalate and 1% saline drinking water, demonstrated an increase in AP not significantly less than the controls. The FI of AT rats was much more enhanced, as were their urine volumes and urine sodium. However, when these rats were fluid-restricted, so that their FI values were similar to those of control rats, there still was no attenuation of AP. Thus, the enhanced FI was not essential for the AP increase.

DISCUSSION

The mechanisms by which AV3V lesions protect against the development of forms of experimental hypertension with diverse etiologies are complex. As reviewed in detail elsewhere [4], the following mechanisms probably participate: loss of the central pressor component of angiotensin, interruption of vasopressin secretion, loss of central osmoreceptors mediating pressor activity, absence of release of a natriuretic factor proposed to exhibit pressor activity, and, in the special case of baroreceptor-mediated hypertension, the presence of long-loop neural connections between the brainstem and the anterior hypothalamus required for full expression of neurogenic hypertension. In the case of renal hypertension, it has been puzzling that hypertension may be sustained despite the fact that circulating plasma renin activity may be normal. The study summarized in the present paper suggests that renal manipulations may elicit sensory discharge to the central nervous system through pathways involving the AV3V that are necessary for the production of high arterial pressure.

This study demonstrated that RANS results in a complex, integrated hemodynamic reflex that requires the integrity of the AV3V and is mediated exclusively via efferent sympathetic nerves. The slight decrease in mean AP and decreased flow in the superior mesenteric and renal vessels, together with a simultaneous increase in flow in the hindquarter vessels, were essentially abolished by an electrolytic lesion in the AV3V. Control experiments demonstrated that the effect of the AV3V lesion could not be attributed to placement of an electrode, passage of current, or effect of time; therefore, abolition of the reflex appeared to be the result of destruction of specific tissue in the anterior hypothalamus.

Previous studies in rats [1], dogs [20], cats [2], and rabbits [18] have shown that physiologic manipulations known to increase interrenal pressure (e.g., renal vein occlusion) increase perfusion pressure; carotid occlusion and application of pressure to the kidney near the hilum increase renal afferent nerve activity. Recordati et al. [19] differentiated between renal chemoreceptors responsive to alterations of the kidney's chemical environment by renal artery occlusion, severe hypotension, or prolonged renal vein clamping, and the previously mentioned renal mechanoreceptors.

In both one- and two-kidney renal hypertension, there is an almost immediate loss of norepinephrine storage and the vasoconstrictor function of the renal sympathetic nerves, yet hypertension does develop [7]. Thus, potential renal neural mechanisms must involve sensory afferent connections rather than efferent sympathetic nerves. Previous studies in spontaneously hypertensive rats (15, 16, 22) and renovascular hypertensive rats (13, 14, 17) demonstrated an attenuation of AP increase by denervation of the kidney. This study also demonstrates a significant delay in the AP rise by AT in 1-K rats. This technique assures that total denervation has occurred. There was no alteration in renal function, re-innervation did not occur, and the renin-angiotensin system was not inadvertently activated. In contrast, AT did not protect DOC-S rats from developing hypertension.

The pathways connecting the kidney to the central nervous system appear to relay through the NTS and parasrachial complex [21]. Although the sensory receptor has not been identified, Barajas and Wang [3] have demonstrated myelinated renal nerves which they presumed to serve an afferent function. The present data suggest that the afferent nerves ascend to the AV3V region and synapse with a descending efferent pathway. In addition to this long-loop reflex arc, it is conceivable that other shorter pathways at the spinal or brainstem level may also exist. Taken together, these data indicate that through connections to the anterior hypothalamus, renal afferent nerves may play an important role in initiating the complex alterations in blood pressure regulation that lead to renal hypertension.

ACKNOWLEDGEMENTS

Supported in part by USPHS grants HLB-14388, HLB-0712, grant NHBLI-1T32-HLO7413-01 and Research Scientist Development Award 1-KOS-MH00064-01.

REFERENCES

1. Astrom A, Crafoord J: Afferent activity recorded in the kidney nerves of rats. Acta Physiol Scand 70: 10–15, 1967
2. Astrom A, Crafoord J: Afferent and efferent activity in the renal nerves of cats. Acta Physiol Scand 74: 69–78, 1968
3. Barajas L, Wang P: Myelinated nerves of the rat kidney. J of Ultrastruct Res 65: 148–162, 1978
4. Brody MJ, Johnson AK: Role of the anteroventral third ventricle region in fluid and electrolyte balance, arterial pressure regulation, and hypertension. In: Martini L, Ganong WF (eds), Frontiers in neuroendocrinology. Raven Press, New York, 1980
5. Buggy J, Fink GD, Johnson AK, Brody MJ: Prevention of the development of renal hypertension by anteroventral third ventricular tissue lesions. Circ Res Supp. I, 40: I–110 – I–117, 1977
6. Davis JO: The pathogenesis of chronic renovascular hypertension. Circ Res 40: 439–444, 1977
7. Fink GD, Brody MJ: Neurogenic control of the renal circulation in hypertension. Federation Proc 37: 1202–1208, 1978
8. Fink GD, Buggy J, Haywood JR, Johnson AK, Brody MJ: Hemodynamic effects of electrical stimulation of forebrain angiotensin and osmosensitive sites. Am J of Physiol 235: H445–H451, 1978
9. Fink GD, Buggy J, Johnson AK, Brody MJ: Prevention of steroidsalt hypertension in the rat by anterior forebrain lesions. Circulation, Supp. III 56: 242, 1977
10. Gavras H, Brunner HR, Larash JH, Vaughan ED Jr, Koss M, Cote LJ, Gavras I: Malignant hypertension resulting from deoxycorticosterone acetate and salt excess. Circ Res 36: 300–309, 1975
11. Hartley CJ, Cole JS: An ultrasonic pulsed Doppler system for measuring blood flow in small vessels. J of Applied Physiol 37: 626–629, 1974

212

12. Haywood JR, Shaffer RA, Fastenow C, Fink GD, Brody MJ: Regional blood flow measurement with pulsed Doppler flowmeter in conscious rat. Am J Physiol. 241: H273–H278, 1981
13. Katholi RE, Whitlow PL, Winternitz SR, Oparil S: Importance of renal nerves in established two-kidney, one-clip Goldblatt hypertension. Hypertension 4 (Suppl II): 166–174, 1982
14. Katholi RE, Winternitz SR, Oparil S: Decrease in peripheral sympathetic nervous system activity following renal denervation or unclipping in the one-kidney, one-clip Goldblatt hypertensive rat. J Clin Invest 69: 55–62, 1982
15. Kline RL, Kelton PM, Mercer PF: Effect of renal denervation on the development of hypertension in SHR. Can J Physiol Pharm 56: 818–822, 1978
16. Liard JF: Renal denervation delays blood pressure increase in the spontaneously hypertensive rat. Experentia 33: 339–340, 1977
17. Ljungquist A: The role of the intrarenal sympathetic innervation in the development of renal hypertension. Acta Pathol et Microbiol Scand, Sect A, 82: 450–454, 1974
18. Niijima A: The effect of efferent discharges in renal nerves on the activity of arterial mechanoreceptors in the kidney in rabbit. J of Physiol (London), 78: 339–369, 1972
19. Recordati GM, Moss NG, Waselkow L: Renal chemoreceptors in the rat. Circ Res 40: 534–543, 1978
20. Uchida Y, Kamisaka K, Ueda H: Two types of renal mechanoreceptors. Jap Heart J 12: 233–241, 1971
21. Webb RL, Boutelle S, Brody MJ: Central relay sites for cardiovascular reflexes elicited by renal afferent nerve stimulation (RANS). Fed Proc 42(3): 1701, 1983
22. Winternitz SR, Katholi RE, Oparil S: Role of the renal sympathetic nerves in the development and maintenance of hypertension in the spontaneously hypertensive rat. J Clin Invest 66: 971–978, 1980

16. NEURONAL SYSTEMS AND THEIR IMPACT ON BLOOD PRESSURE REGULATION

WALTER LOVENBERG, DONALD KUHN, JUDITH JUSKEVICH

INTRODUCTION

The primary focus of this meeting is a discussion of the fundamental fault(s) in human essential hypertension. I believe we all agree that a number of different physiologic systems contribute to both long-term and short-term regulation of blood pressure. The nervous system undoubtedly plays a particularly important role in maintaining blood pressures within normal limits, and it would appear that perhaps an inbalance in the various systems could result in blood pressure exceeding limits. The information concerning the physiologic state of the organism is transmitted to the central nervous system (CNS) via afferent neuronal pathways. In the CNS the information appears to be processed in a number of centers and responses are transmitted via peripheral efferent pathways to the heart, kidneys and vasculature. Because of the complexity of the system a malfunction of any one of a number of circuits in the brain could be hypothesized as contributing to or comprising the fundamental fault in essential hypertension. In the following discussion we will review briefly our current knowledge of CNS-blood pressure regulation and describe some of our recent experimentation on the role of the central serotonergic neurons in regulating arterial blood pressure. Finally, we will speculate on the longterm effect of (altered or increased) sympathetic activity on the vasculature.

CENTRAL BLOOD PRESSURE REGULATION SYSTEM

An understanding of how the CNS processes and stores information has been described by many scientists as the last big frontier in our understanding of the human organism. The complexity of the CNS presents a formidable challenge, although numerous neurotransmitters and neuromodulators have been identified and we now have a rudimentary understanding of some of the circuitry relating to blood pressure regulation. In considering the role of the CNS one can arbitrarily divide the process of blood pressure regulation into three components. These are: (1) The sensor afferent system which provides the brain with information concerning the blood pressure and metabolic state of the organism; (2) the integra-

Sambhi, M.P. (ed.) Fundamental fault in hypertension
© *1984, Martinus Nijhoff Publishers. Boston/The Hague/Dordrecht/Lancaster.*
ISBN 978-94-010-9006-3

tion of the information and the initiation of regulatory responses and (3) the efferent pathways carrying the designated responses back to the periphery.

The two major sensor systems are the baro- and chemoreceptors located in the heart and major arterial conduits. The information from these receptors is carried along afferent pathways in the carotid sinus and aortic depressor nerve. Although early studies suggested that the baro-reflex was a relatively simple reflex mediated through pressor and depressor centers in the lower brainstem, it is now apparent that this system is vastly more complex. Afferents project directly or indirectly to many parts of the brain and a number of known modulatory systems from higher regions in the brain have an input into the 'reflex centers' of the brainstem. Finally the information to adjust blood pressure is distributed to the peripheral organs and vasculature via the sympathetic nervous system.

While no one nucleus or region dominates the central regulation of blood pressure perhaps the area most thoroughly studied is the nucleus tractus solitarius (NTS). Considerable evidence [24, 25, 14, 37] suggests that the first synapse in the CNS from the sensor afferent system occurs in the NTS although little is known about the nature of the transmitter at this synapse. A number of other brain areas also appear to have primary input from the periphery. These include the medulla oblangata centralis, (MOC) [24], parahypoglossal area [37] and possibly the paramedian reticular nucleus (PRN) [24, 14]. The carotid sinus nerve also appears to carry multisynaptic afferent pathways to both the PRN and raphe nuclei [24]. Examination of single unit responses in the hypothalamus to carotid nerve stimulation suggest that baroreceptor afferents have an inhibitory, and chemoreceptor afferents an excitatory effect on firing rate [38].

The NTS, which appears to be the primary point of entry of peripheral blood pressure information, has connections with other brain regions that have an impact on blood pressure. These include the MOC [7], the nucleus ambiguus, dorsal motor nucleus of the vagus, the medial reticular formation, the nucleus intercalatus [8], anterior hypothalamus, [15], the bed of the nucleus stria terminalis, the central nucleus of the amygdala and the posterior hypothalamus [30].

In recent years we have become increasingly aware that the hypothalamus plays an important role in the regulation of blood pressure. Two major pressor pathways are known to pass through the hypothalamus: one appears to originate in the posterior hypothalamus and the other traverses the lateral hypothalamus [10, 11]. The origin of the lateral pathway is in several areas rostral to the hypothalamus including orbital cortex, septal nuclei, the preoptic area and the limbic system. The neurons pass through this tract in the nucleus mesencephalus profundus (NMP). The other pressor pathway appears to originate in the posterior hypothalamus and it travels to the periaqueductal gray and superior colliculi and then on to the NMP. This pressor pathway is diffuse having input to a number of other brain centers [17]. The functional connections with the sympathetic outflow are unknown, although Saper et al. [33] provided evidence that this pathway may have direct connections to the spinal cord.

215

Either by lesioning or electrophysiologic studies, a number of other brain nuclei have been demonstrated to participate in cardiovascular regulation. These potential sites of regulation have been reviewed recently [17]. In that review we attempted to integrate our current knowledge of CNS regulation into a single wiring diagram (Figure 1). It should be emphasized that this diagram represents an interpretation of current literature and that many of the putative connections are controversial and subject to future revision. It should also be noted that despite its complexity, the diagram is undoubtedly incomplete.

SCHEMATIC OF SOME OF THE CONNECTIONS OF CENTRAL
NERVOUS SYSTEM AREAS INVOLVED IN BLOOD PRESSURE
REGULATION

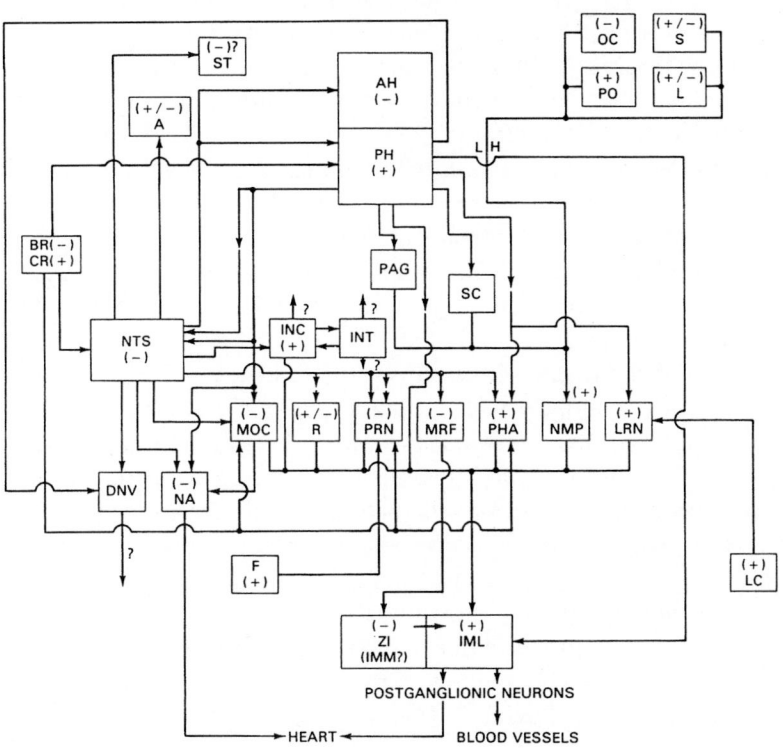

Figure 1. Interconnections of some of the central nervous system areas involved in cardiovascular regulation. Symbols: (+): stimulation of an area results in an increase in blood pressure; (−): stimulation results in a decrease in blood pressure; (+/−): both increases and decreases in blood pressure have been reported following stimulation of an area. Abbreviations: *A*, amygdala; *AH*, anterior hypothalamus; *BR*, baroreceptors; *CR*, chemoreceptors; *DNV*, dorsal motor nucleus of the vagus; *F*, fastigial nucleus; *IML*, intermediolateral nucleus; *IMM*, intermediomedial nucleus; *INC*, intercalatus nucleus; *INT,* intermediate nucleus; *L*, limbic system; *LC*, locus coeruleus; *LH*, lateral hypothalamus; *LRN*, lateral reticular nucleus; *MOC*, medullae oblongatae centralis; *MRF*, medial reticular formation; *NA*, nucleus ambiguus; *NMP,* nucleus mesencephalus profundas; *NTS*, nucleus tractus solitarius; *OC*, orbital cortex; *PAG*, periaqueductal gray; *PHA*, parahypoglossal area; *PO*, preoptic area; *PRN*, paramedian reticular nucleus; *R*, raphé nuclei; *S*, septal nuclei; *SC*, superior colliculus; *ST*, stria terminalis; *ZI*, zona intermedia. (From Juskevich and Lovenberg [17].)

The neuronal pathways depicted in Figure 1 are comprised of a variety of neurotransmitter containing cells. The catecholamine and indoleamine neurotransmitters, in particular, have been extensively studied with regard to CNS-blood pressure regulation probably because of the relative analytical ease with which they can be quantified. These studies have included determination of synthesis, content, and turnover of the central biogenic amines in brain regions of a variety of experimental hypertension animal models. Norepinephrine and epinephrine have also attracted much attention partly because of their well known peripheral cardiovascular effects.

The epinephrine containing neurons are all located in the cell groups C_1 and C_2 of the brainstem. The strategic location of these cells near the blood pressure regulatory centers of the baro-reflex suggest a possible role for neurons utilizing this transmitter. Interest in this neurotransmitter system was further advanced by the observation of Saavedra et al. [31] that spontaneously hypertensive rats appear to have increased amounts of phenylethanolamine N-methyl transferase a marker enzyme for epinephrine cells in the brainstem. This observation has been confirmed by other laboratories including our own. A recent study [16] shows that the genetically hypertensive rats have an increased number of epinephrine containing cells in the brainstem. While such studies suggest a role for epinephrine neurons in blood pressure regulation, no direct evidence for the participation of this system exists at this time.

Examination of noradrenergic systems in the CNS has perhaps been even more extensive. Increases and decreases of norepinephrine in a number of brain regions or nuclei have been reported for a variety of experimental animal models. Considerable circumstantial evidence now exists suggesting that central, norepinephrine containing neurons participate in blood pressure regulation. However, the exact neuronal connections remain to be defined.

The cell bodies of the neurons utilizing serotonin as a neurotransmitter lie in clusters in the mesencephalon known as the raphe nuclei. Recent biochemical and electrophysiologic studies in our laboratory suggest that serotonergic cells in certain of these raphe nuclei may participate in a specific pressor system. These studies will be reviewed in detail in the succeeding section.

PRESSOR RESPONSES IN A CENTRAL SEROTONERGIC SYSTEM

In this section we will briefly review the role of the brain serotonergic system in the regulation of blood pressure. It is obviously difficult, if not impossible, to attribute the control of such a complex process as blood pressure regulation to a single neurochemical system. However, neurochemical and neurophysiological studies of blood pressure regulation are still in their infancy and we remain somewhat dependent on these 'undimensional' studies for information that will certainly serve as the foundation for an increased understanding of neural contributions to cardiovascular control in the future. As evidenced by this chapter, as well as by numerous other chapters in this volume, there are a number of central nervous system components that influence arterial blood pressure. The serotonergic neuronal system is one such component which is of great interest in our laboratory. We will summarize the involvement of the brain serotonergic system in blood pressure control and present the results of some recent experiments on this subject from our laboratory. For an extensive treatment of the role of the central serotonergic system in blood pressure regulation, the interested reader is referred to our recent review article [19].

Although the general neuroanatomical pathways that influence blood pressure have been known for some time, it was not until Dahlstrom and Fuxe (1964) actually demonstrated the occurrence of neurotransmitter containing cells in the brain that specific neurochemical systems could be implicated and studied in blood pressure regulation. The cells of interest for the present discussion are the serotonin-containing neurons located in the mesencephalon. These cell bodies send projections to the forebrain as well as to the spinal cord and neurotransmission along these pathways is subserved presumably by serotonin. Perhaps the most prominent and most extensively studied serotonin-containing cell bodies are the dorsal and median raphe nuclei, designated B7 and B8, respectively, by Dahlstrom and Fuxe [9]. Within these cell bodies, the essential amino acid tryptophan is converted by enzyme action first to 5-hydroxytryptophan then to 5-hydroxytryptamine (serotonin). This biosynthetic pathway is shown in Figure 2. Some amount of serotonin is transported along axons arising from B7 and B8 to other parts of the brain as are the enzymes necessary for producing serotonin. In this fashion, serotonin can be synthesized and released throughout the brain.

A variety of methods have been employed to determine how the serotonergic system contributes to the control of blood pressure. For example, systemic injections of tryptophan or 5-hydroxytryptophan will produce large increases in brain serotonin. However, the effects of such treatments on blood pressure are not completely understood and the variability often observed can be attributed in part to a lack of specificity of action of these compounds, the methods of injection, species tested, and anesthetic agents used. In general, it is often observed that increases in brain serotonin will lead to increases in blood pressure in normotensive animals. Conversely, reductions in the levels of brain serotonin produced by injections of the tryptophan hydroxylase inhibitor para-chlorophenylalanine (PCPA) or by the neurotoxic agents 5,6- or 5,7-dihydroxytryptamine can lower the blood pressure of normotensive and hypertensive

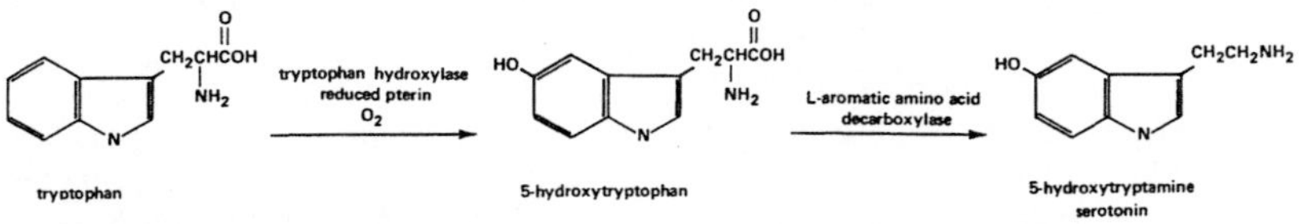

Figure 2. Biosynthetic pathway of serotonin.

animals. Detailed discussions of these results can be found in Kuhn et al. [19].

In an effort to learn more about how the central serotonergic neuronal system affects blood pressure we decided to stimulate electrically either the dorsal or median raphe nucleus in anesthetized rats and record mean arterial blood pressure. It had been shown previously by Adair et al. (1977) that stimulation of those serotonergic cell bodies which project to the spinal cord could produce either increases or decreases in the blood pressure of cats. More recently, Smits et al. [36] demonstrated that electrical stimulation of either the dorsal or median raphe in rats produced a large pressor effect and our initial studies were aimed at repeating these very interesting observations. Although electrical stimulation of the brain obviously has certain drawbacks, we felt that the control which we could exert over the stimulus parameters as well as the specificity with which certain small brain structures could be reliably stimulated more than outweighed the disadvantages of electrical stimulation. In fact, electrical stimulation offers substantially more specificity than most pharmacological agents which are used to alter brain serotonin levels (e.g., 5-hydroxytryptophan).

Our initial experiments [20] with raphe stimulation were successful in repeating the original observations of Smits et al. [36]. If the stimulating electrodes were placed either in the dorsal or median raphe nucleus, stimulation produced large pressor effects. The blood pressure response to dorsal raphe stimulation was usually much larger in magnitude than the pressor response to median raphe stimulation. An example of the blood pressure response to raphe stimulation is shown in Figure 3. Heart rate was also recorded throughout the blood pressure experiments. Although tachycardia and bradycardia were observed on occasion, heart rate remained relatively constant during electrical stimulation and in a few

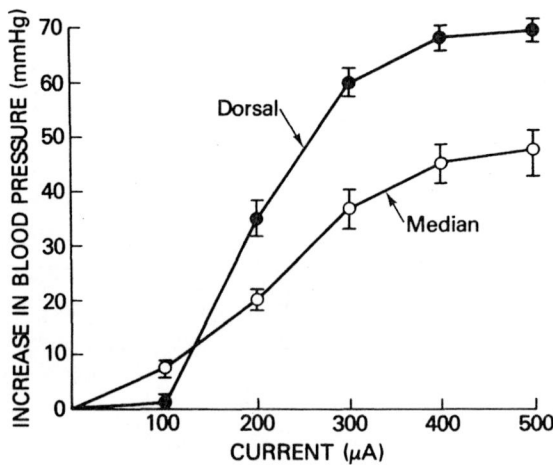

Figure 3. Effects of electrical stimulation of the raphe nuclei on arterial blood pressure. Anesthetized rats were stimulated in the dorsal or median raphe nucleus at 50 Hz, 0.3 msec pulse duration, 5.0 sec train duration at the current levels indicated on the abscissa. Blood pressure was recorded directly from one femoral artery.

cases it appeared that pulse pressure widened after some episodes of electrical stimulation. Perhaps heart rate did not respond reflexly with the pressor responses because the pressor response was of such short duration; the increase in blood pressure was evident as soon as current was applied and the pressure remained elevated for the duration of the 5-second stimulus train. Recovery was also quite rapid.

The midbrain site which subserves these pressor responses is apparently quite selective. Serial coronal sections through the raphe nuclei are shown in Figure 4. It can be seen that pressor areas are located primarily in both raphe nuclei.

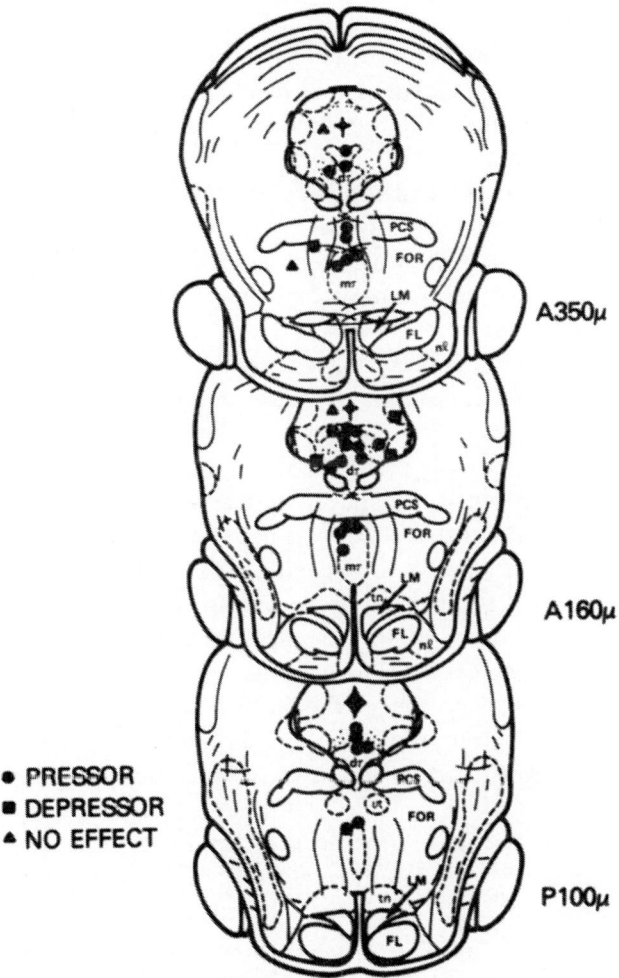

Figure 4. Rat brain sections demonstrating the locations of electrode sites at which electrical stimulation produced pressor, depressor, or no effect on blood pressure. Abbreviations: *dr,* nucleus dorsalis raphe; *mr,* nucleus medianus raphe; *PCS,* pedunculus cerebellaris superior; *FOR,* formatio reticularis; *LM,* lemniscus medialis; *FL,* fasciculus longitudinalis; *pl,* nucleus pontis pars lateralis; *tp,* nucleus tegmenti pontis.

Stimulation in various regions of the periaqueductal gray failed to alter blood pressure reliably. However, in some instances, stimulation of the fasciculus longitudinalis dorsalis (Schutz) pars tegmenti did produce a pressor effect. Stimulation of the superior cerebellar peduncle in the same anterior-posterior plane with the raphe nuclei was without effects on blood pressure. It was also noted in a few rats that stimulation of the substantia grisea centralis, pars ventralis led to a depressor effect.

Preliminary attempts were also made to determine which serotonergic pathway mediated the pressor effects. To accomplish this, knife transections were made in various parts of the mesencephalan or diencephalon.

Transections rostral to both raphe nuclei effectively prevented the pressor response to dorsal raphe stimulation. Similarly, transections caudal to the raphe nuclei blocked the pressor response. These results indicate that the pressor effect is mediated neuronally and that the primary axonal pathway mediating the pressor effect is ascending.

Pharmacological studies were also carried out to determine more conclusively whether or not serotonin was actually mediating the pressor response. First, rats were depleted of serotonin by treating them with PCPA (350 mg/kg, i.p.). Blood pressure experiments were carried out three days after treatment when brain serotonin is reduced to its lowest levels. At this time, the pressor response to dorsal or median raphe stimulation was significantly reduced. PCPA did not alter resting blood pressure. Restoration of brain serotonin by injecting rats with 5-hydroxytryptophan (5-HT) (50 mg/kg) plus the decarboxylase inhibitor Ro 4-4602 was effective in partially restoring the pressor response to only median raphe stimulation. There was a tendency toward reversal of the PCPA effect after dorsal raphe stimulation but this effect was not statistically significant.

Second, rats were pretreated with a specific serotonin uptake inhibitor, fluoxetine, in an effort to increase synaptic serotonin. Fluoxetine (10 mg/kg, i.p.) produced a short lived decrease in blood pressure and slightly increased the magnitude of the pressor response to dorsal raphe stimulation. More significantly, fluoxetine markedly prolonged the duration of the pressor responses. For example, at 100 μA of current, the recovery time for blood pressure to return to prestimulation levels was 25 sec. whereas after fluoxetine the recovery time was 45 sec.

Third, rats were pretreated with the serotonin receptor antagonist bromolysergic acid diethylamide (BOL) in an attempt to attenuate the raphe pressor effect. We found that this antagonist was most effective if injected directly into the brain. Specifically, the injection of 25 μg of BOL into the anterior hypothalamus/preoptic area significantly attenuated the pressor response to dorsal raphe stimulation.

Finally, rats were injected with bretylium (4.0 mg/kg, i.v.), a drug that selectively blocks sympathetic preganglionic neurons. The pressor response to dorsal raphe stimulation was significantly attenuated by sympathetic blockade. The effects of these various pharmacological treatments on the blood pressure response to electrical stimulation of the raphe nuclei are presented in Table 1.

In summary, it seems clear that activation of the central serotonergic neuronal system can profoundly alter blood pressure. Our conclusion is that stimulation of the raphe nuclei leads to the evoked release of 5-HT in most forebrain areas receiving a 5-HT input from the raphe nuclei. For several reasons, the anterior hypothalamus-preoptic area may be the most important 'target' for released 5-HT with respect to influence on the cardiovascular system. First, this brain area contains rather large concentrations of 5-HT [32] and apparently receives a prominent input from the raphe nuclei [2, 23, 28]. Second, Smits and Struyker-Boudier [36] demonstrated that microinjections of 5-HT directly into the anterior hypothalamus-preoptic area produce significant increases in the arterial blood pressure of anesthetized rats. Third, microinjections of the 5-HT antagonist BOL into the anterior hypothalamus/preoptic area partially blocks the stimulation induced pressor effect [20]. Finally, it has also been demonstrated that injections of angiotensin II into the cerebral ventricles leads to a pressor effect in rats [26] and this increase in blood pressure has been attributed to an angiotensin II-induced release of 5-HT in the hypothalamus. Without question, other neurotransmitters are involved in mediating the raphe pressor effect but the initating step certainly involves serotonin. The experiments described earlier with breytilium suggest that raphe stimulation culminates with a change in sympathetic outflow. In fact, it has been demonstrated recently that central 5-HT neurons facilitate transmission in central sympathetic pathways [22]. Thus a transient

Table 1. Effects of pharmacological manipulation of the serotonergic neuronal system on the dorsal raphe pressor effect

Treatment	Current (μA)	Blood pressure		Recovery time* (sec)
		Resting	Stimulation	
Control	100	84	102	24
	300		136	62
	500		159	72
PCPA	100	80	98	
	300		120	
	500		130	
Fluoxetine	100	83	101	45
	300		162	110
	500		175	145
BOL	100	80	80	
	300		95	
	500		120	
Bretylium	100	84	87	
	300		109	
	500		109	

* Recovery time was measured as the interval between stimulus offset and the return of blood pressure to pre-stimulation values.

increase in sympathetic outflow as a result of an increase in serotonergic tone could cause the phasic increase in blood pressure seen after raphe stimulation.

It has been demonstrated that electrical stimulation of the posterior hypothalamus produces increases in both blood pressure and sympathetic activity in both normotensive and in spontaneously hypertensive rats [6, 18]. It will be of interest to determine whether there is a relationship between the pressor responses produced by raphe stimulation and by posterior hypothalamic stimulation. The interfacing of 5-HT release in the area of the anterior hypothalamus (subsequent to raphe stimulation) with increases in impulse flow out of the posterior hypothalamus (which leads to increases in sympathetic outflow) will probably be the most critical but most difficult aspect of the circuitry to study, assuming that these two systems interface.

It seems clear from the foregoing discussions that the serotonergic neuronal system can influence blood pressure in normotensive animals; the next obvious question is whether the development or maintenance of hypertension is influenced by brain serotonin. Based on those few studies done thusfar, some preliminary answers to this question can be offered. Before discussing these experiments, however, an important species difference with respect to serotonin-blood pressure interactions must be re-emphasized. It is generally observed that 5-HT (centrally injected) is a pressor agent in rats and rabbits, whereas it is a depressor agent in cats and dogs. This species difference has been discussed in detail in our previous review [19, 20].

Treatment of prehypertensive (4 week old) spontaneously hypertensive rats (SHR) with the serotonin neurotoxin 5,6-dihydroxytryptamine delays the onset of hypertension [5] and either 5,6-dihydroxytryptamine or PCPA can reduce the blood pressure of rats with established hypertension [12, 13]. Similarly, prior treatment of rabbits with 5,6-DHT prevents the rise in blood pressure observed after sino-aortic denervation and sharply reduces the blood pressure of rabbits with established neurogenic hypertension [39]. More recently, Smith et al. [34] observed that the *in vivo* rate of serotonin synthesis was higher in pre-hypertensive SHR than in controls. This difference was no longer evident in SHR with established hypertension.

Thus, it appears that 5-HT can play a role in both the development and maintenance of hypertension in various experimental animals. Lown and colleagues [29, 4] have also recently suggested that increases in cerebral 5-HT can protect the heart against ventricular fibrillation. These investigators noted a significant increase in the repetitive extrasystole threshold (electrical current necessary to cause ventricular fibrillation) after pharmacologically inducing increases in brain 5-HT levels of anesthetized dogs. It was suggested that the ability of 5-HT to depress efferent sympathetic outflow is responsible for the results observed [29, 4]. Too few studies have been completed on the role that 5-HT may play in regulating blood pressure in man, therefore substantive conclusions cannot be made at this time. It is probably significant, nevertheless, that the platelets of hypertensive individuals apparently take up and store less 5-HT than do the platelets of normotensive individuals [3].

In conclusion, the central serotonergic neuronal system can apparently exert powerful influence on the cardiovascular system. Although there are significant species differences, it appears that 5-HT modulates blood pressure by a phasic influence (increase or decrease) on efferent sympathetic nerve traffic. It will be of interest to determine through further research whether the 5-HT system is a contributing factor in the development and maintenance of hypertension.

SYMPATHETIC ACTIVITY AND VASCULAR PROTEIN SYNTHESIS

While it is clear that the central nervous system can have a major role in the short-term regulation of blood pressure there remains a question as to whether it could also have a role in sustained hypertension. In other words, how could a malfunction in the central nervous system be translated into the pathological events that are associated with the disease. It is known that significant changes in peripheral resistance and vascular structure occur in most hypertensive models and in essential hypertension. While it was thought that this was simply a hypertrophic response due to the mechanical stress of the increased pressure, we examined the possibility of its being a trophic response due to increased sympathetic activity.

In our initial experiments [40] we attempted to establish a system in rats to evaluate the rate at which vascular proteins were synthesized. In this study the small mesenteric arteries were removed following an iv injection of radioactive lysine. The proteins from these arteries were fractionated into three major groups, elastin, collagen, and non-collagen protein. We were particularly interested in the non-collagen fraction that included the contractile elements and might be indicative of a pathogenic process. On the other hand, collagen and elastin might be more indicative of adaptive responses to the increased arterial pressure.

With this system we observed that the incorporation of lysine into the vascular non-collagen protein of young spontaneously hypertensive rats occurs at a rate about twice that of control Wistar-Kyoto rats (Table 2). The results in this table were obtained with 33 day old rats. At this age, the blood pressure in the SHR is only slightly higher than in the control strain, and not in what is usually considered to be the hypertensive range. This suggested that the apparent increase in vascular protein synthesis in the SHR might be related to factors other than mechanical stress.

In a subsequent study [41] we examined the potential impact of the sympathetic nervous system on vascular protein synthesis. To summarize, this study indicated that if the sympathetic input into vessels was reduced by either denervation of the vessels or ganglionic blockade, the rate of lysine incorporation into vascular protein was reduced to the level of that seen in control animals. Conversely if the

Table 2. Lysine incorporation into non-collagen protein of heart and vasculature*

	SHR/N (dpm/mg)	WK/N (dpm/mg)	
Heart	360 ± 15	325 ± 24	NS
Aorta	49 ± 3	40 ± 7	
Mesenteric arteries			
Main	12.0 ± 0.9	5.1 ± 0.5**	
Intestinal branches	22.2 ± 2.3	12.3 ± 1.8†	
Liver	873 ± 99	975 ± 66	NS

* Data taken from Yamabe and Lovenberg [40]
** $p < 0.001$
† $p < 0.01$

blood pressure was reduced in these animals by a vasodilator there was no decrease in the rate of amino acid incorporation into non-collagen protein. Since it is thought that sympathetic activity is increased following vasodilation, the data would suggest that the increase in protein synthesis in the small resistance vessels of these rats might result from a trophic effect of the sympathetic nerves.

In order to investigate further the role of the sympathetic nerves, we attempted to perform a series of pharmacological interventions [27]. In these studies we found that treating animals with hypotensive doses of clonidine significantly reduced the rate of amino acid incorporation into the non-collagen proteins. Clonidine is thought to exert its antihypertensive effect by activating certain α-receptors in the central nervous system and in this way modify sympathetic outflow. In other experiments, the effect of α-and β receptor blockers was also examined. Phenoxybenzamine was effective in reducing amino acid incorporation whereas propranolol was ineffective. From these amino acid incorporation studies we suggest the following scenario for the SHR. It has been suggested that the sympathetic tone in the SHR is slightly enhanced even during the prehypertensive phase. If so, the increased nerve activity arriving at the small arterial vessels interacts with α-receptors, which in turn modify vascular protein synthesis. In this way, one of the early events in the pathogenic process might be a stimulation of protein synthesis in the vessel wall. A thickening of the vessel wall in turn would cause an increase in peripheral resistance and consequently hypertension.

CONCLUSIONS

It is clear that the fundamental fault in the initiation of human essential hypertension is not defined. The above discussion does not attempt to make the definition, but rather to provide a hypothesis to which further experimentation can be directed. To recapitulate, it is suggested that the central regulation of blood pressure can occur on both a short-term and a long-term basis. Our experiments suggest that serotonin neurons participate in one of these regulatory circuits. It appears that sensory inputs are integrated with environmental and emotional inputs in the higher centers of the brain. This results in moment to moment regulation of blood pressure with the information traveling to the periphery via the sympathetic nervous system. Perhaps from a pathogenic point of view it may be more important to consider possible prolonged subtle changes in sympathetic nerve activity. These changes may be below the threshold for acute changes in blood pressure, but may have trophic effects on blood vessels. Our experiments suggest that a significant portion of the increased non-collagen protein synthesis observed in the small vessels of spontaneously hypertensive rats is mediated by the sympathetic nervous system. Therefore, it is possible that changes in central regulation of sympathetic outflow over long periods of time may have an impact on vascular structure, and thus the increased peripheral resistance often observed in essential hypertension.

REFERENCES

1. Adair JR, Hamilton BL, Scappaticci KA, Helke CJ, Gillis RA: Cardiovascular responses to electrical stimulation of the medullary raphe area of the cat. Brain Res 128: 141–145, 1977
2. Azmitia EC, Segal M: An autoradiographic analysis of the differential ascending projections of the dorsal and median raphe nuclei in the rat. J Comp Neur 179: 641–668, 1978
3. Bhargava KP, Raina N, Misra N, Shanker K, Vrat S: Uptake of serotonin by human platelets and its relevance to CNS involvement in hypertension. Life Sci 25: 195–200, 1979
4. Blatt CM, Rabinowitz SH, Lown B: Central serotonergic agents raise the repetitive extrasystole threshold of the vulnerable period of the canine ventricular myocardium. Circ Res 44: 723–730, 1979
5. Buckingham RE, Hamilton TC, Robson D: Effect of intracerebroventricular 5,6-hydroxytryptamine on blood pressure of spontaneously hypertensive rats. Eur J Pharmacol 36: 431–437, 1976
6. Buñag RD, Eferakeya AE, Langdon DS: Enhancement of hypothalamic pressor responses in spontaneously hypertensive rats. Am J Physiol 228: 217–222, 1975
7. Calaresu FR, Thomas MR: Electrophysiological connections in the brainstem involved in cardiovascular regulation. Brain Res 87: 335–338, 1975
8. Cottle MKW, Calaresu FR: Projections from the nucleus and tractus solitarius in the cat. J Comp Neurol 161: 143–158, 1975
9. Dahlstrom A, Fuxe K: Evidence for the existance of monoamine neurones in the central nervous system: I. Demonstration of monoamines in the cell bodies of brain stem neurons. Acta Physiol Scand 62 Suppl 232, 1964
10. Enoch DM, Kerr FWL: Hypothalamic vasopressor and vesicopressor pathways. I. Functional Studies. Arch Neurol 16: 290–306, 1967
11. Enoch DM, Kerr FWL: Hypothalamic vasopressor and vesicopressor pathways. II. Anatomic study of their course and connections. Arch Neurol 16: 307–320, 1967
12. Finch L: The cardiovascular affects of intraventricular 5,6-dihydroxytryptamine in conscious hypertensive rats. Clin Exp Pharmacol Physiol 2: 503–508, 1975

226

13. Gothert M, Klupp N: Cardiovascular effects of neurotoxic indolethylamines. Ann NY Acad Sci 305: 457–477, 1978
14. Hildebrandt JR: Central connections of aortic depressor and carotid sinus nerves. Exptl Neurol 45: 590–605, 1974
15. Hilton SM, Spyer KM: Participation of the anterior hypothalamus in the baroreceptor reflex. J Physiol 218: 271–293, 1971
16. Howe PRC, Lovenberg W, Chalmers JP: Increased number of PNMT-immuno-fluorescent nerve cell bodies in the medulla oblongata of strokeprone hypertensive rats. Brain Res 205: 123–130, 1981
17. Juskevich JC, Lovenberg W: Neuronal Regulation of Blood Pressure. In: Biochemical Actions of Hormones, Litwack, J. (Ed.), Academic Press, New York, 8: 117–165, 1981
18. Juskevich JC, Robinson DS, Whitehorn D: Effect of hypothalamic stimulation in spontaneously hypertensive and Wistar-Kyoto rats. Eur J Pharmacol 52: 429–439, 1978
19. Kuhn DM, Wolf W, Lovenberg W: The role of the central serotonergic neuronal system in blood pressure regulation. Hypertension 2: 243–255, 1980
20. Kuhn DM, Wolf W, Lovenberg W: Pressor effects of electrical stimulation of the dorsal and median raphe nuclei in rats. J Pharmacol Exp Ther 214: 403–409, 1980
21. Lambert GA, Friedman E, Buchweitz E, Gershon S: Involvement of 5-hydroxy-tryptamine in the central control of respiration, blood pressure and heart rate in the anesthetized rat. Neuropharmacol 17: 807–813, 1978
22. McCall RB, Humphrey SJ: Involvement of serotonin in the central regulation of blood pressure: Evidence for a facilitating effect on sympathetic nerve activity. J Pharmacol Exp Ther 222: 94–102, 1982
23. Moore RY, Halaris AE, Jones BE: Serotonin neurons of the midbrain raphe: ascending projections. J Comp Neurol 180: 417–438, 1978
24. Miura M, Reis DJ: Termination and secondary projections of carotid sinus nerve in the cat brain stem. Am J Physiol 217: 142–153, 1969
25. Miura M, Reis DJ: The role of the solitary and paramedian ventricular nuclei in mediating cardiovascular reflex responses from carotid baro- and chemoreceptors. J Physiol 223: 525–548, 1972
26. Nahmod VE, Finkielman S, Benarroch EE, Pirola CJ: Angiotensin regulates release and synthesis of serotonin in brain. Science 202: 1091–1093, 1978
27. Nakada T, Lovenberg W: Lysine incorporation in vessels of spontaneously hypertensive rats: Effects of adrenergic drugs. Eur J Pharmacol 48: 87–96, 1978
28. Palkovits M, Saavedra JM, Jacobowitz DM, Kizer JS, Zaborszky L, Brownstein MJ: Serotonergic innervation of the forebrain: effect of lesions on serotonin and tryptophan hydroxylase levels. Brain Res 130: 121–134, 1977
29. Rabinowitz SH, Lown B: Central neurochemical factors related to serotonin metabolism and cardiac ventricular vulnerability for repetitive electrical activity. Am J Cardiol 14: 516–522, 1978
30. Ricardo JA, Koh ET: Anatomical evidence of direct projections from the nucleus of the solitary tract to the hypothalamus amygdala, and other forebrain structures in the rat. Brain Res 153: 1–26, 1978
31. Saavedra JM, Grobecker H, Axelrod J: Adrenaline – forming enzyme in brainstem: Elevation in genetic and experimental hypertensive rats. Science 191: 483–484, 1976
32. Saavedra JM, Palkovits M, Brownstein MJ, Axelrod J: Serotonin distribution in the nuclei of the rat hypothalamus and preoptic region. Brain Res 77: 157–165, 1974
33. Saper CB, Loewy AD, Swanson LW, Cowan WM: Direct hypothalamus-autonomic connections. Brain Res 117: 305–312, 1976
34. Smith ML, Browning RA, Myer JH: In vivo rate of serotonin synthesis in brain and

spinal cord of young, spontaneously hypertensive rats. Eur J Pharmacol 53: 301–305, 1979
35. Smits JF, Struyker-Boudier HA: Intrahypothalamic serotonin and cardiovascular control in rats. Brain Res 111: 422, 1976
36. Smits JFM, Van Essen H, Struyker-Boudier HAJ: Serotonin mediated cardiovascular responses to electrical stimulation of the raphe nuclei in the rat. Life Sci 23: 173, 1978
37. Spyer KM: Organization of baroreceptor pathways in the brain skin. Brain Res 87: 221–226, 1975
38. Thomas MR, Calaresu FR: Responses of single units in the medial hypothalamus to electrical stimulation of the carotid sinus nerve in cat. Brain Res 44: 49–62, 1972
39. Wing LMH, Chalmers JP: Effects of p-chlorophenylalanine on blood pressure and heart rate in normal rabbits and rabbits with neurogenic hypertension. Clin Exp Pharmacol Physiol 1: 219, 1972
40. Yamabe H, Lovenberg W: Increased incorporation of ^{14}C-lysine into vascular proteins of the spontaneously hypertensive rat. Eur J Pharmacol 29: 109–116, 1974
41. Yamori Y, Nakada T, Lovenberg W: Effect of antihypertensive therapy on lysine incorporation into vascular protein of the spontaneously hypertensive rat. Eur J Pharmacol 38: 349–355, 1976

17. BRAIN CATECHOLAMINERGIC MECHANISMS AND HYPERTENSION

WYBREN DE JONG, DIRK H.G. VERSTEEG

Brain catecholaminergic neuronal systems play an important role in the control of arterial blood pressure [1, 9]. A role can be attributed to norepinephrine and epinephrine in this respect, while some evidence for the involvement of dopamine is also available. Neuronal systems employing norepinephrine and epinephrine as neurotransmitters appear to be located in strategic positions in the brainstem, thereby enabling these substances to participate in cardiovascular control [5, 15, 14, 21]. An inhibiting role for catecholamines in blood pressure regulation is supported by the fact that antihypertensive drugs such as clonidine and α-methyldopa appear to exert their central blood pressure lowering action via activation of catecholaminergic receptors in the brain [9, 11, 20, 29]. Malfunction of the central nervous control of blood pressure, in particular of the catecholaminergic systems, may be a cause of essential hypertension [7]. In this paper we will briefly review the hypotensive effects of microinjections of catecholamines into the nucleus of the solitary tract in the medulla oblongata. In addition, altered CNS catecholaminergic neurotransmission in spontaneously hypertensive rats will be considered in relation to hypertension.

NUCLEUS TRACTUS SOLITARII (NTS) AND ARTERIAL BLOOD PRESSURE

The nucleus of the solitary tract is an elongated paired nucleus located dorsally in the medulla oblongata. It extends from the transition zone of spinal cord and medulla to the border of the pons. Various physiological functions appear to be influenced by the NTS (for literature see Zandberg et al. [31]). The major role of the NTS in arterial blood pressure regulation has been studied most extensively. Due to the fact that the afferent baroreceptor fibers have their first synapse in the NTS, a limited number of brain cells in the NTS play a key role in cardiovascular regulation. The activity of these cells is also modulated by higher brain structures. Excellent reviews of the neuroanatomy of the NTS and of baroreceptor pathways became recently available [15, 14]. The perikarya of the baroreceptor neurons are located in the ganglion nodosum. Axons of these cell bodies reach the NTS via the glossopharyngeal and vagal nerves, and terminate in the medio-caudal part of the NTS. In this way, instant information about the arterial blood pressure is pro-

Sambhi, M.P. (ed.) Fundamental fault in hypertension
© *1984, Martinus Nijhoff Publishers. Boston/The Hague/Dordrecht/Lancaster.*
ISBN 978-94-010-9006-3

vided to the CNS. One of the major effector systems concerned with blood pressure control is the sympathetic nervous output to the resistance vessels. Although direct connections between the NTS and the intermediolateral nucleus (IML) of the thoraco-lumbar spinal cord do exist, the majority of the efferent pathways involve various nuclei of the pons-medulla, the hypothalamus, and the limbic system. It appears that complicated multisynaptic pathways convey the influence of the CNS to the output of the autonomic nervous system.

As illustrated in Figure 1, electrical stimulation of the NTS causes hypotension and bradycardia, thus mimicking the effect of baroreceptor stimulation. In contrast, electrical stimulation of the reticular formation below the NTS results in an increase in blood pressure. Interestingly, the most pronounced pressor response can be observed with electrode positions just below the NTS. The pressor response appears to be absent in neonatally sympathectomized rats [16], while the hypotension and bradycardia can still be observed (Figure 1). Following vagotomy, the decrease in heart rate is almost absent, while the decrease in blood pressure is attenuated. Differences in threshold current intensity and, in particular, the difference in frequency characteristic for the depressor and pressor response indicate that two separate fiber systems are involved [12]. Recently, Ferrario et al. [4] reported that electrical stimulation of the adjacent area

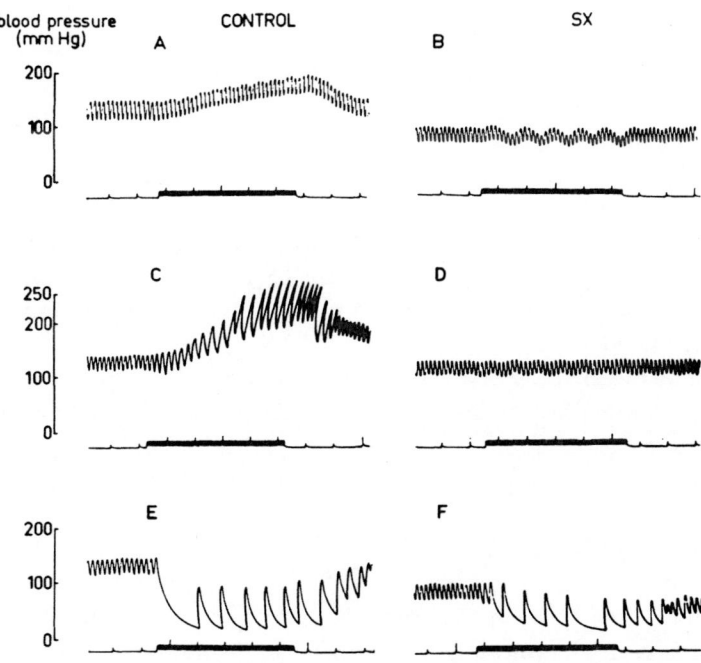

Figure 1. Effect of electrical stimulation of the medulla oblongata just caudally of the obex in an anesthetized intact rat (left panel) and in an anesthetized neonatally sympathectomized rat (SX; right panel). Electrode locations were 0.5 mm lateral of the midline at a depth of 1.8 mm (A, B), 0.9 mm (C, D) and 0.6 mm (E, F; the NTS). For details, Provoost et al. [16].

postrema in dogs caused a pressor response.

The depressor influence of the NTS as illustrated by the effect of electrical stimulation is also indicated by an opposite effect, i.e., an increase in blood pressure and heart rate following elimination of the NTS structures at the level of the obex by bilateral lesions [3, 11]. The acute hypertension thus caused in rats is usually lethal within 4 to 8 hr, probably due to heart failure and development of pulmonary edema. When the severe acute hypertension is inhibited by reserpine pretreatment, chronic hypertension is observed [31]. Removal of the area postrema causes no hypertension, either acutely or chronically [30]. Acute hypertension also occurs after elimination of baroreceptor input by transection of the IXth and Xth fibers in the medulla oblongata [10]. These data emphasize the key role of the structures in the NTS in blood pressure regulation and its potential importance in the development of hypertension. The dense catecholaminergic innervation of the NTS and the presence of two major catecholaminergic cell body regions in this nucleus (see below) may be indicative of an interaction of catecholamines with blood pressure regulation at the level of the NTS.

CATECHOLAMINES AND THE NTS

Catecholaminergic neurotransmission probably has a role in blood pressure regulation by the NTS. Relatively high concentrations of dopamine, norepinephrine, and epinephrine are present in the different parts of the NTS [22]. The noradrenergic cell bodies – the A2 region according to the nomenclature of Dahlström and Fuxe [2] – are for a major degree contained within the mediocaudal NTS caudal of the obex and in the pars commissuralis. The epinephrine-containing perikarya (C2 region) have a slightly more rostral distribution. The abundant noradrenergic innervation of the NTS is derived from different cell body regions. Important contributions come from the A2 region and the locus coeruleus [15, 14, 18].

The NTS may be one of the sites playing a role in the blood pressure decrease induced by catecholamines. It has been postulated that centrally acting antihypertensive drugs such as clonidine and α-methyldopa act by stimulation of receptor sites in the NTS (for review, see van Zwieten [20]). It is likely, however, that these drugs act at a more widely distributed system in the CNS, and that the NTS is one of the sites involved.

Following microinjections of volumes of 0.4–1.0 μl given into the NTS, methylene blue and radioactivity are found to be distributed in a longitudinal fashion along the NTS. Norepinephrine given in this way decreases blood pressure and heart rate [6]. An important metabolite of α-methyldopa, α-methylnorepinephrine, causes a similar effect, but the decrease in blood pressure is longer lasting. Stereospecificity appears to be required, since the (+)-isomers of both norepinephrine and α-methylnorepinephrine are practically devoid of activity in this respect. We have postulated that α-methylnorepinephrine might be a more effective transmitter in the CNS than the endogenous catecholamine and, in contrast, in some peripheral tissue may be less effective than norepinephrine [8]. The effective sites for α-methylnorepinephrine are restricted to the medio-caudal NTS and appear to correspond to the distribution of the noradrenergic perikarya of the A2 region [27, 29]. This is further supported by the finding that destruction of more rostral or more caudal parts of the NTS fails to affect the decrease in blood pressure caused by α-methylnorepinephrine. Similarly, removal of the area postrema is without effect [29]. Whereas catecholamines cause a hypotensive effect, increases in blood pressure are observed following microinjections of physostigmine into the same area of the NTS [28], while acetylcholine and carbachol induce biphasic changes of blood pressure. Up to now the catecholaminergic receptor sites in the NTS that mediate an inhibitory influence on blood pressure have not been characterized. The β-mimetic agent isoprenaline in various doses is ineffective. This is also the case for phenylephrine, oxymetazoline, and amidephrine [29]. A recent autoradiographic study showed the presence of a high density of $α_2$-receptors, as indicated by binding of ^{3}H-para-amino-clonidine [26]. Although clonidine is effective in decreasing blood pressure following administration into the NTS, it has to be given in a much higher (approximately 100-fold) dose than epinephrine, and no clear dose-response relationship has been established [29].

REGIONAL BRAIN CATECHOLAMINES AND HYPERTENSION

Alterations in the activity of groups of catecholaminergic neurons related to particular functions can be better studied in small brain regions than in larger brain parts. In the latter case, changes are often not detected due to 'dilution' of the alterations by the presence of other catecholaminergic neurons with unrelated functions, or of neurons showing opposite changes. For example, the relative small increase in the concentration of norepinephrine in the pons-medulla of spontaneously hypertensive rats (SHR), as compared to normotensive Wistar Kyoto rats (WKY), was found to be due mainly to a marked increase in norepinephrine concentration in particular regions such as the A2 region of the NTS [9, 2]. The development of a very reproducible technique for collecting small brain regions by Palkovits [13] and of a specific sensitive radiometric catecholamine assay [19] enabled us to study the relationship between catecholamines in individual brain nuclei and hypertension in SHR employing WKY as controls. A two-fold increase in the concentration of dopamine, norepinephrine, and epinephrine of the A2 region was observed at age 16 weeks in SHR [21]. At a younger age (3–10 weeks), no striking changes in catecholamine concentrations were found in various nuclei [25, 24]. Changes in noradrenergic neuronal activity were detected, however, using the α-methyl-paratyrosine (α-MPT) technique to

232

study noradrenaline turnover. A diminished α-MPT-induced norepinephrine disappearance was observed in the pars commissuralis of the NTS of SHR at 10 weeks of age. A transient decrease in the activity of noradrenergic neurons appeared to occur in SHR in the anterior hypothalamus, as a lowered disappearance of norepinephrine was detected at 3 weeks of age in different nuclei (nucl. paraventricularis, nucl. periventricularis, and the anterior hypothalamic nucleus) of the hypothalamus [25, 24]. Such changes were absent at age 7 weeks. Epinephrine levels of the hypothalamic periventricular and paraventricular nuclei and of the nucleus interstitialis striae terminalis of SHR appeared to increase with the development of hypertension [25, 24, 23]. Injection of adrenaline into this region causes a decrease in blood pressure [17]. As discussed before [25], it remains to be determined whether the gradual increase in hypothalamic epinephrine concentration reflects changes in the activity of adrenergic neurons opposing the increase in blood pressure, or whether it contributes to the development of hypertension. In contrast to this gradual increase in epinephrine level in the hypothalamus, elevated epinephrine levels in nuclei in the medulla oblongata were already pronounced at an early age. The rostral NTS and the A1 region of SHR showed such increases in epinephrine concentration at age 2–4 weeks. It is of interest that direct neuronal connections between the NTS and the nuclei in the anterior hypothalamus do exist. It is possible that the altered epinephrine levels in the medulla and the decreased α-MPT-induced norepinephrine disappearance in the anterior hypothalamus at an early age of SHR may be related to the same dysfunction.

CONCLUSIONS

Alterations in the activity of neurons containing norepinephrine and epinephrine in the hypothalamus and the medulla oblongata of SHR may reflect a dysfunction in brain catecholaminergic systems involved in the regulation of arterial blood pressure. It is of interest that local administration of norepinephrine or epinephrine in the anterior hypothalamus and in the NTS causes a decrease in blood pressure, and that biochemical changes related to these catecholamines were found to be most pronounced in these two regions of the brain of SHR.

REFERENCES

1. Chalmers JP: Brain amines and models of hypertension. Circ Res 36: 469–480, 1975
2. Dahlström A, Fuxe K: Evidence for the existence of monoamine containing neurones in the central nervous system. I. Demonstration of monoamines in the cell bodies of brain stem neurons. Acta Physiol Scand 62, suppl 232: 1–55, 1964
3. Doba N, Reis DJ: Acute fulminating neurogenic hypertension produced by brainstem lesions in the rat. Circ Res 32: 584–593, 1973

233

4. Ferrario CM, Barnes KL, Szilagyi JE, Conomy JP: Hemodynamic characteristics of acute electrical stimulation and chronic ablation of the area postrema. In: Meyer P, Schmitt H (eds), Nervous system and hypertension. Wiley-Flammarion, Paris, 1979, pp 85–101
5. Fuxe K, Hökfelt T, Bolme P, Goldstein M, Johansson O, Jonsson G, Lidbrink P, Ljungdahl O, Sachs Ch: The topography of central catecholamine pathways in relation to their possible role in blood pressure control. In: Davies DS, Reid JS (eds), Central action of drugs in blood pressure regulation. Pitman Medical, London, 1975, pp 8–33
6. de Jong W: Noradrenaline: central inhibitory control of blood pressure and heart rate. Eur J Pharmacol 29: 179–181, 1974
7. de Jong W: Brain and hypertension. Trends Neurosci 2: 71–72, 1979
8. de Jong W, Nijkamp FP: Centrally induced hypotension and bradycardia after administration of α-methylnoradrenaline into the area of the nucleus tractus solitarii of the rat. Br J Pharmacol 58: 593–598, 1976
9. de Jong W, Nijkamp FP, Bohus B: Role of noradrenaline and serotonin in the central control of blood pressure in normotensive and spontaneously hypertensive rats. Arch Intern Pharmacodyn Ther 213: 272–284, 1975
10. de Jong W, Palkovits M: Hypertension after localized transection of brainstem fibres. Life Sci 18: 61–64, 1976
11. de Jong W, Zandberg P, Bohus B: Central inhibitory noradrenergic cardiovascular control. Progr Brain Res 42: 285–298, 1975
12. de Jong W, Zandberg P, Palkovits M, Bohus B: Acute and chronic hypertension after lesions and transections of the rat brain stem. Progr Brain Res 47: 189–197, 1977
13. Palkovits M: Isolated removal of hypothalamus or other brain nuclei of the rat. Brain Res 59: 449–450, 1973
14. Palkovits M, Mezey E, Záborzky L: Neuroanatomical evidences for direct neural connections between the brain stem baroreceptor centers and the forebrain areas involved in the neural regulation of the blood pressure. In: Meyer P, Schmitt H (eds), Nervous system and hypertension. Wiley-Flammarion, Paris, 1979, pp 18–30
15. Palkovits M, Záborzky L: Neuroanatomy of central cardiovascular control. Nucleus tractus solitarii: afferent and efferent neuronal connections in relation to the baroreceptor reflex arc. Progr Brain Res 47: 9–34, 1977
16. Provoost AP, Bohus B, de Jong W: Differential influence of neonatal sympathectomy on the development of DOCA-salt and spontaneous hypertension in the rat. Progr Brain Res 47: 417–424, 1977
17. Struyker Boudier HAJ, Bekers A: Adrenaline-induced cardiovascular changes after intrahypothalamic administration into rats. Eur J Pharmacol 31: 153–155, 1975
18. Takahashi Y, Satoh K, Sakumoto T, Tohyama M, Shimizu N: A major source of catecholamine terminals in the nucleus tractus solitarii. Brain Res 172: 372–377, 1979
19. van der Gugten J, Palkovits M, Wijnen HJLM, Versteeg DHG: Regional distribution of adrenaline in rat brain. Brain Res 107: 171–175, 1976
20. van Zwieten PA: Antihypertensive drugs with a central action. Progr Pharmacol 1: 1–63, 1975
21. Versteeg DHG, Palkovits M, van der Gugten J., Wijnen HLJM, Smeets GWM, de Jong W: Catecholamine content of individual brain regions of spontaneously hypertensive rats (SH-rats). Brain Res 112: 429–434, 1976
22. Versteeg DHG, van der Gugten J, de Jong W, Palkovits M: Regional concentration of noradrenaline and dopamine in rat brain. Brain Res 113: 563–574, 1976
23. Versteeg DHG, Wijnen HJLM, de Jong W: Changes in hypothalamic adrenaline during hyper- and hypotensive states. In: Fuxe K, Goldstein A, Hökfelt T, Hökfelt F

234

(eds), Central adrenaline neurons: basic aspects in their role in cardiovascular functions. Pergamon Press, New York, 1980, pp 245–257

24. Wijnen HJLM, Palkovits M, de Jong W, Versteeg DHG: Elevated adrenaline content in nuclei of the medulla oblangata and the hypothalamus during the development of spontaneous hypertension. Brain Res 157: 191–195, 1978
25. Wijnen HJLM, Versteeg DHG, Palkovits M, de Jong W: Increased adrenaline content of individual nuclei of the hypothalamus and the medulla oblongata of genetically hypertensive rats. Brain Res 135: 180–185, 1977
26. Young WS III, Kuhar MJ: Noradrenergic α_1 and α_2 receptors: autoradiographic visualization. Eur J Pharmacol 58: 317–319, 1979
27. Zandberg P, de Jong W: α-Methylnoradrenaline-induced hypotension in the nucleus tractus solitarii of the rat: a localization study. Neuropharmacology 16: 219–222, 1977
28. Zandberg P, de Jong W: Localization of catecholaminergic receptor sites in the nucleus tractus solitarii involved in the regulation of arterial blood pressure. Progr Brain Res 47: 117–122, 1977
29. Zandberg P, de Jong W, de Wied D: Effect of catecholamine-receptor stimulating agents on blood pressure after local application in the nucleus tractus solitarii of the medulla oblangata. Eur J Pharmacol 55: 43–56, 1979
30. Zandberg P, Palkovits M, de Jong W: The area postrema and control of arterial blood pressure; absence of hypertension after excision of the area postrema in rats. Pflügers Arch 372: 169–173, 1977
31. Zandberg P, Palkovits M, de Jong W: Effect of various lesions in the nucleus tractus solitarii of the rat on blood pressure, heart rate and cardiovascular reflex responses. Clin Exp Hypert 1: 355–379, 1978

18. CONTINUOUS INTRA-ARTERIAL BLOOD PRESSURE RECORDING IN HUMAN HYPERTENSION

GIUSEPPE MANCIA, ALBERTO FERRARI, LUISA GREGORINI, GIANFRANCO PARATI, PIERO CIOFFI, MARCO DI RIENZO, ANTONIO PEDOTTI

Interest in direct and continuous blood pressure recording in human beings stems from the recognition that the method generally employed so far for measuring blood pressure, i.e., the cuff method [25], is encumbered with at least two major limitations. First, as the cuff method makes use of signs indirectly related to the pressure phenomena, it cannot guarantee under all circumstances an accurate estimation of the blood pressure values, in particular of diastolic blood pressure. Second, and more important, the cuff method, even when measurements are frequently repeated in the same subject, provides only a minute fraction of the thousands of blood pressure values that are extant day and night and compose a pressure profile characterized by a considerable degree of variability [16].

We will discuss some aspects of the research related to direct and continuous blood pressure recording in unrestrained human beings, concentrating on the following specific items: (1) The information provided by this method on the effects of various spontaneous behaviors on blood pressure, (2) the blood pressure variability (capable of being evaluated in great detail by this method) in subjects with different blood pressure levels, and (3) the clinical applications that can be foreseen with regard both to the diagnosis of human hypertension and to evaluation of the efficacy and duration of any given antihypertensive treatment [21].

We realize that this may not add much to this meeting's provocative topic, i.e., the fundamental fault in essential hypertension (if there is a single foundamental fault). Nevertheless, it may focus on an approach that has great potential and may help to understand some of the pathophysiological mechanisms that derange blood pressure in this so frequent and etiologically elusive human disease.

Let us begin with a description of the most widely adopted method for direct and continuous blood pressure measurements in man, developed mainly by investigators in Oxford [3] (Figure 1). In brief, it consists of a small catheter placed under local anesthesia in a brachial or a radial artery (we use a radial artery) to be connected via a rigid polyethylene tube to a small rigid box bound to the subject's chest. The box contains a battery-operated constant-flow pump and a 40 ml reservoir of sterile saline that provide a continuous drip into the catheter and keep it patent for 24 hours without disturbing by any measurable amount the pressure generated by the arterial system. It also contains a pressure transducer,

Sambhi, M.P. (ed.) Fundamental fault in hypertension
© *1984, Martinus Nijhoff Publishers. Boston/The Hague/Dordrecht/Lancaster.*
ISBN 978-94-010-9006-3

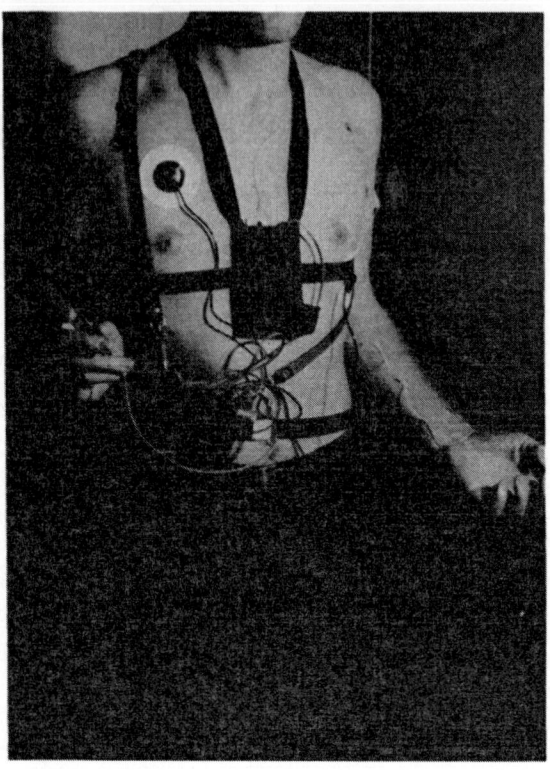

Figure 1. Components of the Oxford method for intra-arterial continuous blood pressure recording in human beings. See text for explanation.

its signal being conveyed to a battery-operated amplifier and a small tape recorder, where it is stored during the 24 hour period. There are two other channels in the tape that can record two EKG leads [14], and an additional channel that can be used in connection with a marker to signal the more important behavioral events taking place during the recording and/or those events that are important for the experimental protocol. The blood pressure signal provided by the Oxford apparatus is of satisfactory quality regarding linearity and the stability of the transducer over the physiological pressure range, and the frequency-response curve of the entire catheter-transducer-tape recorder system. Equally important, the pressure signal can be obtained without any gross interference with the subject's physical activity, his sleep, or in general with his pattern of life.

The blood pressure recording can be displayed at variable speed on a poligraph, along with the EKG trace and the heart rate measurements obtained by connecting the pressure or the electrocardiographic signal with a tachograph. This has provided detailed information on the pressure changes that occur during various behavioral events, and in several instances has allowed correlation of these changes with concomitant alterations in heart rate and in the electrocardiographic pattern [15]. For example, it has been established that there are behaviors (eating, digestion, mental work, etc.) that do not alter blood pressure by much, whereas several other behaviors usually induce pressure rises [3, 24]. Among the latter, special consideration must be given to emotional events, not only because the emotionally induced pressure rises can be very marked and prolonged, but also because they may materialize during the doctor's examination of the subject, thus interfering with his correct estimation of the real basal blood pressure values. Figure 2 illustrates how marked and prolonged a pressure rise induced by an emotional condition can be. From top to bottom, the traces show pulsatile blood pressure, mean arterial pressure, blood pressure integrated over consecutive 37.5–sec. periods, and heart rate measured by a tachograph. At the time indicated by the first arrow, the subject began to play poker, and continued playing for several hours, to end at the second arrow. It is clear that this playful but certainly not totally relaxed activity was capable of inducing a rise in blood pressure and heart rate, and to maintain both these variables at the new high level as long as it lasted. The rise was indeed very marked during the poker game, as blood pressure (also showing greater oscillations than in the preceding and following periods) was elevated by an average of about 50 mmHg, and heart rate increased on the average about 30 b/min.

Figure 3 shows what may happen in the other stressful event mentioned above, the doctor's measurement of the subject's blood pressure. Again from top to bottom, the traces represent pulsatile arterial blood pressure, mean arterial pressure, integrated blood pressure, and heart rate. The period between the two arrows represents the time the doctor spent measuring the subject's blood pressure; it can clearly be seen that blood pressure was higher during this interval than during the preceding and following periods. We have observed a pressure rise in the majority of the normotensive and hypertensive subjects in whom this phenomenon was studied, the rise being in some cases very marked and stable. It is obvious that in these latter subjects the blood pressure values provided by the doctor's measurement may represent a gross overestimation of the pressure values in most of the subjects' daily life. This observation may be the basis of a diagnostic application for continuous blood pressure recording, as will be discussed later.

At the opposite end of the spectrum, there are behaviors that induce a fall in blood pressure; sleep is certainly the best known in this regard. Knowledge of the hypotensive action of sleep in man goes back to the beginning of the century [4], but direct and continuous blood pressure recording has added two important findings [12, 22]. First, the hypotensive action of sleep has proved to be very marked, falls in blood pressure during this condition being often 20% or more of the values recorded during wakefulness. Second, it has been clearly shown that in the majority of hypertensive subjects the hypotension induced by sleep is quite evident, and certainly no less than that observed in normotensive subjects. Figure 4, a record taken on a subject with a marked degree of hypertension, illustrates this point. The record represents a computerized analysis of the mean arterial

238

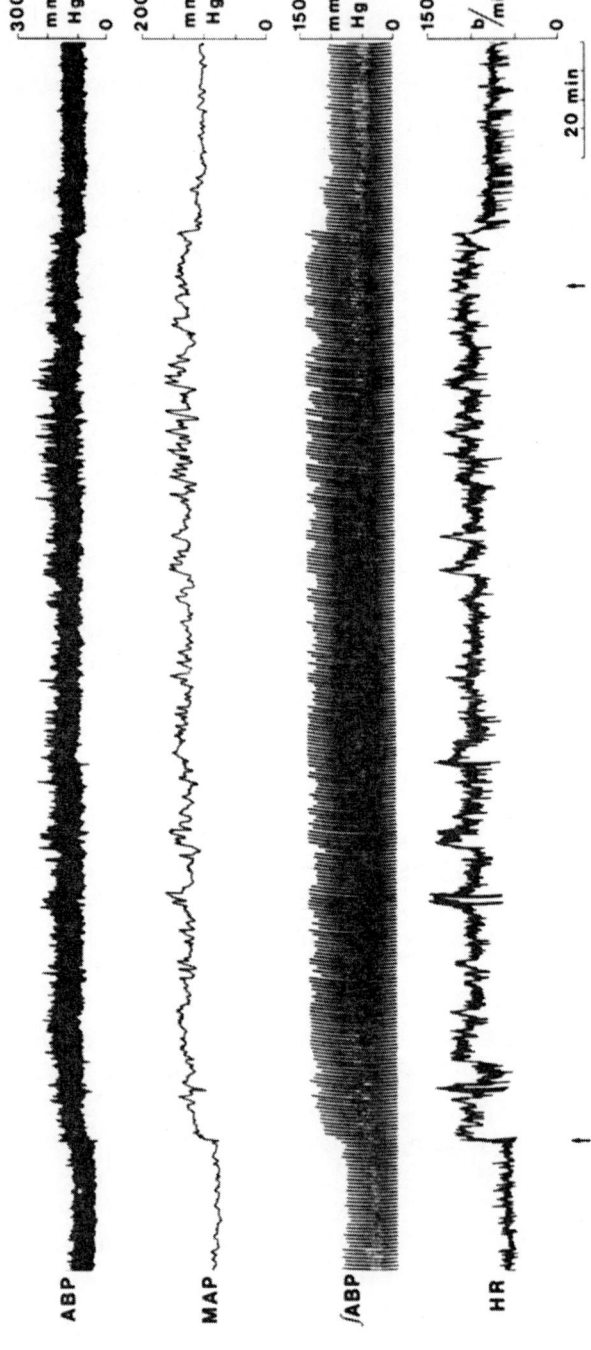

Figure 2. Original record, taken from a 24-hour blood pressure recording in one of our patients, displayed on a Grass polygraph. *ABP*: pulsatile arterial blood pressure; *MAP*: mean arterial pressure; *∫ABP*: blood pressure integration over consecutive 37.5-sec. intervals; *HR*: heart rate. The subject played poker during the time between arrows.

239

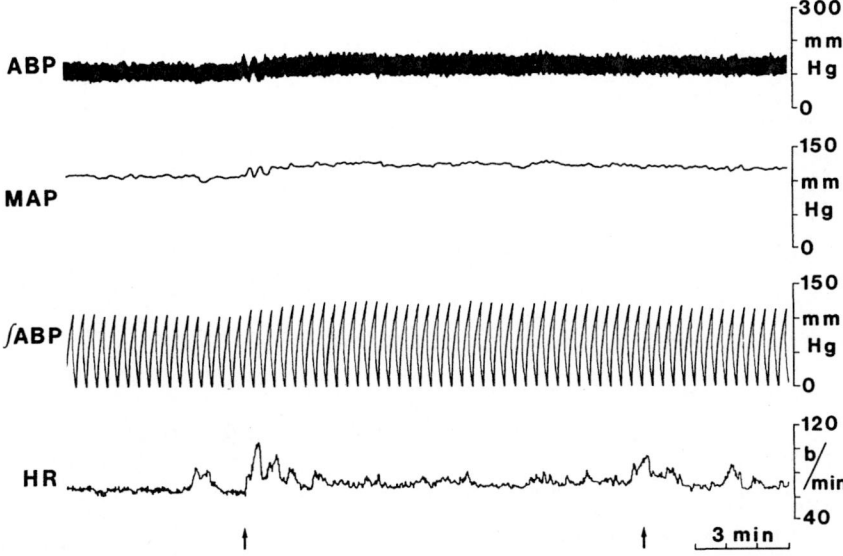

Figure 3. Original record, taken from a 24-hour blood pressure recording in one of our patients, displayed on a Grass polygraph. Symbols as in Fig. 2. The interval between arrows shows the time the doctor spent measuring the patient's blood pressure by the cuff method.

pressure trace of the subject, the data being expressed as averages ± standard deviations for each of the 48 different half-hours in which the recording period was divided. The mean arterial pressure values during wakefulness oscillated around 140 mmHg. During sleep, blood pressure showed a marked reduction, falling to less than 100 mmHg, a value within the normotensive range according to current standards. We would like to point out that this may be regarded as another example of the phenomenon described yesterday by Professor Doyle, i.e., the importance of sympathetic activity in the maintenance of the high blood pressure levels of many hypertensive subjects, which can be assessed by the hypotensive effect of pharmacological abolition of sympathetic tone [6]. It can also be assessed, and perhaps in a more physiological way, by the magnitude of the hypotensive action of sleep, which reduces blood pressure by performing a sort of 'functional sympathectomy' [2, 22]. It must also be pointed out that cardiovascular phenomena during sleep are more complex than simple hypotension because of reduction in sympathetic vasoconstrictor tone. Excitatory as well as inhibitory vascular effects of sleep have been described in animals and man, particularly during REM sleep [18, 10, 22]. It has been reported that the hypotensive effect of sleep in man tends to wane during the latter part of the night, when an arterial pressure value that may be the highest of the 24 hours can be reached. This has been ascribed to a cyrcadian rhythm inherent to blood pressure [23] a conclusion that has been strongly criticized, however [26].

Blood pressure variability has been widely investigated [5] for several good

```
NOME E COGNOME DEL SOGGETTO TRIVELLATO FABIO     BALE
CONDIZIONI DEL SOGGETTO:        ------    2-2-79
DATA REGISTRAZIONE:             13-6-79
                                        20        40        60        80       100       120       140       160       180       2
IN ORDINATA:[MMHG]                       !         !         !         !         !         !         !         !         !
IN ASCISSE:[TEMPO]               0-!-------------------------------------------------------------------------------------------------
V.M.= 140.91    D.S.=12.28       1-!         !         !         !         !         !       ***0***   !         !         !
V.M.= 143.86    D.S.= 9.04       2-!         !         !         !         !         !        **0**    !         !         !
V.M.= 141.01    D.S.=10.03       3-!         !         !         !         !         !       ***0***   !         !         !
V.M.= 143.05    D.S.= 9.61       4-!         !         !         !         !         !        **0**    !         !         !
V.M.= 142.20    D.S.= 6.34       5-!         !         !         !         !         !        **0**    !         !         !
V.M.= 141.35    D.S.= 7.12       6-!         !         !         !         !         !        **0**    !         !         !
V.M.= 145.08    D.S.=11.03       7-!         !         !         !         !         !       ***0***   !         !         !
V.M.= 145.18    D.S.= 8.32       8-!         !         !         !         !         !        **0**    !         !         !
V.M.= 138.80    D.S.= 7.70       9-!         !         !         !         !         !       **0**     !         !         !
V.M.= 136.90    D.S.= 8.29      10-!         !         !         !         !         !       **0**     !         !         !
V.M.= 141.26    D.S.= 8.48      11-!         !         !         !         !         !        **0**    !         !         !
V.M.= 134.68    D.S.=19.60      12-!         !         !         !         !         !   *****0*****    !         !         !
V.M.= 122.44    D.S.=10.96      13-!         !         !         !         !       ***0***   !         !         !
V.M.= 108.59    D.S.= 7.04      14-!         !         !         !         !  **0**  !         !         !         !
V.M.= 102.14    D.S.= 3.50      15-!         !         !         !         ! *0*     !         !         !         !
V.M.= 103.11    D.S.= 5.78      16-!         !         !         !         ! *0*     !         !         !         !
V.M.= 100.73    D.S.= 3.81      17-!         !         !         !         !*0*      !         !         !         !
V.M.= 104.04    D.S.= 4.58      18-!         !         !         !         ! *0*     !         !         !         !
V.M.= 106.04    D.S.= 6.31      19-!         !         !         !         ! **0**   !         !         !         !
V.M.= 107.28    D.S.= 6.80      20-!         !         !         !         ! **0**   !         !         !         !
V.M.= 125.09    D.S.= 7.63      21-!         !         !         !         !         ! **0**   !         !         !
V.M.= 141.64    D.S.=12.53      22-!         !         !         !         !         !        ***0***  !         !         !
V.M.= 121.83    D.S.=10.00      23-!         !         !         !         !         ! ***0***  !         !         !
V.M.= 117.07    D.S.= 5.05      24-!         !         !         !         !         !*0*      !         !         !
V.M.= 115.53    D.S.= 7.01      25-!         !         !         !         !         !**0**    !         !         !
V.M.= 115.65    D.S.= 8.37      26-!         !         !         !         !         !**0**!   !         !         !
V.M.= 113.24    D.S.= 8.02      27-!         !         !         !         !         !**0**!   !         !         !
V.M.= 105.93    D.S.= 4.98      28-!         !         !         !         !        !*0*      !         !         !
V.M.= 110.22    D.S.= 7.84      29-!         !         !         !         !         ! **0**   !         !         !
V.M.= 140.90    D.S.=15.39      30-!         !         !         !         !         !       ****0****  !         !         !
V.M.= 126.48    D.S.= 6.72      31-!         !         !         !         !         !!**0**   !         !         !
V.M.= 130.46    D.S.= 5.85      32-!         !         !         !         !         ! *0*     !         !         !
V.M.= 130.92    D.S.= 8.34      33-!         !         !         !         !         ! **0**   !         !         !
V.M.= 122.88    D.S.= 4.89      34-!         !         !         !         !         !*0*      !         !         !
V.M.= 148.11    D.S.=12.14      35-!         !         !         !         !         !       !***0***   !         !
V.M.= 134.88    D.S.=12.44      36-!         !         !         !         !         ! ***0***  !         !         !
V.M.= 129.60    D.S.= 9.67      37-!         !         !         !         !         ! **0**   !         !         !
V.M.= 121.86    D.S.= 4.26      38-!         !         !         !         !         !*0*      !         !         !
V.M.= 132.60    D.S.=14.84      39-!         !         !         !         !         ! ****0****  !         !         !
V.M.= 136.93    D.S.=18.27      40-!         !         !         !         !         ! *****0*****     !         !         !
V.M.= 146.76    D.S.= 7.91      41-!         !         !         !         !         !       !**0**     !         !         !
V.M.= 169.19    D.S.=18.34      42-!         !         !         !         !         !         !       *****0*****  !
V.M.= 157.47    D.S.= 7.95      43-!         !         !         !         !         !         !       **0**   !         !
V.M.= 127.16    D.S.=10.30      44-!         !         !         !         !         !!***0***  !         !         !
V.M.= 116.92    D.S.= 6.02      45-!         !         !         !         !         ! **0**   !         !         !
V.M.= 112.46    D.S.=12.19      46-!         !         !         !         !         ! ***0***! !         !         !
```

Figure 4. Computerized analysis of a day and night blood pressure recording in a subject with severe essential hypertension. The data refer to mean arterial pressure and were analyzed by calculating averages and standard deviations of values occurring during each half-hour period. The computer considered one value every 50 msec, making averages of all points within each 3-sec. interval.

reasons. First, variability may represent a risk factor, as subjects in whom blood pressure shows marked rises and falls throughout the day and night may be more prone to strokes and heart attacks, particularly if they are hypertensive and have atherosclerotic lesions in their arteries. Second, as the cuff method reads only a few pressure values, it is clear that its validity is in some way related to blood pressure variability: the more blood pressure varies and the more it varies differently among subjects, the less chance the cuff method has to provide a fair and matched representation of the subjects' pressure profile. Third, assessment of blood pressure variability may help understand some of the mechanisms that control blood pressure in the normal unrestrained man, and to find out whether these mechanisms are deranged in hypertension.

Table 1 shows our results on blood pressure variability in human beings of similar ages but with different blood pressure levels [19]. The data were analyzed as in Figure 4, that is, by computer calculation of average values and standard deviations of 48 different half-hour values within the 24-hour recording period. The 48 different averages allowed us to obtain mean blood pressure values for the 24 hours, whereas the 48 different standard deviations allowed us to obtain an average measure of the tendency of mean arterial pressure to vary within these short half-hour spans. This tendency was expressed either in absolute terms (average of the 48 different standard deviations) and as a variation coefficient (average standard deviation as a percentage of the 24-hour mean blood pressure level). A similar analysis was carried out for heart rate. It can be seen that, when expressed in absolute terms, blood pressure variability was significantly greater in subjects with mild or borderline essential hypertension than in normotensive subjects, and that a further significant increase was present in subjects with more

Table 1. Variability of mean arterial pressure (MAP) and heart rate (HR) in subjects with different blood pressure levels

	24 hour MAP (mm Hg)	Standard deviation (mm Hg)	Variation coefficient (%)
Normotensive subjects (n = 22)	88.1 ± 1.7	6.54 ± 0.27	7.43 ± 0.28
Mildly hypertensive subjects (n = 26)	107.8 ± 0.8	8.06 ± 0.28	7.47 ± 0.29
More severely hypertensive subjects (n = 41)	137.9 ± 3.1	9.24 ± 0.38	6.70 ± 0.29

	24 hour HR (b/min)	Standard deviation (b/min)	Variation coefficient (%)
Normotensive subjects (n = 22)	75.0 ± 1.8	8.94 ± 0.90	11.92 ± 0.63
Mildly hypertensive subjects (n = 26)	77.5 ± 1.9	7.89 ± 0.49	10.17 ± 0.63
More severely hypertensive subjects (n = 41)	79.5 ± 1.5	7.97 ± 0.56	10.00 ± 0.61

Data are expressed as means ± SE. Mean age (± SE) was 38.6 ± 2.9 for the normotensive, 39.8 ± 1.8 for the mildly hypertensive, and 44.8 ± 1.5 for the more severely hypertensive group. See text for further details.

severe essential hypertension. This pattern was not reproduced by using the variation coefficient, however, as in this instance the values were similar in normotensive and mildly hypertensive subjects and, if anything, reduced in the more severely hypertensive subjects. No significant differences were observed among the three groups as far as absolute or percentage heart rate variability was concerned. Thus, absolute blood pressure values tend to have greater oscillations in essential hypertension; this may have clinical implications and consequences. On the other hand, relative blood pressure oscillations around the mean are in fact similar in hypertensive and in normotensive subjects; this may suggest that the factors responsible for blood pressure changes (central autonomic influences) and homeostasis (baroreflexes) may not be deranged in human hypertension. Our data also suggest that as far as blood pressure variability is concerned, subjects with borderline hypertension do not represent a separate group, as their variability falls exactly between that of the normotensive and the severely hypertensive subjects. This conclusion supports previous studies [8] and underlines the inappropriateness of calling this form of hypertension 'labile,' a term that may misleadingly imply that only in these subjects is blood pressure variable.

As for the diagnostic applications of continuous blood pressure recording in hypertension, two aspects merit mention. One is related to the hyperactive subjects described above, in whom blood pressure readings taken by a doctor are probably higher than the subject's true daily blood pressure. This has actually been reported in a study by Littler [13], in which average blood pressure values obtained by daily continuous blood pressure recording were compared with those reported by a general practioner in an outpatient clinic. In several instances, subjects under treatment who were considered to have severe hypertension on the basis of indirect measurements turned out to have much lower blood pressure values on continuous recording. According to Littler et al. [13] these were patients who presented little sign of target organ damage, which suggests continuous blood pressure values to be a more important prognostic determinant than the greater values occasionally occurring at the time of the indirect measurements. A similar suggestion has been made by Sokolow et al. [27], who found that repeated blood pressure estimations through the day (obtained by an automatic indirect recorder) correlated more closely than casual measurements with the extent of the complications induced by hypertension. It is very important that this issue be clarified, for, in our experience as well as in others [9], differences between casual blood pressure values and values measured during continuous blood pressure recording (the latter being lower) occur in a fairly large number of cases.

Continuous and direct blood pressure recording may also be usefully applied to the diagnosis of cases of pheocromocytoma in which paroxismal symptoms, although suggestive of the disease, are too brief to allow indirect blood pressure measurements or to cause measurable alterations in urinary and plasma catecholamines [20]. Figure 5A shows a recording from a normotensive subject who

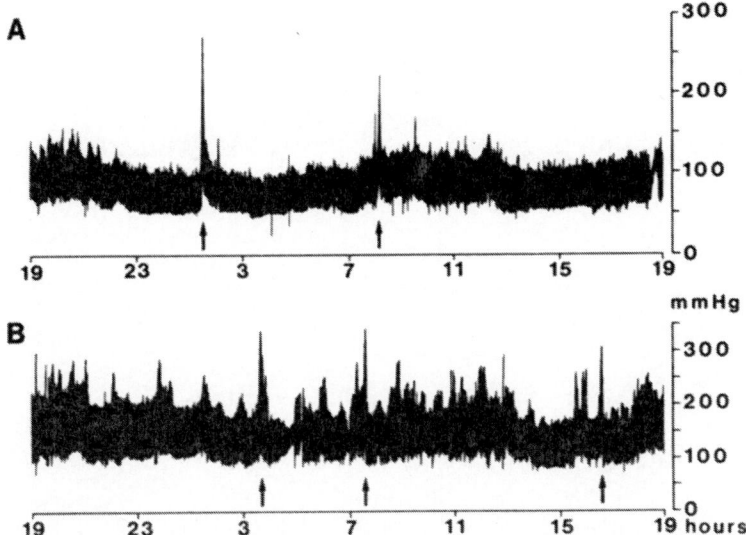

Figure 5. Direct blood pressure recordings (24 hr) in 2 patients with pheochromocytoma. Arrows refer to brief episodes of palpitation (subject A) and headache (subject B), which were identified by the marker and turned out to be accompanied by huge pressure rises (From Mancia et al., [20], by permission).

complained of having 3-5 minute long episodes of palpitation. Two of these episodes were reported by the subject during the recording, and both were revealed to be accompanied by huge increases in arterial blood pressure. The first episode is illustrated at higher speed in Figure 6, and it can be seen that not only did blood pressure rise to extremely high values (systolic pressure approaching 300 mmHg), but that the subject's perception of the beginning and the end of the episode (indicated by the two arrows) was not related to the height of the pressure values, but to the appearance and disappearance of the marked heart rate irregularities indicated in the bottom trace. A further display at an even greater speed, this time with the addition of the electrocardiographic trace (Figure 7), showed the heart rate disturbances to consist of a large number of ventricular premature beats and of runs of ventricular tachycardia that put the subject's life at a particularly great risk. The existence of a pheochromocytoma in the left adrenal gland was later confirmed by further examinations, and surgical treatment was followed by disappearance of all symptoms. Another case of phechromocytoma with several short huge rises in blood pressure during continuous recording (sometimes not signalled by the subject) is shown in Figure 5B.

The role of continuous blood pressure recording in the evaluation of antihypertensive drugs is another important field of application of this method, as knowledge of all pressure values during a period of relatively normal life pattern can obviously provide a better appreciation of the effectiveness of a given antihypertensive treatment than a few isolated pressure measurements in a standard condition. Figure 8 shows the results we obtained by performing 24-hour blood

244

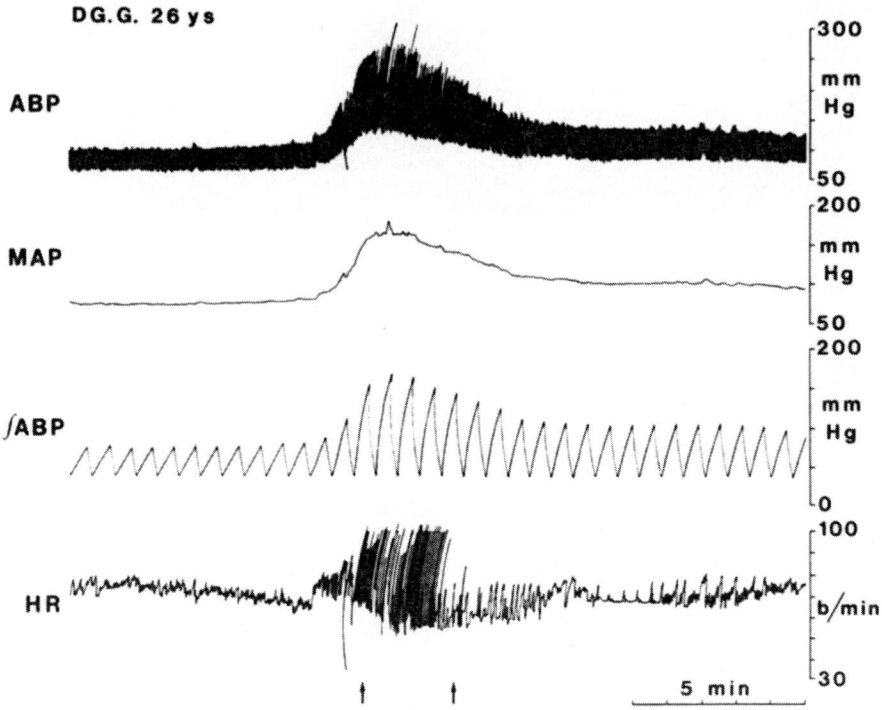

Figure 6. Original record, displaying at higher speed the first pressure rise observed in subject A (Fig. 5). Symbols as in Fig. 2. The arrows indicate the beginning and the end of the episode as perceived by the subject (From Mancia et al., [20], by permission).

pressure recordings in seven hypertensive subjects under control conditions and after 15 days of treatment with labetalol, at doses of 600–1200 mg per day divided into three administrations. The recordings were plotted by the computer as frequency-distribution histograms for all patients, a separate analysis being performed for morning, afternoon, and night values. It can be seen in the no-drug recordings (upper panel) that blood pressure values covered similar spectra during the morning and afternoon periods, while lower values were clearly evident at night. All spectra moved to the left during treatment with labetalol (lower panel), demonstrating the effective antihypertensive action of this alpha- and beta-blocking drug. Interestingly, in the latter condition the morning, afternoon, and night values were no longer different, suggesting that labetalol reduced sympathetic tone so as to diminish the further reduction due to sleep influence.

This alteration in the sleep pattern was not observed for heart rate, however. As shown in Figure 9, frequency-distribution histograms related to the heart rate of the same patients as in Figure 8 also moved to the left in the control night period because of the bradycardic influence exerted by sleep (left panel). This was also the case during treatment with labetalol, indicating that (a) at clinically effective doses the blood pressure effect of the drug may be independent of its

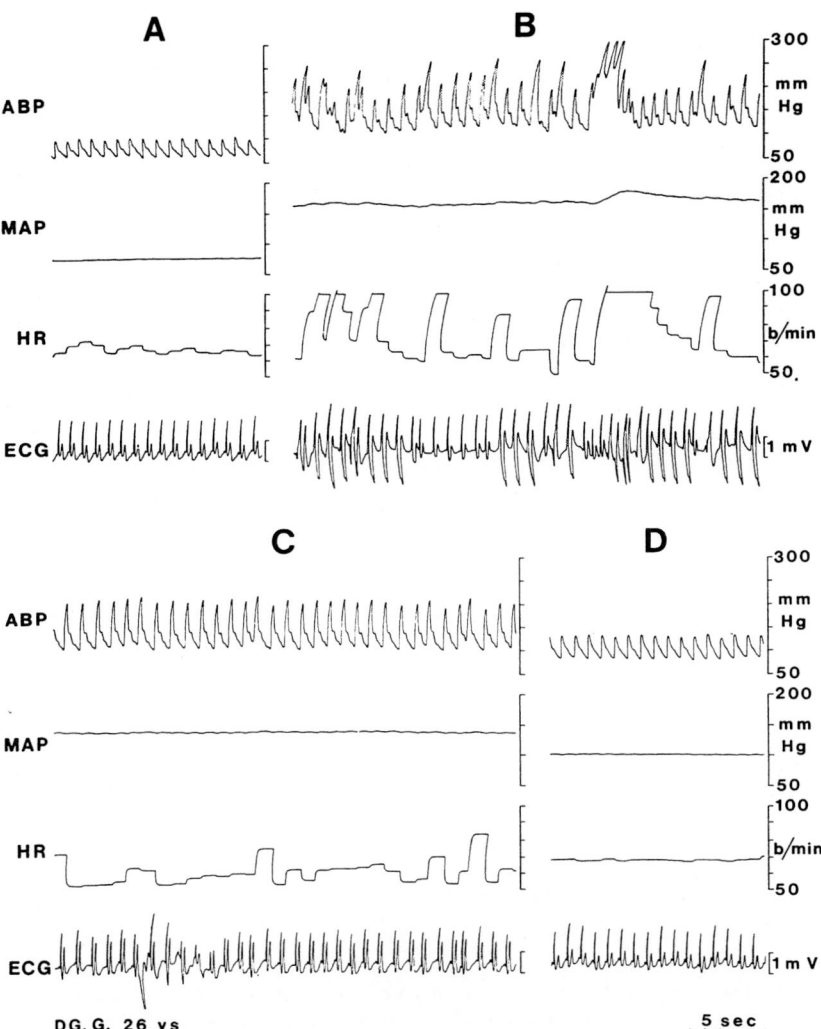

Figure 7. Original record of the pressor episode in Figs. 5 and 6, displayed at a still higher speed, with the addition of the electrocardiogram trace. Symbols as in Fig. 2. *A*: Control period before the episode; *B*: period during the maximal pressor response during the episode; *C*: towards the end of the episode; *D*: after the end of the episode (From Mancia [17], by permission).

effect on heart rate, and (b) the beta-blocking action of labetalol does not interfere with neural control of heart rate, probably because under normal circumstances and during sleep this depends to a large extent on vagal cardiac influence. This is an example of the concept mentioned above, i.e., the usefulness of continuous blood pressure recording to obtain additional information on some aspects of hemodynamic regulation under various normal and abnormal circumstances.

Continuous blood pressure recording represents a particularly suitable method

246

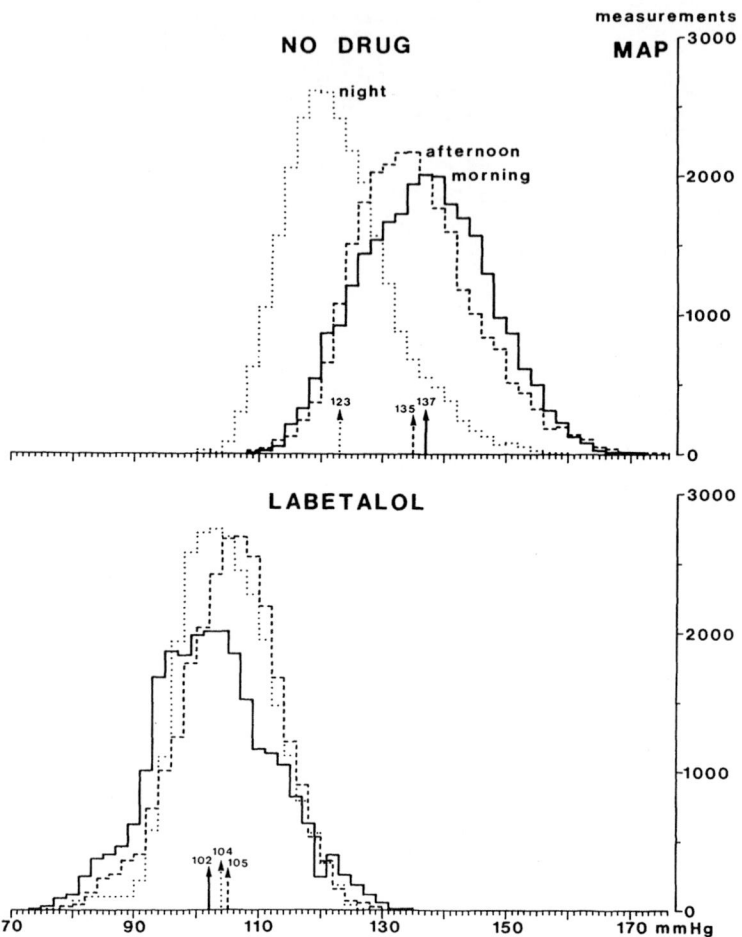

Figure 8. Frequency distribution histograms (mean arterial pressure) from 7 subjects with essential hypertension before and during treatment with labetalol. See text for further explanation.

for evaluating slow-acting antihypertensive drugs because of its ability to measure all pressure values in the periods that may be farther apart from the drug administration (and harder for use of the cuff). Figure 10 shows the effects of a short-acting clonidine preparation in three different subjects after administration of a single daily dose of 0.250 mg. The symbols represent mean arterial pressure for half-hour periods for the three patients, the vertical line indicating pressure values with placebo, and the horizontal line pressure values (related to the same half-hour) after about a week of clonidine treatment. As can be seen, most of the points are above the line of identity, showing that almost all values recorded during the 24 hours were lower after than before drug administration. A confirmation oof the effectiveness of this clonidine preparation was obtained by examination of heart rate values in the same way, almost all the values being

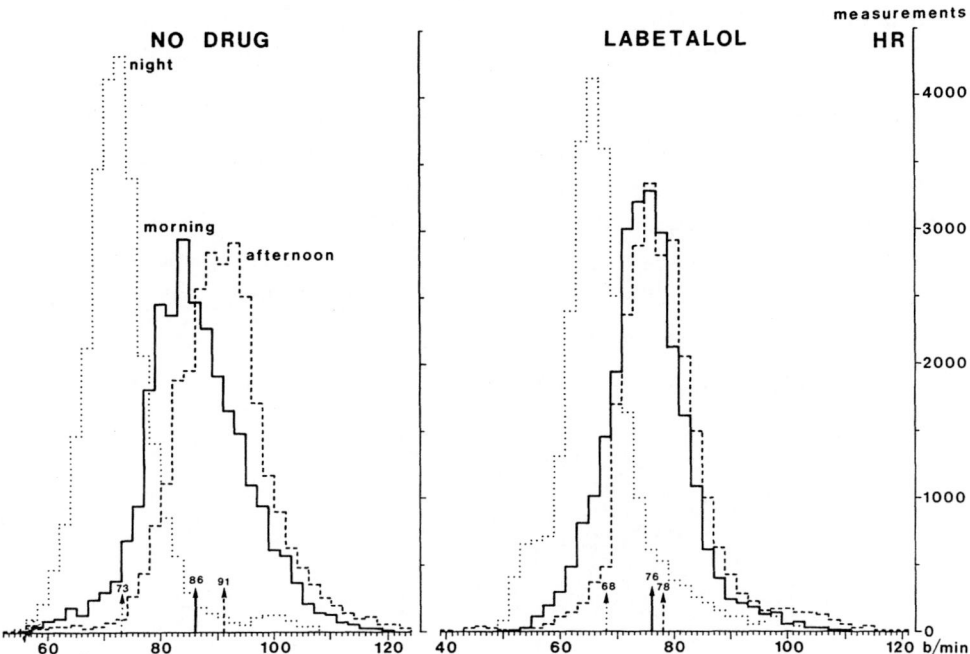

Figure 9. Frequency distribution histograms (heart rate) from the patients in Fig. 8 before and during treatment with labetalol. See text for further explanation.

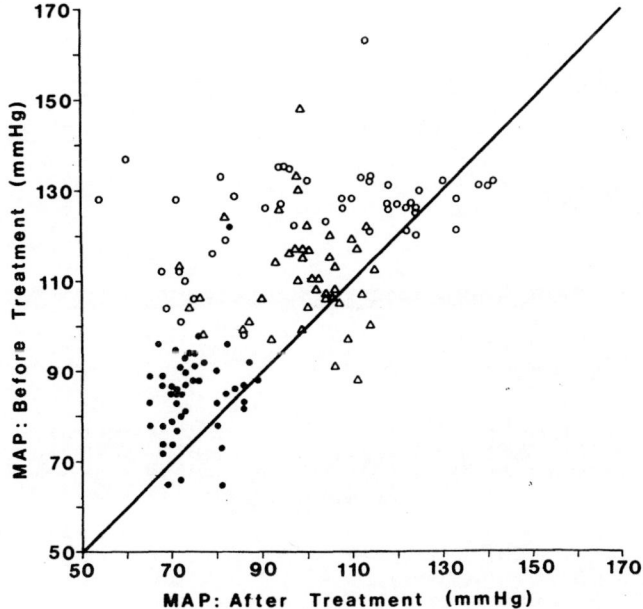

Figure 10. Effects of a slow-acting clonidine preparation on mean arterial pressure (MAP). Black circles, white circles, and triangles represent average half-hour values from 3 different patients, plotting before and during treatment being made for corresponding half hours.

248

lower after the single administration of the drug (Figure 11).

Finally, it must be mentioned that continuous blood pressure recording also demonstrates clearly the disadvantages of antihypertensive treatment, as shown in Figure 12, taken from a study by Goldberg and Raftery [7]. The recording is concerned with an hypertensive patient under treatment with guanethidine; it can be seen that this drug impaired cardiovascular homeostatic mechanisms to such a large extent that dramatic hypotension occurred while the patient was micturating. In several instances, these hypotensive episodes were accompanied by EKG changes, indicating their ability to induce myocardial ischemia.

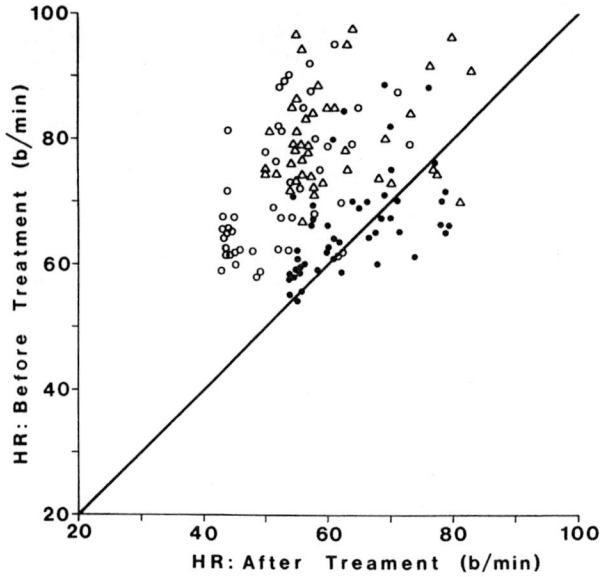

Figure 11. Effects of a slow-acting clonidine preparation on heart rate (HR) in the same 3 patients as in Fig. 10. Symbols as in Fig. 10.

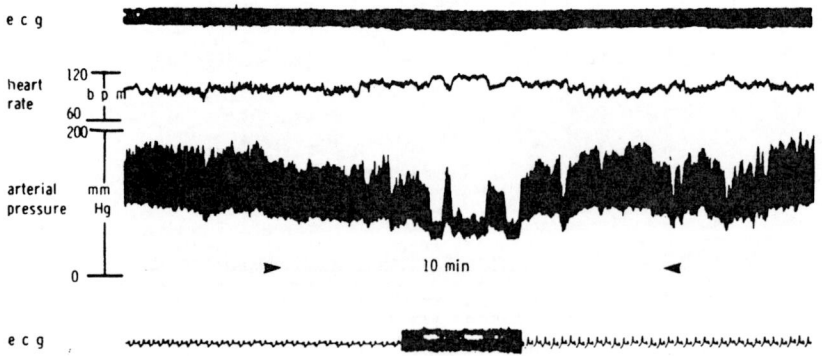

Figure 12. Hypotension during micturition in a patient under treatment with guanethidine (From Goldberg and Raftery [7], by permission).

ACKNOWLEDGEMENTS

This research has been supported in part by the Finalized Project on Hypertension of the National Research Council. Computerized analyses of the data have been performed at the Centro di Bioingegneria, Fondazione Don Gnocchi, Milano.

REFERENCES

1. Baccelli G, Albertini R, Mancia G, Zanchetti A: Central and reflex regulation of sympathetic vasoconstrictor activity of limb muscle during desynchronized sleep in the cat. Circ Res 35: 625, 1974
2. Baccelli G, Guazzi M, Mancia G, Zanchetti A: Neural and non-neural mechanisms influencing circulation during sleep. Nature 223: 184, 1969
3. Bevan AT, Honour AJ, Holt FM: Direct arterial blood pressure recording in unrestricted man. Clin Sci 36: 329, 1969
4. Brush CE, Fayerweather R: Observations on changes in blood pressure during normal sleep. Am J Physiol 5: 199, 1901
5. Clement DL: Blood pressure variability. MTP, Lancaster, 1978
6. Doyle A: This book.
7. Goldberg AD, Raftery EB: Patterns of blood-pressure during chronic administration of post-ganglionic sympathetic blocking drugs for hypertension. Lancet 2: 1052, 1976
8. Goldberg AD, Raftery EB, Cashman PMM, Stott FD: Study of untreated hypertensive subjects by means of continuous intra arterial blood pressure recordings. Brit Heart J 40: 656, 1978
9. Irwing JB, Kerr F, Ewing DJ, Kirby J: Value of prolonged recording of blood pressure in assessment of hypertension. Brit Heart J 38: 859, 1974
10. Khatri IM, Freis ED: Hemodynamic changes during sleep. J Appl Physiol 22: 867, 1967
11. Littler WA: Sleep and blood pressure: further observations. Am Heart J 97: 35, 1979
12. Littler WA, Honour AJ, Carter RD, Sleight P: Sleep and blood pressure. Brit Med J 3: 346, 1975
13. Littler WA, Honour J, Pugsley DJ, Sleight P: Continuous recording of direct arterial pressure in unrestricted patients. Circulation 51: 1101, 1975
14. Littler WA, Honour AJ, Sleight P, Stott FD: Continuous recording of direct arterial pressure and electrocardiogram in unrestricted man. Brit Med J 3: 76, 1972
15. Littler WA, Honour AJ, Sleight P, Stott FD: Direct arterial pressure and the electrocardiogram in unrestricted patients with angina pectoris. Circulation 48: 125, 1973
16. Littler WA, West MJ, Honour AJ, Sleight P: The variability of arterial pressure. Am Heart J 95: 180, 1978
17. Mancia G: Registrazione diretta e continua della pressione arteriosa nell'uomo. In: Attività in campo cardiologico. Corso di Aggiornamento in Cardiologia, Centro De Gasperis, Milano, L Pozzi, 381, 1980
18. Mancia G, Baccelli G, Zanchetti A: Vasomotor regulation during sleep in the cat. Am J Physiol 220: 1086, 1971
19. Mancia G, Ferrari A, Gregorini L, Parati G, Pomidossi G, Bertinieri G, Grassi G, Zanchetti A: Arterial blood pressure variability in man: its relation to high blood pressure, age and baroreflex sensitivity. Clin Sci, 59, 401s, 1980

20. Mancia G, Ferrari A, Gregorini L, Parati G, Pomidossi G, Zanchetti A: Prolonged intra-arterial blood pressure recording in the diagnosis of pheochromocytoma. Lancet 2: 1193, 1979
21. Mancia G, Zanchetti A: Arterial blood pressure recording in human hypertension: a methodological approach. Atherosclerotic Rev 7: 247, 1980
22. Mancia G, Zanchetti A: Cardiovascular regulation during sleep. In: Orem and Barnes (eds), Physiology of sleep, Academic Press, New York, 1, 1980
23. Millar-Craig MW, Bishop CN, Raftery EB: Circadian variation in blood pressure. Lancet 2: 795, 1978
24. Raftery EB: Hypertension day by day. The Practitioner 223: 166, 1979
25. Riva Rocci S: Un nuovo sfigmomanometro. Gazz Med Torino 47: 981, 1896
26. Rowlands DB, Shallard TJ, Watson RDS, Littler WA: The influence of physical activity on arterial pressure during ambulatory recordings in man. Clin Sci 58: 115, 1980
27. Sokolow M, Werdegar D, Kain HK, Hinman AT: Relationship between level of blood pressure measured casually and by portable recorders and severity of complications in essential hypertension. Circulation 34: 279, 1966

19. ROLE OF VASOPRESSIN IN BLOOD PRESSURE REGULATION
THROUGH ITS MODULATORY EFFECT ON BARORECEPTOR
REFLEX

YUTAKI IMAI, PETER L. NOLAN, COLIN I. JOHNSTON

INTRODUCTION

Both the antidiuretic (volume) and vasoconstrictor (pressor) action of vasopressin can be considered as important biological properties in maintaining blood
pressure [12]. These physiological effects are mediated by two different types of
receptors; renal receptors coupled to adenylate cyclase mediating antidiuretic
action, and vascular receptors coupled to a calcium dependent mechanism mediating vasoconstriction. The pressor action of vasopressin, previously thought to
be a pharmacological effect, has recently been shown to be physiologically
important in blood pressure homeostasis [20, 12]. Vasopressin was shown *in vitro*
to be the most powerful vasoconstrictor agent known, more potent even than
angiotensin [2]. Low infusion rates of vasopressin which produce plasma levels
that are close to the physiologic range can elevate blood pressure [33, 27]. Several
authors have recently provided evidence that vasopressin plays a crucial and
quantitative role in maintaining blood pressure after haemorrhage [15, 10] or
dehydration [1, 3]. Furthermore the vasoconstrictor properties of vasopressin
have been considered to be important in the pathophysiology of various forms of
experimental hypertension [12]. However, elevation of the blood pressure by
vasopressin *in vivo* is limited by secondary compensatory mechanisms, including
a direct negative chronotropic effect, modulation of the baroreceptor reflex, the
modulation of autonomic nervous system and inhibition of renin release from the
kidney by the vasopressin. Thus, vasopressin can influence blood pressure by
several different mechanisms including an action on the central nervous system,
modulation of the baroreceptor reflex or by potentiating the action of the
sympathetic nervous system, catecholamines and other vasoactive hormones as
well as direct vasoconstriction of the vasculature.

This review will present evidence and discuss the modulatory effect of vasopressin on the baroreceptor reflex. Elimination of the baroreflex buffering
mechanisms remarkably potentiates the pressor response to vasopressin [9, 27].
Furthermore the pressor response to vasopressin is augmented more than to
phenylephrine or norepinephrine after elimination of baroreflex buffering [9, 18].
It has also recently been reported that even small elevations in plasma vasopressin
can cause considerable bradycardia without a change in arterial pressure [12, 21].

Sambhi, M.P. (ed.) Fundamental fault in hypertension
© *1984, Martinus Nijhoff Publishers. Boston/The Hague/Dordrecht/Lancaster.*
ISBN 978-94-010-9006-3

Möhring et al. [21] also suggested that heart rate fell more for a given increase in arterial pressure during infusion of vasopressin than during an infusion of phenylephrine or norepinephrine. These results imply that vasopressin specifically modulates the baroreflex pathway and that even under normal conditions, endogenous vasopressin may have a circulatory effect through a baroreflex mechanism. Recent evidence suggests that vasopressin may also act centrally to alter the function of the baroreflex [5, 8, 4, 19] and that cardiovascular reflex activity is specifically enhanced during an infusion of vasopressin [21]. These reports all suggest that endogenous vasopressin may participate in the control of baroreflex in physiological and pathophysiological conditions.

In the present study the role of vasopressin in influencing the baroreflex mechanism has been examined by comparing baroreflex function in Brattleboro rats (DI rat) with that in the Long-Evans rats (LE rats). The homozygous Brattleboro rat has a genetic total deficiency in vasopressin with hypothalamic diabetes insipidus. It thus provides a good model to quantitate the cardiovascular role of vasopressin. As a result, we observed that the reflex bradycardia caused by pressor stimuli in DI rats was remarkably suppressed when compared to control LE rat. To evaluate the mechanism of the suppressed baroreflex sensitivity in DI rats, we have examined the modulation of baroreflex function by vasopressin administered intravenously (i.v.) or intracerebroventricularly (i.c.v.). We have also compared the heart rate response in LE and DI rats to stimulation of the parasympathetic nervous system caused by pathophysiological and pharmacological manoeuvers between LE and DI rats.

COMPARISON OF BAROREFLEX SENSITIVITY BETWEEN LE AND DI RATS

Male homozygous brattleboro rats (DI rat; 23.8 ± 1.2 weeks) and male Long-Evans rats (LE rats 26.5 ± 1.2 weeks) of 200–400 g were used.

Baroreflex function was assessed in conscious unrestrained rats by pharmacological increases of blood pressure with phenylephrine (200 μg/kg min^{-1} for 10 seconds) according to the method of [31]. The slope of the baroreflex function line was used as baroreflex sensitivity and expressed as follows : Slope $= \Delta \log$ PP/ΔSBP, where PP is pulse period (msec) and SBP is systolic blood pressure (mmHg).

As shown in Figure 1, the baroreflex sensitivity in LE rats [$(19.0 \pm 1.4) \times 10^{-4}$] was significantly higher than that in DI rats [$(6.9 \pm 0.6) \times 10^{-4}$, $p < 0.001$]. Thus, for any given rise in blood pressure, there is less bradycardia seen in DI rats than LE rats.

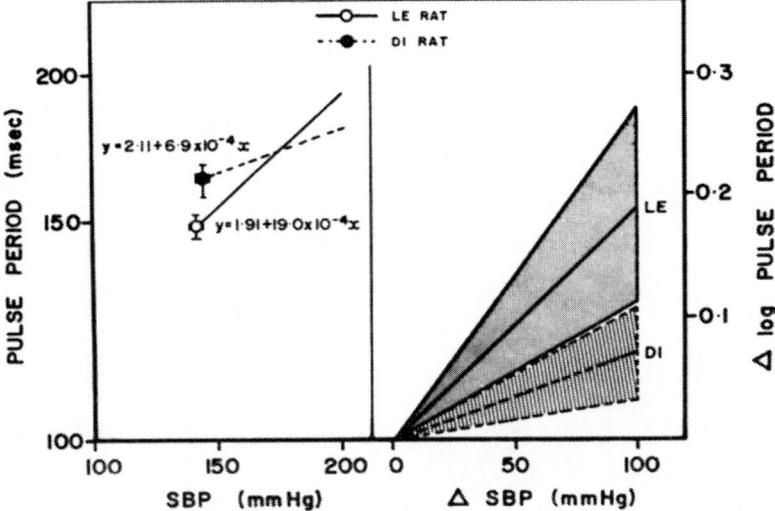

Figure 1. The baroreflex sensitivity in Long-Evans rats (LE: ○) and Brattlevoro rats with hereditary hypothalamic diabetes insipidus (DI: ●). Baroreflex sensitivity is expressed as the slope of baroreflex function line, ΔlogPP/ΔSBP, where PP is pulse period (msec) and SBP is systolic blood pressure (mmHg).

EFFECT OF INTRAVENOUS (I.V.) OR INTRACEREBROVENTRICULAR (I.C.V.) VASOPRESSIN ON BAROREFLEX SENSITIVITY

Effect of i.v. vasopressin

To determine whether the suppressed baroreflex function in DI rats was due to the specific loss of vasopressin, baroreflex function was reassessed in DI rats during an infusion of exogenous vasopressin.

The baroreflex function was examined in 9 DI rats before and during i.v. infusion of arginine[8]-vasopressin (AVP, Calbiochem, n = 7). After establishing a control baroreflex function line, a subpressor dose of AVP was infused at a rate of $2n$/kg min^{-1} for 2 hr and the baroreflex function was re-examined during these infusions.

Alternatively the baroreflex function was examined in 14 DI rats before and during i.c.v. infusion of AVP. Cerebroventricular cannulae were implanted chronically into the left lateral ventricle with the aid of a stereotaxic instrument. After establishing a control baroreflex function line, AVP was infused i.c.v. at a rate of 2 ng/kg min^{-1} in a volume of 1.4 μl/min for 1 hr and the baroreflex function was re-examined during these infusions.

Arginine-vasopressin infused i.v. at a rate of 2 ng/kg min^{-1} for 2 hrs did not significantly change the mean arterial pressure (98 ± 3 vs 101 ± 2 mmHg). However, it did significantly prolong the pulse period (165 ± 9 vs 183 ± 11 msec, $p < 0.01$). DI rats had no measurable vasopressin in their plasma. The AVP infusion, $2\,\text{ng/kg min}^{-1}$, produced a plasma AVP level of $48.1 \pm 6.8\,\text{pg/ml}$ after two hrs in DI rats. Figure 2 (left) shows the baroreflex sensitivity before and during i.v. infusion of AVP. The baroreflex sensitivity during AVP infusion $[(17.0 \pm 0.8) \times 10^{-4}]$ was significantly higher than that before AVP infusion $[(7.5 \pm 1.0) \times 10^{-4}, p < 0.001]$. During AVP infusion the baroreflex sensitivity fell within the range of mean $\pm 1\text{SD}$ to that found in LE rats.

Effect of i.c.v. vasopressin

Intracerebroventricular infusion of saline vehicle alone did not cause any cardiohaemodynamic changes. Vasopressin infused i.c.v. at a rate of $2\,\text{ng/kg min}^{-1}$ caused transient hypertension and tachycardia from $101 \pm 5\,\text{mmHg}$ and 186 ± 10 msec to $115 \pm 8\,\text{mmHg}$ ($p < 0.05$) and 148 ± 8 msec ($p < 0.01$), respectively. One hour after infusion, both parameters returned to the initial levels ($104 \pm 8\,\text{mmHg}$ and 182 ± 9 msec, respectively).

Figure 2 (right) shows the modification of baroreflex sensitivity by i.c.v. infusion of AVP. Baroreflex sensitivity during AVP infusion $[(13.3 \pm 1.9) \times 10^{-4}]$ was significantly higher than that before infusion $[(8.5 \pm 1.0) \times 10^{-4}, n = 14, p < 0.01]$. However, the baroreflex sensitivity during i.c.v. infusion of AVP was significantly lower than that during i.v. infusion of AVP. DI rats had no measurable plasma vasopressin after one hour infusion. Centrally administered AVP, therefore, did not leak into the periphery at this infusion rate. Infusion of saline vehicle alone did not affect baroreflex sensitivity $[(8.5 \pm 1.0) \times 10^{-4}$ vs $(9.0 \pm 1,1) \times 10^{-4}]$.

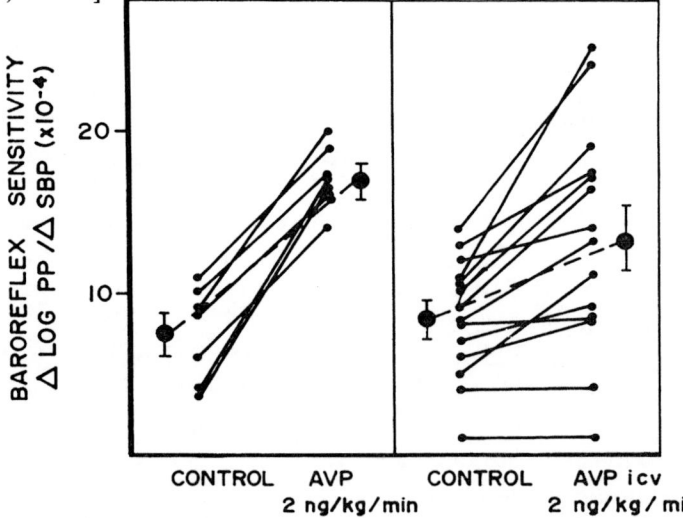

Figure 2. Modification of baroreflex sensitivity by intravenous infusion of vasopressin (left panel) and intracerebroventricular (i.c.v.) infusion of vasopressin (right panel) in DI rats. Remainings are the same as Figure 1.

EFFECT OF ATROPINE ON BAROREFLEX FUNCTION IN LE AN DI RATS

To determine the parasympathetic contribution to the baroreflex function in rats, the effect of atropine was examined in 6 LE and 6 DI rats. After testing the control baroreflex function, 1 mg/kg of atropine sulphate (David-Bull Laboratories) was injected intravenously. Fifteen minutes later, baroreflex function was re-examined.

Atropine significantly shortened the resting pulse period both in LE (163 ± 8 to 125 ± 4 msec, p<0.01) and DI rats (166 ± 6 to 129 ± 3 msec, p<0.01) but did not affect mean arterial pressure.

Atropine nearly abolished the baroreflex function slope in both LE [(18.0 ± 2.1) × 10^{-4} to (1.0 ± 0.3) × 10^{-4}, p<0.001] and DI rats [(6.3 ± 1.3) × 10^{-4} to (0.8 ± 0.3) × 10^{-4}, p<0.001].

THE DIFFERENCE OF CARDIAC RESPONSE AGAINST RAPID HAEMORRHAGE BETWEEN LE AND DI RATS

Haemorrhage in rats is often associated with bradycardia despite a fall in blood pressure. This bradycardia in mainly due to a result of increase in central parasympathetic tone [7, 24]. To see whether this bradycardia could also involve vasopressinergic pathways haemorrhage was studied in DI rats.

The cardiac response against rapid haemorrhage was examined in 6 LE and 5 DI rats. The blood was withdrawn from the arterial catheter at a rate of 1 ml/100 g within 30 sec. The pulse period one minute after the start of haemorrhage was compared between LE and DI rats.

There was no difference in pulse period between LE (159 ± 5 msec) and DI rat (154 ± 4 msec) in the control period. One minute after the start of haemorrhage, pulse period prolonged in both strains of rat. Prolongation of pulse period in LE rat (93.7 ± 21.7 msec) was significantly greater than that in DI rat (11.4 ±6.1 msec, p<0.02).

INTERACTION OF THE SYMPATHETIC NERVOUS SYSTEM AND CENTRAL VASOPRESSINERGIC SYSTEM. STUDIES WITH CLONIDINE

Clonidine administered i.v. or i.c.v. causes bradycardia. This bradycardia is mainly mediated by stimulation of parasympathetic nervous system [30, 14]. The bradycardic effects of clonidine were compared between LE (i.v. n = 12, i.c.v. n = 17) and DI (i.v. n = 12, i.c.v. n = 7) rats. Clonidine at a rate of 30 μg/kg was injected i.v. or i.c.v. The change in pulse period was examined 5 and 10 min after administration of clonidine.

In the other series of experiments, cardiac response against i.c.v. clonidine

($30\,\mu$g/kg) was examined with and without i.v. infusion of subpressor dose of AVP in DI rats. At least 24 hr after establishing the control experiment, a subpressor dose of AVP at a rate of $2\,$ng/kg min^{-1} was infused intravenously. One hour after the start of infusion, clonidine was injected again i.c.v. and cardiac response was re-examined.

Effect of i.v. clonidine

The pulse period in the control period was not significantly different between LE and DI rats (167 ± 5 vs $160 \pm 3\,$msec). As shown in Figure 3 (left), 5 and 10 min after i.v. administration of clonidine, pulse period prolonged significantly in LE rats. However clonidine did not cause significant change in the pulse period in DI rats. Thus i.v. clonidine did not cause bradycardia in DI rats, whereas it caused significant bradycardia in LE rats.

Effect of i.c.v. clonidine

As shown in Figure 3 (middle), 5 and 10 min after i.c.v. administration of clonidine, pulse period prolonged significantly both in LE and DI rats. However, prolongation of pulse period in DI rats was significantly less than that in LE rats at both times.

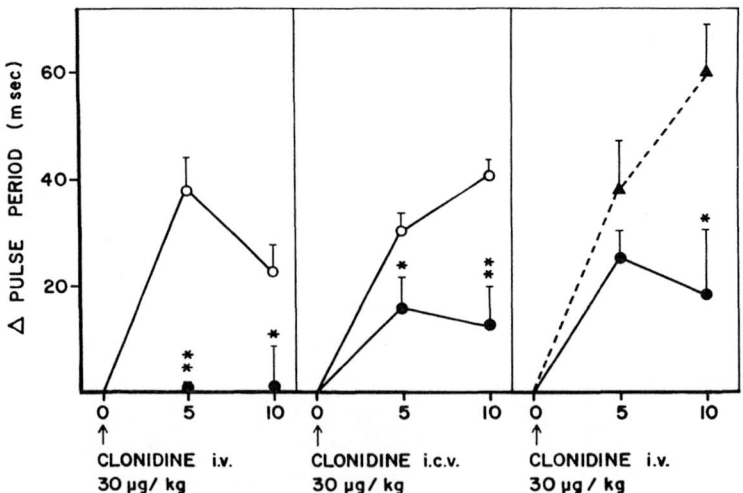

Figure 3. Difference of bradycardic response to clonidine administered intravenously (i.v.) (left panel) and intracerebroventricularly (i.c.v.) (middle panel) between LE and DI rats, and its modification by exogenous vasopressin in DI rat (right panel).
  ○: LE rats, ●: DI rats
  Dotted line: during vasopressin infusion in DI rats
  * $p<0.05$, * * $p<0.01$

Modification of cardiac effect of i.c.v. clonidine by vasopressin in DI rats.

Although vasopressin infused for 2 hr did not change the basal mean arterial pressure, the basal pulse period was prolonged significantly by vasopressin infusion from 168 ± 5 msec to 181 ± 2 msec ($p \pm 0.05$). As shown in Figure 3 (right) the bradycardic effect of i.c.v. clonidine was greatly potentiated during vasopressin infusion.

DISCUSSION

The present studies show that in Brattleboro rat with hereditary hypothalamic diabetes insipidus and completely lacking endogenous vasopressin, baroreflex sensitivity is greatly suppressed and bradycardia mediated by the parasympathetic nervous system is less when compared to that in normal Long-Evans rats.

Heart rate change in response to transient increases in arterial pressure depends mainly upon the vagus nerve [36, 29, 34, 25]. Bradycardia caused by clonidine is also mediated by stimulation of parasympathetic nervous system [30, 14]. In addition several authors have reported that the heart rate lowering effect following rapid haemorrhage in the rat is abolished by vagotomy [7, 24] indicating a parasympathetic contribution to the bradycardia. In the present study, atropine completely abolished the reflex bradycardia induced by pressor stimuli both in LE and DI rats. Furthermore it was shown that baroreflex sensitivity and bradycardic response to clonidine and haemorrhage in DI rats are significantly less than in LE rats, suggesting a suppressed response of parasympathetic nervous system against stimulation. Intravenous administration of AVP at a subpressor rate, which achieved plasma levels within the physiological range, resulted in bradycardia and restored baroreflex sensitivity. Such a dose of vasopressin also potentiated the bradycardic response to clonidine in DI rats.

There is now considerable evidence that vasopressin acts within the central nervous system to affect vasomotor regulatory mechanism [35, 5, 8, 19]. In this context i.c.v. administration of AVP also restored the baroreflex sensitivity in DI rats without leaking to the periphery. Izdebska et al. [11] also reported that i.c.v. injection of lysine-vasopressin into the anaesthetized rats enhanced reflex bradycardia induced by a blood pressure rise. Such an effect is mimicked by vasopressin administered intravenously, as shown in the present study, suggesting that restoration of baroreflex sensitivity and potentiation of bradycardic response to clonidine by i.v. vasopressin is probably mediated by its central action. However, it is interesting that AVP infused i.v. was more effective on restoration of baroreflex sensitivity than that infused i.c.v. This suggests that peripheral as well as central pathways of the baroreflex could be modulated by vasopressin. It has been reported that local application of a variety of drugs to the carotid sinus, or stimulation of sympathetic fibres innervating the sinus wall, results in a fall in blood pressure through stimulation of the afferent limb of the reflex [13]. Although the effect of vasopressin on the baroreflex afferent pathway has not yet been studied, the possibility remains that vasopressin may also modulate the baroreflex function via this route.

It is widely recognized that systemic administration of vasopressin causes considerable bradycardia in various species of animals. Since a direct chronotropic effect of vasopressin is observed only when pharmacological doses of vasopressin are administered [23], the chronotropic effect of vasopressin in low concentration must be due to an indirect action mediated by the autonomic nervous system and/or baroreceptor reflex [22]. In the present study we also observed that intravenous infusion of AVP resulted in bradycardia. On the contrary, the same dose of AVP caused tachycardia when administered centrally. Tachycardia mediated by a central effect of AVP in rats was also reported by Matsuguchi et al. [19] who injected AVP into the nucleus tractus solitarius. Such results indicate that the cardiovascular effects of centrally administered vasopressin are different from those observed after i.v. administration at least in the rat. There are now several pieces of evidence that vasopressin administered peripherally can act in the central nervous system [16, 17, 37]. However, it is difficult to postulate which part of the central loci of the baro reflex pathways may be affected by i.v. administration of vasopressin. Since vasopressin may act at several loci within the central nervous system, the discrepancy of cardiovascular effect of vasopressin via administration routes may be due to the precise anatomical site of action in the central nervous system.

Recent anatomical studies support the notion of an interaction between vasopressin and central cardiovascular control centres. Extra-hypothalamic projection of pituitary vasopressinergic neuron to some of the central cardiovascular regulatory center have been described [28, 6, 32]. Centrally·administered AVP caused transient tachycardia, while it also restored to suppressed baroreflex sensitivity in DI rats. This suggests the existence of differential pools of vasopressinergic neurones which are responsible for different functions of cardiovascular control. There is some controversy regarding the central effect of vasopressin on cardiovascular control mechanism. The discrepancy may be due to species, anaesthesia and precise antomical site of action [35, 5, 8, 4, 11, 19, 26].

In conclusion, endogenous vasopressin makes an important contribution to the homeostasis of cardiohaemodynamics through the maintenance of baroreflex function. The maintenance of baroreflex function by AVP is mainly mediated by the parasympathetic nervous system through its modulatory action on baroreflex pathway, both centrally and peripherally.

ACKNOWLEDGEMENTS

This study was supported by grant-in-aid from the National Health and Medical

Research Council of Australia and the Australian Kidney Foundation of Australia. The expert technical assistance of J. Abrahams in measuring the plasma vasopressin is gratefully acknowledged.

REFERENCES

1. Aisenbrey GA, Handelman WA, Arnold P, Manning M, Schrier RA: Vascular effects of arginine vasopressin during fluid deprivation in the rat. J Clin Invest 67: 961–968, 1981
2. Altura BM, Altura BT: Vascular smooth muscle and neurohypophyseal hormones. Fed Proc 36: 1853–1860, 1977
3. Andrews, CEJr, Brenner BM: Relative contributions of arginine vasopressin and angiotensin II to maintenance of systemic arterial pressure in the anaesthetized water-deprived rat. Circ Res 48: 254–258, 1981
4. Berecek KH, Webb RL, Barron KW, Brody MJ: Vasopressin projections and central control of cardiovascular function. Ann NY Acad Sci 394: 729–734, 1982
5. Brattström A, Kalkoff W: Der Einfluss intracisternal applizierten Vasopressins auf Höhe und Einstellung des arteriellen Druckes. Arch Int Pharmacodyn 183: 190–198, 1970
6. Buijs RM, Swaab DF, Dogterom J, Van Leeuwen FW: Intra- and extrahypothalamic vasopressin and oxytocin pathways in the rat. Cell tissue Res 186: 423–433, 1978
7. Castenfors J, Sjöstrand T: Circulatory control via vagal afferents. Acta Physisol Scand 84: 347–354, 1972
8. Ciriello J, Calaresu FR: Role of paraventricular and supraoptic nuclei in central cardiovascular regulation in the cat. AM J Physiol 239: R137–R142, 1980
9. Cowley AWJr, Monos E, Guyton AC: Interaction of vasopressin and the baroreceptor reflex system in the regulation of arterial blood pressure in the dog. Circ Res 34: 505–514, 1974
10. Cowley AW Jr, Switzer SJ, Guinn MM: Evidence and quantification of the vasopressin arterial pressure control system in the dog. Circ Res 46: 58–67, 1980
11. Izdebska E, Jodkowski J, Trzebski A: Central influence of vasopressin on baroreceptor reflex in normotensive rats and its lack of spontaneously hypertensive rats (SHR). Experientia 38: 594–595, 1982.
12. Johnston CI, Newman M, Woods RL: Role of vasopressin in cardiovascular homeostasis and hypertension. Clin Sci 61: 129s–139s, 1981
13. Kirchheim HR: Systemic arterial baroreceptor reflexes. Physiol Rev 56: 100–176, 1976
14. Kobinger W: Central α-adrenergic systems as targets for hypotensive drugs. Rev Physiol Biochem Pharmacol 81: 39–100, 1978
15. Laycock JF, Penn W, Shirley DG, Walter SJ: The role of vasopressin in blood pressure regulation immediately following acute haemorrhage in the rat. J Physiol 296: 267–275, 1979
16. LeMoal M, Koob GF, Koda LY, Bloom FE, Mannin M, Sawyer WH, Rivier J: Vasopressor receptor antagonist prevents behavioural effects of vasopressin. Nature 291–491–493, 1981
17. Liard JF, Deriaz O, Tschopp M, Schoun J: Cardiovascular effects of vasopressin infused into the vertebral circulation of conscious dogs. Clin Sci 61: 345–347, 1981
18. Matsuguchi H, Schmid PG: Pressor response to vasopressin and impaired baroreflex function in DOC-salt hypertension. Am J Physiol 242:H44–H49, 1982
19. Matsuguchi H, Sharabi FM, Gordon FJ, Johnson AK, Schmid PG: Blood pressure

and heart rate responses to microinjection of vasopressin into the nucleus tractus solitarius region of the rat. Neuropharmacology 21: 687–693, 1982

20. Möhring J, Arbogast R, Dusting R, Glanzer K, Kintz J, Liard J-F, Maciel JAJr, Montani JP, Shoun J: Vasopressor role of vasopressin in hypertension. In: Wuttkew, Weindl A, Voigt KH, Dreis RR. (eds), Brain and Peptides, Fierring Symposium, Munich 1979, Karger, Basel, 1980, pp 157–167
21. Möhring J, Kintz J, Schoun J, McNeill JR: Pressor responsiveness and cardiovascular reflex activity in spontaneously hypertensive and normotensive rats during vasopressin infusion. J Cardiovasc Pharmacol 3: 948–957, 1981
22. Nakano J: Cardiovascular responses to neurohypophysial hormones. In: Knobil E, Sawyer WH (eds), Handbook of Physiology, Section 7, Endocrinology, vol 4, American Physiol Soc, Washington DC, 1974, pp 395–468
23. Nakashima A, Angus J, Johnston CI: Chronotropic effects of angiotensin I, angiotensin II, bradykinin and vasopressin in guinea pig atria. Eur J Pharmacol 81: 479–485, 1982
24. Pendleton RG, McCafferty JP, Roesler JH: The effects of PNMT inhibitors upon the cardiovascular changes induced by haemorrhage in the rat. Eur J Pharmacol 66: 1–10, 1980
25. Pickering TG, Gribbin B, Petersen ES, Cunningham DJC, Sleight P: Effects of autonomic blockade on the baroreflex in man at rest and during exercise. Circ Res 30: 177–185, 1972
26. Pittman QJ, Lawrence D, McLean LC: Central effect of vasopressin on blood pressure in rats. Endocrinology 110: 1058–1060, 1982
27. Pullan PT, Johnston CI, Anderson WP, Korner PI: Plasma vasopressin in blood pressure homeostasis and in experimental renal hypertension. Am J Physiol 239: H81–H87, 1980
28. Saper CB, Loewy AD, Swanson LW, Cowan WM: Direct hypothalamo-autonomic connections. Brain Res 117: 305–312, 1976
29. Scher AM, Young AC: Reflex control of heart rate in the unanaesthetized dog. Am J Physiol 218: 780–789, 1970
30. Schmitt H: The pharmacology of clonidine and related products. In: Gross H. (ed), Handbook of Experimental Pharmacology Vol 39, Springer-Verlag, Berlin, Heidelberg, New York, 1977, pp 299–296
31. Smyth HS, Sleight P, Pickering GW: Reflex regulation of arterial pressure during sleep in man. Circ Res 24: 109–121, 1969
32. Sofroniew MV: Projections from vasopressin, oxytocin and neurophysin neurons to neural targets in the rat and human. J Histochem Cytochem 28: 475–478, 1980
33. Szczepanska-Sadowska E: Hemodynamic effects of a moderate increase of the plasma vasopressin level in conscious dogs. Pflügers Arch 338: 313–322, 1973
34. Thames MD, Kontos HA: Mechanisms of baroreceptor-induced changes in heart rate. Am J Physiol 218: 251–256, 1970
35. Varma S, Jaju BP, Bhargava KP: Mechanism of vasopressin-induced bradycardia in dogs. Circ Res 24: 787–792, 1969
36. Warner HR, Cox A: A mathematical model of heart rate control by sympathetic and vagus efferent information. J Appl Physiol 17: 349–355, 1962
37. Weingartner H, Gold P, Ballenger JC, Smallberg SA, Summers R, Rubinow DR, Post RM, Goodwin A: Effects of vasopressin on human memory functions. Science 211: 601–603, 1981

VII. ALTERED HEMODYNAMICS: A CAUSE OR A CONSEQUENCE?

20. CONTROVERSIES IN THE RESEARCH ON HEMODYNAMIC
    MECHANISMS IN THE DEVELOPMENT OF HYPERTENSION

STEVO JULIUS

Regardless of the underlying cause or causes, a permanent elevation of blood
pressure must, by definition, represent a derangement of homeostatic mechanisms that under ordinary conditions maintain normotension. Two major hypotheses have been proposed to explain the events that lead to established hypertension. The first presumes that hypertension develops as a summation of repeated
pressor episodes, the other that hypertension stems from a failure of counter-
regulatory mechanisms that tend to restore normality to temporary blood pressure elevations. Both of these concepts are plausible and are supported by animal
experimentation, but their applicability to human essential hypertension is still
conjectural. In this presentation I will outline some problems with both of these
concepts and then present our data, which lend themselves to yet another
interpretation of the chain of events leading to the development of hypertension.

HYPERTENSION VIEWED AS ENHANCED POSITIVE FEEDBACK

According to this concept, best represented by works from Folkow's laboratory
[12], repeated pressor episodes lead to arteriolar medial hypertrophy and to
changes in the wall-to-lumen ratio. Increased wall-to-lumen ratio renders blood
vessels more responsive to pressor stimuli and sets in motion a positive feedback
for further increases in vascular hypertrophy and in pressor responsiveness. Over
a period of time, this leads to inevitable acceleration of hypertension. Based on
this view, one would expect patients destined to develop hypertension to either a)
show increased pressor responsiveness to naturally occurring pressor stimuli, or
b) have a history of more frequent exposure to such stimuli. On the whole, the
evidence for increased pressor responsiveness in the early phases of hypertension
is negative. Blood pressure variability is not increased in patients with mild and
borderline hypertension [23]. Blood pressure responses to dynamic [20, 31, 37]
and static [38] exercise are similar in patients with borderline hypertension and in
normotensive subjects. Blood volume expansion elicits similar modest blood
pressure elevations in patients with borderline hypertension as in normotensive
subjects [27, 31]. In spite of the original claim by Hines and Brown [18], blood
pressure responses to the cold pressor test are not increased in patients with

Sambhi, M.P. (ed.) Fundamental fault in hypertension
© *1984, Martinus Nijhoff Publishers. Boston/The Hague/Dordrecht/Lancaster.*
ISBN 978-94-010-9006-3

264

borderline hypertension [7, 16, 48]. Some patients with borderline hypertension may be hyperresponsive to tilting. Whereas we could not find such a hyperresponsiveness [39], excessive blood pressure responses to orthostasis have been reported by others [13, 19]. Borderline hypertension is considered to be a precursor of future hypertension, but there is no evidence that these patients typically have a tendency for increased pressor responses. The lack of a propensity for blood pressure hyperresponsiveness is reflected in the absence of increased spontaneous blood pressure variability in borderline hypertension [23]. It is therefore unlikely that in human essential hypertension an innate tendency to overrespond to pressor stimuli leads to frequent transient blood pressure elevations which then cause medial arteriolar hypertrophy, eventually leading to established, accelerated hypertension.

The other possibility, that patients with a tendency toward hypertension respond normally but are exposed to more frequent pressor stimuli, must also be considered. It has been reported that patients with borderline hypertension may be hyperresponsive to mental stress [32]. In a recent study, Falkner et al. [10] found hyperresponsiveness to mental stress to be characteristic for normotensive and hypertensive children of hypertensive parents. Personality tests given to patients with borderline and mild hypertension tend to show a distinct personality characterized by submissiveness and suppressed hostility combined with a need to be socially active and accepted [8, 15]. One could easily construe that such a personality leads to conflict and to repeated pressor episodes. As indicated earlier, however, the overall blood pressure variability in borderline hypertension appears to be normal. This could happen if the increased variability were present only in a minority of patients with borderline hypertension – those with a specific personality type [15]. An equally plausible alternative is that characteristic personality traits in borderline hypertension are not associated with paroxysmal blood pressure elevation but are characterized by a state of persistent intense alertness, a continuous mental 'engagement' that leads to chronic elevation of the sympathetic tone and a slow increase in blood pressure. This possibility will be discussed later.

HYPERTENSION VIEWED AS DERANGEMENT IN THE NEGATIVE FEEDBACK

Guyton and Coleman [14] have developed a model of evolution for hypertension that experimentally supports and gives a detailed qualitative assessment of principles set out by Borst and Borst-de Geus [1]. Basic to this concept is the notion that the average pressure levels are controlled by powerful negative feedback mechanisms, of which the kidney is most important. Under normal circumstances, an increase in blood pressure will cause enhanced diuresis; this will decrease the blood volume and thereby the blood pressure will return to usual levels. The gain of this negative feedback is linear and infinite, so that the kidneys possess the capacity to respond with diuresis, normalizing the blood pressure across a wide range of elevations. Hypertension develops if the threshold for the renal pressure diuresis is increased and a higher pressure is required to attune the volume to the blood pressure. If the renal threshold is increased, a volume expansion and an increase of the cardiac output ensues. The high output triggers an autoregulatory increase in vascular resistance and in blood pressure through the longterm 'total body autoregulation.' The time constant of these processes in humans is not known. Coleman et al. [2] have shown that in anephric humans autoregulation of the cardiac output during volume expansion occurs within a week. Onesti et al. [33], however, suggest that the time may be rather variable. Some of their volume-expanded normotensive anephric patients failed to increase the vascular resistance. Previously hypertensive anephric patients, equally volume-expanded, and observed over the same period of time, did respond with a high resistance.

These studies are not fully informative, but they suggest that the phase of volume expansion prior to normalization of the cardiac output may last a variable amount of time and could in some instances be rather lengthy. It is therefore reasonable to assume that, at least in some subjects destined to have hypertension, one may find volume expansion and elevation of the cardiac output. In a study employing a large number of subjects with borderline hypertension [25], however, we could not find a single patient with expanded blood volume; the majority had decreased blood and plasma volumes. I realize that measurement of the blood volume per se is not fully satisfactory: these patients may have a 'relative' hypervolemia if their capacitance space is reduced. A redistribution of blood from the peripheral to the central portion of the capacity space has been reported in borderline hypertension [36, 46], but this occurs in a minority of patients, at best in 30% overall. These patients may indeed have an expansion of the blood volume in relation to the restricted capacity. Thus, the human data are only partially supportive for a phase of volume expansion in early hypertension. Absolute expansion of the blood volume is never found, and a relative expansion may exist in a minority of patients with borderline hypertension [9]. These patients with a relative volume expansion have a higher cardiac output and conform to the sequence of events as described by Guyton's group. The sequence, however, apparently does not conform with a primary fluid and volume retention, as suggested by Borst and Borst-de Geus [1]; rather, a primary restriction in the venous capacity may be responsible for a relative hypervolemia.

Whereas the absence of absolute volume expansion in early phases of hypertension leaves a number of questions unanswered, it is even more difficult to find data supportive of the cornerstone of Guyton's concept for the development of hypertension, i.e., the increased renal threshold for pressure diuresis. To be sure, the basic experiment has never been performed in human beings, and in view of increasing restrictions placed upon invasive experimentation, it is not likely that this will ever be accomplished. Nevertheless, the existing body of evidence clearly shows that, in response to volume load, patients with hypertension and prehypertension excrete more urine than normotensive control subjects [4]. This apparent discrepancy is often explained as a consequence of the high blood pressure: the diuresis is higher because the pressure is higher. This argument is acceptable only if blood pressure *changes* after volume expansion are larger in hypertensive subjects. After a careful review of the literature, I am satisfied that there is no evidence whatsoever that patients with hypertension have larger blood pressure increases, either during or after volume expansion. The case is particularly convincing in borderline hypertension, where the blood pressure levels are lowest, so that a primary abnormality of volume excretion should be easier to demonstrate. Cottier et al. [4] found excessive diuresis but a normal blood pressure increase during volume expansion. Their work did not focus on precise blood pressure measurements, but later precise determinations of intraarterial blood pressure by Lund-Johansen [31] and by ourselves [27] confirmed that the blood pressure increase to acute volume expansion in borderline hypertension is normal.

SEQUENCE OF EVENTS IN THE DEVELOPMENT OF HYPERTENSION: A VIEW BASED ON HUMAN EXPERIMENTS

It is not my purpose to construct a full alternative concept of the development of hypertension. Rather, I would like to review our data and point out that some major assumptions of both theories of the development of hypertension cannot be demonstrated in patients with borderline hypertension who, we believe, are in the early developmental stage of hypertension. It will be shown that data on these patients allow postulation of an alternative sequence of events in the development of human hypertension. I will limit the discussion to patients with 'hyperkinetic' borderline hypertension. No claim will be made that the proposed sequence also occurs in all other patients with borderline hypertension. Our data support the feasibility of the hypothesis, but the experiments to test the hypothesis have not been designed.

There is very good evidence that the hyperkinetic state in borderline hypertension is neurogenic [8, 21]. The hypothesis is that a *tonic* increase in sympathetic discharge sets into motion processes that lead to conversion from 'hyperkinetic borderline' to 'normokinetic established' hypertension without excessive pressor episodes, without volume expansion, and without an autoregulatory return of the cardiac output to the normal range. The hypothesis assumes that steady sympathetic stimulation leads to decreased cardiac but increased arteriolar responsiveness, so that eventually the cardiac output decreases and vascular resistance increases. We postulate that excessive sympathetic stimulation ultimately leads to decreased responsiveness of adrenergic receptors. In the heart, the decreased beta-adrenergic responsiveness combines with structural changes to decrease the cardiac output, returning it to the normal range. In the arterioles, the decreased receptor sensitivity is offset by the ensuing structural alteration of the wall-to-lumen ratio. The result is a positive feedback of ever-increasing vascular responsiveness to sympathetic stimulation.

To support the feasibility of this concept, one must show that a) hyperkinetic borderline hypertension evolves into a normal cardiac output established hypertension, b) that patients with borderline hypertension have an increased sympathetic tone, c) that classic autoregulation of the increased cardiac output does not occur in human beings, and d) that the cardiac responsiveness is decreased and the vascular responsiveness is increased in borderline hypertension.

Does hyperkinetic borderline hypertension lead to 'normokinetic' hypertension?

Whereas it is generally known that patients with borderline hypertension tend to develop later established hypertension more than the general population, the incidence of future hypertension among patients with borderline hypertension is not overwhelming; the majority will remain normotensive [23]. It is therefore appropriate to ask whether patients with hyperkinetic borderline hypertension are particularly prone to develop later hypertension. The question is not fully answered, but a few lines of evidence suggest that the hyperkinetic state may be a precursor of hypertension. Faster heart rates are associated with higher blood pressure values in population studies [35, 40, 41]. Furthermore, in longitudinal studies, a faster heart rate at youth predicts the future development of hypertension [30, 34, 43, 47]. This predictive effect is independent of the blood pressure. When subjects with normal blood pressure and tachycardia are compared to those with normal blood pressure and a normal heart rate, those with the faster heart rate develop twice the rate of later hypertension. If tachycardia is combined with mild hypertension, the risk of future hypertension is four times greater than in normotensive-normal heart rate subjects [30]. Longitudinal hemodymamic data are available on only two sparsely populated studies; when patients developed hypertension the cardiac output and heart rate decreased [6, 49]. Cross-sectional data in hemodynamic laboratories also support the notion of transition from a hyperkinetic to a normokinetic state in hypertension. We find that patients with increased cardiac output and tachycardia exhibit signs of increased cardiac sympathetic drive and decreased cardiac vagal inhibition [26]. In patients with normal cardiac output, one can demonstrate decreased vagal inhibition [28]. Decreased vagal inhibition has also been described in patients with moderately severe established hypertension [29]. This similarity suggests that patients with normal cardiac output may have had an initially hyperkinetic circulation, but with the passage of time the effective cardiac sympathetic drive diminished while the vagal inhibition remained decreased.

Evidence for increased sympathetic tone in hyperkinetic borderline hypertension

The elevation of the cardiac output in hyperkinetic borderline hypertension can be abolished with a combination of intravenous propranolol and atropine [26], suggesting that the elevation in cardiac output is entirely neurogenic. Interestingly, when the cardiac output is normalized, the blood pressure still remains elevated through a higher vascular resistance. In patients with hyperkinetic borderline hypertension, after cardiac blockade with propranolol and atropine, an additional alpha-adrenergic blockade with phentolamine removes this continued elevation of vascular resistance [24]. Since complete autonomic blockade normalizes the blood pressure in these patients only, they can be considered to have a true neurogenic hypertension. A further study indicated that a neurogenic elevation of blood pressure can also be found in patients with established, but mild, hypertension who still demonstrate a hyperkinetic circulation and who also characteristically have elevated plasma renin and plasma norepinephrine values [8].

The pathophysiology of this neurogenic blood pressure elevation in the hyperkinetic state is not fully understood. The magnitude of cardiac responses to propranolol and atropine indicates that the sympathetic drive to the heart is increased and the cardiac parasympathetic inhibition is decreased [26]. Such a reciprocal relationship between the sympathetic and parasympathetic 'tone' points to an abnormal integration of the autonomic control of the circulation, probably originating in the medulla oblongata. What could cause these changes in the central integration? Decreased baroreceptor sensitivity has been described in borderline hypertension [45] but it is unlikely to be the primary problem. Eckberg [5] believes that decreased baroreceptor function is secondary to the increase in blood pressure in these patients; we concur, since baroreceptor sensitivity tended to be normal in our patients with true borderline hypertension [22]. A more likely explanation for the abnormal central integration of the cardiovascular autonomic tone in borderline hypertension is to be found in the general area of psychosomatics. Profound changes in cardiovascular autonomic tone have been described during the defense reaction [17], and it is not unlikely that persons who are prone to perceive more stress also have a chronic alteration of the central autonomic cardiovascular integration. We have found that patients with borderline hypertension have a characteristic conflict-and-stress-prone personality [8, 15].

Is there evidence for autoregulation of the cardiac output in hypertension?

Even though the elevation of cardiac output in hyperkinetic borderline hypertension is not associated with an obviously expanded blood volume, as expected from Guyton's model [14], the neurogenic elevation of cardiac output could independently trigger an autoregulatory increase of the peripheral vascular resistance, which could then lead to the establishment of a high resistance-normal output hypertension. The specific mechanism that mediates local tissue auto-regulation is not clear, but it is accepted that autoregulation occurs only if the flow exceeds or is below the prevailing metabolic needs of the tissue. By analogy, total body autoregulation will occur only if the cardiac output exceeds the total metabolic needs of the body. In the resting state, the cardiac output is closely attuned to oxygen consumption. For autoregulation to occur in hypertension, one would expect to find 'luxurious perfusion,' a cardiac output inappropriately elevated over the prevailing oxygen consumption. This is not the case, however (Figure 1). In borderline hypertension, both the cardiac output and oxygen consumption are elevated; patients with borderline hypertension cluster at the right end of a normal cardiac output-oxygen consumption regression line. High cardiac output in borderline hypertension was associated with an elevated oxygen consumption in two other studies [31, 37]. Consequently, the condition of hyper-kinetic borderline hypertension does not meet the theoretic criteria for total body autoregulation.

At this point it is interesting to speculate about the nature of the increased oxygen consumption in borderline hypertension, and whether this increase may be the primary event causing an elevation of the cardiac output. A high cardiac output in hypermetabolic states, such as in hyperthyroidism or during exercise, is associated with a decrease of the vascular resistance. In borderline hypertension, however, the vascular resistance is not appropriately decreased for the prevailing levels of cardiac output (Figure 2). I view this as hypothetical evidence for increased sympathetic activity in hyperkinetic borderline hypertension; an in-creased beta-adrenergic drive could be responsible for increased cardiac output and for the increase in oxygen consumption, whereas the alpha-adrenergic vascu-lar effect could account for the inappropriately elevated vascular resistance.

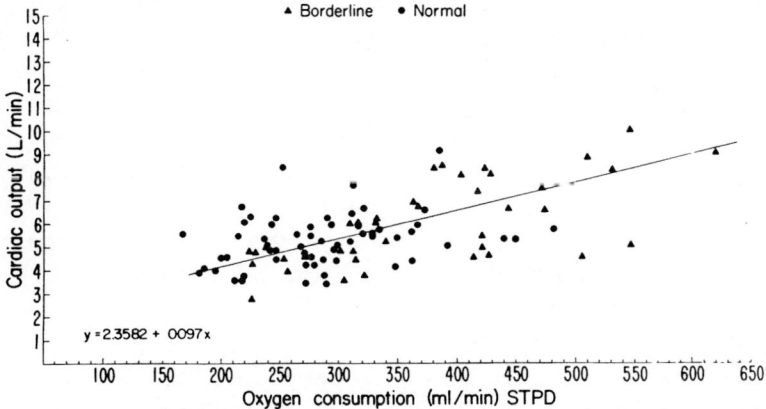

Figure 1. Relationship between cardiac output and oxygen consumption in normotensive control subjects (circles) and patients with bordeline hypertension (triangles). Note that patients with a higher cardiac output also had a high oxygen consumption. * p<0.05. (From Julius and Conway [20]; reprinted by permission from the American Heart Association.)

270

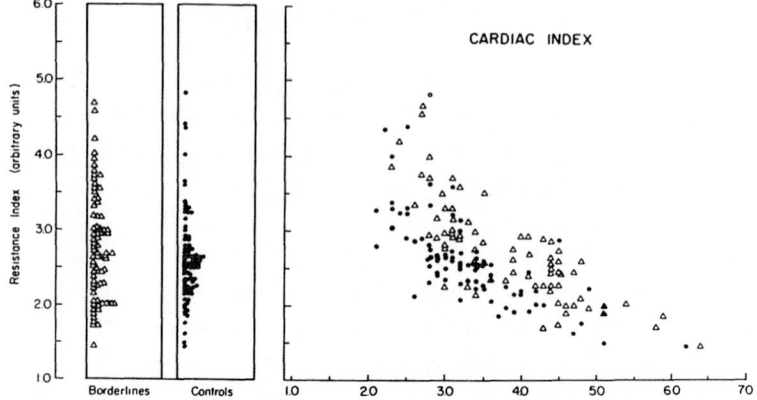

Figure 2. Relationship between cardiac output and vascular resistance in normotensive control subjects (circles) and patients with borderline hypertension (triangles). Note that the resting vascular resistance in patients and control subjects overlapped, but, when the resistance was analyzed in relation to the cardiac output, patients with borderline hypertension always showed a higher resistance. Resistance in borderline hypertension is inappropriately adjusted to the cardiac output. (From Julius et al. [27]; reprinted by permission from the American Heart Association.)

Evidence for decreased cardiac responsiveness in normokinetic borderline hypertension

As indicated earlier, my hypothesis is that increased sympathetic stimulation of the heart leads to decreased receptor responsiveness which, combined with structural changes in the heart, leads to limitation of the cardiac output and to its eventual return to the normal range. The hypothesis further assumes that increased sympathetic stimulation leads to increased arterial responsiveness due to wall-to-lumen ratio changes. At the Ann Arbor laboratory we have data to support the first part of the hypothesis. Evidence for the other part, the vascular hyperresponsiveness, is only inferential and based on the work of others.

In 1975, we demonstrated that patients with a normal cardiac output type of borderline hypertension exhibit alterations in cardiac responsiveness and regulation [28]. It was noted that these patients had a decreased resting stroke volume but maintained a normal cardiac output through a higher heart rate. When this elevation of heart rate was abolished with cardiac receptor blockade, the patient's cardiac output was significantly lower than in control subjects (figure 3). At this point the decrease of the stroke volume in borderline hypertension became even more significant. In normotensive subjects, the resting cardiac output is under a predominant restraining influence of the autonomic nervous system; an injection of propranolol and atropine causes an increase in cardiac output. This restraint was substantially less pronounced in patients with normokinetic borderline hypertension. In this regard, patients with normokinetic borderline hypertension resembled the patients with hyperkinetic borderline hypertension; they too

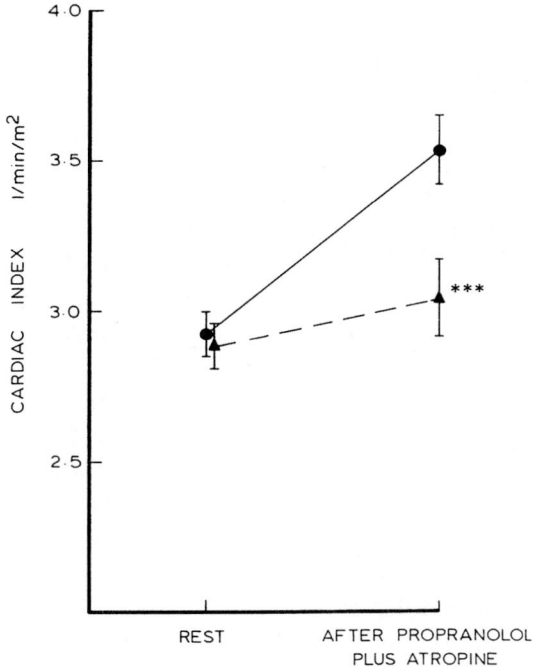

Figure 3. Cardiac index in normotensive control subjects (circles) and patients with a normal cardiac output type of borderline hypertension (triangles) before and after autonomic blockade. Note that upon blockade with 0.2 mg/kg of propranolol and 0.04 mg/kg of atropine, the patients' cardiac outputs were significantly lower than the control subjects. * * * $p < 0.001$. (From Julius et al. [28]; reprinted by permission from the American Heart Association.)

showed a decreased resting autonomic restraint of the heart. Why then is the cardiac output normal in one group and elevated in the other? Clearly, one of the reasons must be the smaller stroke volume. This decrease of the stroke volume in patients with normokinetic borderline hypertension is not due to a decreased cardiac preload. For reasons explained elsewhere, we believe that the cardiopulmonary blood volume is a good indirect index of cardiac filling [28]. Patients and control subjects had similar cardiopulmonary blood volumes, yet the patients' stroke volumes were significantly decreased. Further evidence that patients with borderline hypertension have a true limitation of the stroke volume was provided by Lund-Johansen [31], who demonstrated a failure of the patients adequately to increase stroke volume with exercise. As these patients average only a 10 mm Hg increase of mean arterial pressure, it is difficult to visualize how this degree of elevation in afterload could produce the decrease in stroke volume. A normal heart is able to maintan a normal stroke volume in the presence of a much higher acute elevation of blood pressure. The most likely explanation for the low stroke volume in borderline hypertension is in the decrease of cardiac compliance. In spite of an apparent normal filling, the end diastolic volumes in these patients may be decreased.

272

Another reason for the failure of the resting cardiac output to be elevated in spite of a decreased autonomic restraint in normokinetic borderline hypertension is decreased responsiveness to sympathetic stimulation, as shown in Figure 4. In response to a graded infusion of isoproterenol, heart rate and cardiac output rose less in borderline hypertension than in normal subjects. At the highest rate of infusion ($3\,\mu g$), the cardiac responses in the borderline hypertensive subjects were substantially less than in normal subjects ($p < 0.01$) for heart rate and $p < 0.05$ for cardiac index). As the isoproterenol was infused in intact subjects, the differences observed in Figure 4 do not necessarily reflect only the direct car-diostimulatory effect of a beta-adrenergic agonist, but could also in part reflect differences in reflex responses. Isoproterenol elicited changes in the patients' peripheral resistance, pulse pressure, and diastolic pressure similar to those seen in control subjects. Apparently, the high-pressure baroreceptors in both groups were exposed to similar fractional stimuli. Nevertheless, the patients responded with a lesser increase in the heart rate, indicative of diminished cardiac respon-siveness to beta-adrenergic stimulation.

The experiments described with normokinetic borderline hypertension lend support to the concept that a decrease in cardiac output from high to normal values in the course of developing hypertension may be due both to structural changes in the heart and to a decreased responsiveness to sympathetic stimula-tion. The decreased responsiveness in these patients is in all likelihood a con-sequence of the prolonged increase in sympathetic tone, leading to changes in the density of beta-adrenergic receptors.

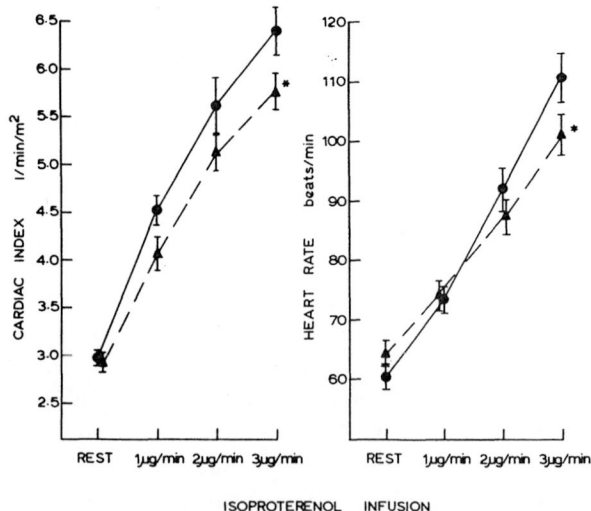

ISOPROTERENOL   INFUSION

Figure 4. Response of the cardiac index and heart rate to graded infusions of isoproterenol (5 min at each dose) in patients (triangles) and control subjects (circles). Note the less steep slope in the patients, and that at the highest dose of isoproterenol the patients' heart rates and cardiac index were significantly lower than those of control subjects. * $p < 0.05$. (From Julius et al. [28]; reprinted by permission from the American Heart Association.)

The other postulate of the hypothesis of 'neurogenic' transition from a high-output to a high-resistance borderline hypertension is that a possible similar decreased sensitivity of alpha-adrenergic receptors would be obscured by ensuing wall-to-lumen ratio changes in resistance vessels. Such changes would tend to lead to an increased vascular responsiveness. Although we have not investigated this part of the hypothesis, studies by Conway [3] and by Sivertsson [42] indicate that such changes do occur in borderline hypertension. Vascular hyperreactivity has also been demonstrated in borderline hypertension [44].

SUMMARY

Hemodynamic investigations in borderline hypertension suggest that an initial high cardiac output may later evolve into a normal output-high resistance state. The hyperkinetic state is entirely neurogenic, and the transition may occur without autoregulation through an entirely neurogenic mechanism where structural and receptor sensitivity changes combine in such a way that the net effect is decreased cardiac and increased vascular responsiveness to sympathetic stimuli.

REFERENCES

1. Borst JGG, Borst-de Geus A: Hypertension explained by Starling's theory of circulatory homeostasis. Lancet 1: 677–682, 1963
2. Coleman TG, Bower JD, Langford HG, Guyton AC: Regulation of arterial pressure in the anephric state. Circulation 42: 509–514, 1970
3. Conway J: A vascular abnormality in hypertension. A study of blood flow in the forearm. Circulation 27: 520–529, 1963
4. Cottier PT, Weller JM, Hoobler SW: Effect of an intravenous sodium chloride load on renal hemodynamics and electrolyte excretion in essential hypertension. Circulation 17: 750–760, 1958
5. Eckberg DL: Carotid baroreflex function in young men with borderline blood pressure elevation. Circulation 59: 632–636, 1979
6. Eich RH, Cuddy RP, Smulyan H, Lyons RH: Hemodynamics in labile hypertension: A follow-up study. Circulation 34: 299–307, 1966
7. Eich RH, Jacobsen ED: Vascular reactivity in medical students followed for 10 years. J Chron Dis 20: 583–592, 1967
8. Esler M, Julius S, Zweifler A, Randall O, Harburg E, Gardiner H, DeQuattro V: Mild high-renin essential hypertension. Neurogenic human hypertension? N Engl J Med 296: 405–411, 1977
9. Esler M, Zweifler A, Randall O, Julius S, Bennett J, Rydelek P: Suppression of sympathetic nervous function in low-renin essential hypertension. Lancet 2: 115–118, 1976
10. Falkner B, Onesti G, Angelakos ET, Fernandes M, Langman C: Cardiovascular response to mental stress in normal adolescents with hypertensive parents. Hemodynamics and mental stress in adolescents. Hypertension 1: 23–30, 1979
11. Folkow B: Role of vascular factors in hypertension. Contrib Nephrol 8: 81–94, 1977

12. Folkow B, Grumby G, Thulasius O: Adaptive structural changes of the vascular wall in hypertension and their relationship to control of the peripheral resistance. Acta Physiol Scand 44: 255–000, 1958
13. Frohlich ED, Tarazi RC, Ulrych M, Dustan HF, Page IH: Tilt test for investigating a neural component in hypertension. Circulation 36: 387–393, 1967
14. Guyton AC, Coleman TG: Quantitative analysis of the pathophysiology of hypertension. Circ Res 24–25 (Suppl. I): 1–19, 1969
15. Harburg E, Julius S, McGinn NF, McLeod J, Hoobler SW: Personality traits and behavioral patterns associated with systolic blood pressure levels in college males. J Chron Dis 17: 405–414, 1964
16. Harlan WR Jr, Osborne RK, Graybiel A: Prognostic value of the cold pressor test and the basal blood pressure: Based on an 18 year follow-up study. Am J Cardiol 13: 683–687, 1964
17. Hilton SM: Inhibition of baroreceptor reflexes on hypothalamic stimulation. J Physiol (Lond) 165: 56–57, 1963
18. Hines EA Jr, Brown GE: The cold pressor test for measuring the reactibility of the blood pressure: Data concerning 571 normal and hypertensive subjects. Am Heart J 11: 1–9, 1936
19. Hull DH, Wolthuis RA, Cortese T, Longo MR Jr, Triebwasser JH: Borderline hypertension versus normotension: differential response to orthostatic stress. Am Heart J 94: 414–420, 1977
20. Julius S, Conway J: Hemodynamic studies in patients with borderline blood pressure elevation. Circulation 38: 282–288, 1968
21. Julius S, Esler M: Autonomic nervous cardiovascular regulation in borderline hypertension. Am J Cardiol 36: 685–696, 1975
22. Julius S, Hansson L: Hemodynamics of prehypertension and hypertension. Verh Dtsch Ges Inn Med 80: 49–58, 1974
23. Julius S, Schork MA: Borderline hypertension-A critical review. J Chron Dis 23: 723–754, 1971
24. Julius S, Esler MD, Randall OS, Ellis CN: Neurogenic maintenance of peripheral resistance in borderline hypertension. Acta Physiol Lat Am 24: 425–431, 1974
25. Julius S, Pascual AV, Reilly K: London R: Abnormalities of plasma volume in borderline hypertension. Arch Intern Med 127: 116–119, 1971
26. Julius S, Pascual AV, London R: Role of parasympathetic inhibition in the hyperkinetic type of borderline hypertension. Circulation 44: 413–418, 1971
27. Julius S, Pascual AV, Sannerstedt R, Mitchell C: Relationship between cardiac output and peripheral resistance in borderline hypertension. Circulation 43: 382–390, 1971
28. Julius S, Randall OS, Esler MD, Kashima T, Ellis CN, Bennett J: Altered cardiac responsiveness and regulation in the normal cardiac output type of borderline hypertension. Circ Res 36–37 (Suppl. I): I-199–I-207, 1975
29. Korner PI, Shaw J, Uther JB, West MJ, McRitchie RJ, Richards JG: Autonomic and non-autonomic circulatory components in essential hypertension in man. Circulation 48: 107–117, 1973
30. Levy RL, White PD, Stroud WD, Hillman CC: Transient tachycardia: Prognostic significance alone and in association with transient hypertension. JAMA 129: 585–588, 1945
31. Lund-Johansen P: Hemodynamics in early essential hypertension. Acta Med Scand 482 Suppl: 1–105, 1967
32. Nestel PJ: Blood pressure and catecholamine excretion after mental stress in labile hypertension. Lancet 1: 692–694, 1969

33. Onesti G, Kim KE, Greco JA, del Guercio ET, Fernandes M, Swartz C: Blood pressure regulation in end-stage renal disease and anephric man. Circ Res 36–37 (Suppl. I): I-145–I-000, 1975
34. Paffenbarger RS Jr, Thorne MC, Wing AL: Chronic disease in former college students-VIII. Characteristics in youth predisposing to hypertension in later years. Am J Epidemiol 88: 25–32, 1968
35. Prior IAM, Harvey HPB, Neave MN, Davidson F: The Health of Two Groups of Cook Island Maoris. Medical Research Council of New Zealand, Medical Statistics Branch of the Department of Health, Wellington, New Zealand, Special Report Series 26, 1966
36. Safar ME, Weiss YA, London GM, Frackowisk RF, Milliez PL: Cardiopulmonary blood volume in borderline hypertension. Clin Sci Mol Med 47: 153–164, 1974
37. Sannerstedt R: Hemodynamic response to exercise in patients with arterial hypertension. Acta Med Scand 458 Suppl.: 1–83, 1966
38. Sannerstedt R, Julius S: Systemic haemodynamics in borderline arterial hypertension: Response to static exercise before and under the influence of propranolol. Cardiovasc Res 6: 398–403, 1972
39. Sannerstedt R, Julius S, Conway J: Hemodynamic response to tilt and beta-adrenergic blockade in young patients with borderline hypertension. Circulation 42: 1057–1064, 1970
40. Simpson FO: β-adrenergic receptor blocking drugs in hypertension. Drugs 7: 85–105, 1974
41. Sive PH, Medalie JH, Kahn HA, Neufeld HN, Riss E: Distribution and multiple regression analysis of blood pressure in 10,000 Israeli men. Am J Epidemiol 93: 317–327, 1971
42. Sivertsson R: The hemodynamic importance of structural vascular changes in essential hypertension. Acta Physiol Scand 79 Suppl 343: 3–56, 1970
43. Stamler J, Berkson DM, Dyer A, Lepper MH, Lindberg HA, Paul O, McKean H, Rhomberg P, Schoenberger JA, Shekelle RB, Stamler R: Relationship of multiple variables to blood pressure-Findings from four Chicago epidemiologic studies. In: Paul O (ed), Epidemiology and Control of Hypertension. Symposia Specialists, Miami, 1975, pp 307–352
44. Suck AF, Mendlowitz M, Wolf RL et al.: Identification of essential hypertension in patients with labile blood pressure. Chest 59: 402–406, 1971
45. Takeshita A, Tanaka S, Kuroiwa A, Nakamura M: Reduced baroreceptor sensitivity in borderline hypertension. Circulation 51: 738–742, 1975
46. Tarazi RC, Ibrahim MM, Dustan HP, Ferrario CM: Cardiac factors in hypertension. Circ Res 34–35 (Suppl. I): I-213–I-243, 1974
47. Thomas CB: Developmental patterns in hypertensive cardiovascular disease: Fact or fiction? Bull NY Acad Med 45: 831–850, 1969
48. Thomas CB, Stanley JA, Kendrick MA: Observations on some possible precursors of essential hypertension and coronary artery disease-VII. The subjective reaction to the cold pressor test as expressed in the verbal response. J Chron Dis 14: 355–365, 1961
49. Weiss YA, Safar ME, London GM, Simon AC, Levenson JA, Milliez PM: Repeat hemodynamic determinations in borderline hypertension. Am J Med 64: 382–387, 1978

21. THE ROLE OF THE HEART IN HYPERTENSION

ROBERT C. TARAZI

INTRODUCTION

The heart has usually been regarded only as a sufferer in hypertension, one of the few organs whose dysfunction was directly related to the elevated arterial pressure. The definition of hypertension as a quantitative rather than a qualitative deviation from the norm [1] fitted well with that concept; cardiac hypertrophy and eventual failure was viewed as a direct function of the level of arterial pressure. This traditional view has been questioned from time to time, more on an intuitive basis than on firm factual evidence [2]. It is only recently, however, that the spectrum of cardiac involvement in hypertension has been demonstrated to be much broader than the hypertrophy and failure of a pump submitted to an excessive load.

The heart is richly innervated [3] and is a potential endocrine organ [4]. It appears ideally placed as a source of information from both the high and low pressure segments of the circulation. Powerful pressor and depressor reflexes can be evoked from the myocardium, coronary arteries and large vessels. Variations in atrial size and pressure can influence blood pressure, renal hemodynamics and the secretion of renin, aldosterone and antidiuretic hormone (ADH). Moreover, if the bloodstream could be likened to a computer tape, as suggested by Page, the heart would be the natural decoder of that information. It is from that central position as producer of energy for the circulation and sensing device for its alterations and needs that the heart can play an essential role in blood pressure regulation and in the evolution of hypertension [5].

This role extends over the whole evolution of the disease; one may discuss its relative importance in the genesis of hypertension, but few would question its profound influence on the evolution of hemodynamic patterns and modulation of neuroendocrine variables as hypertension progresses. Just as vascular hypertrophy will influence the mosaic of factors that sustain hypertension [6], cardiac hypertrophy can alter the balance of these factors, albeit in different ways. The clinical implications of these changes extend not only to the multifaceted aspects which hypertension may present to the physician but also to its varied responses to different treatments.

ROLE OF THE HEART IN THE INITIATION OF HYPERTENSION

Cardiogenic hypertension is not a term frequently used in either clinical or experimental studies of high blood pressure. This is not because the term is

Sambhi, M.P. (ed.) Fundamental fault in hypertension
© *1984, Martinus Nijhoff Publishers. Boston/The Hague/Dordrecht/Lancaster.*
ISBN 978-94-010-9006-3

obscure or unfamiliar; the difficulty in accepting it stems from another source, namely, the widely held belief that a cardiogenic hypertension must be a high output state [7]. Since the hemodynamic characteristic of hypertension is an increase in total peripheral resistance [7–9], and since so many high output conditions are not associated with systemic arterial hypertension, the obvious conclusion was to belittle the role of the heart as a cause of hypertension.

This conclusion has recently been challenged on two bases, the frequency increased cardiac output in the early phases of both essential and secondary hypertension [8–13] and recognition of the importance of pressor reflexes originating from the heart and great vessels. Characterization of a hypertension by a high systemic resistance does not necessarily rule out a possible cardiac origin, since the high resistance might have been triggered by some cardiac dysfunction [7, 10].

The notion of a cardiogenic hypertension is, therefore, much wider than a high output state; for a discussion of its various aspects, a clarification of the terms used is therefore, essential. Cardiogenic hypertension can be defined as a hypertension in which the heart plays a major role either by initiating an increased in output or as the source of pressor reflexes [5]. In the former situation, however, the term is acceptable only as an approximation, since the mechanism increasing cardiac performance may have its origin outside the heart (Table 1).

Hypertension with increased cardiac output

Pathology: The first mechanism that is spontaneously evoked in discussions of cardiogenic hypertension is an increase in cardiac output. Fries [7] first used the term in describing the increased cardiac action produced by stellate stimulation; later Ledingham [14] reported his finding of an increased cardiac output in experimental renovascular hypertension under the title of 'role of the heart in hypertension'. Since studies of the past 10 years have revealed that, contrary to earlier impressions, cardiac output was not infrequently elevated in various types of hypertension, how far could one label as cardiogenic the many types of hyperkinetic hypertension [9, 15]? The question is particularly pertinent since increased cardiac action is not the only, and possibly not even the most frequent cause of a high output [16]. In fact, Guyton has repeatedly stressed the importance of peripheral factors in that regard; he considers the heart as an autonomic

Table 1. Definition of cardiogenic hypertension

1. Literal: hypertension initiated by or from the heart
2. Extended:
    a) Hypertension initiated by cardiac reflexes
    b) Hypertension initiated by reflexes from the coronary arteries or from the aorta
    c) Hypertension initiated via increased heart action due to neurohumoral stimuli

pumping station whose output is determined by its venous filling, which is controlled by peripheral conditions.

However, it is possible to demonstrate under controlled conditions that increased myocardial contractility can initiate an increase in output by the combined effect of increased ejection fraction and of redistribution of blood from the cardiopulmonary area to the systemic circulation [17–19]. However, that source is limited; after its initiation, maintenance of the high output requires peripheral circulatory adjustments to ensure an adequate venous return. Under ordinary conditions, the enhanced myocardial contractility that could initiate these events is the result of an increased cardioadrenergic drive [19–21], although the serum electrolyte and humoral disturbances of some steroid types of hypertensions can play a similar inotropic role [22]. The interdependence of peripheral and cardiac factors is obvious; just as a 'cardiogenic' increase in output depends on a participation of peripheral mechanisms, the increase in systemic flow secondary to peripheral conditions demands a competent heart to respond to the increased load.

The list of types of hypertension associated with a high cardiac output (Table 2) includes some with an obvious explanation for the increased flow, but in most cases the mechanism responsible is not immediately obvious. Hypervolemia has not proven to be *per se* a common or indeed even a necessary cause of a high output hypertension [18]. A volume overload of the magnitude encountered in most forms of hypertension can easily by accommodated by minor adjustments of the capacitance vessels or within the interstitial space [23]. Hypervolemic essential hypertension is not characterized by an increase in cardiac output but by marked elevation in peripheral resistance similar to hypervolemic hypertension [18]. Thus, the postulated subdivision of hypertension into a 'vasoconstrictive' and a 'high flow' type dependent on volume and renin status [24] did not prove hemodynamically possible, since both groups shared an equivalent level of systemic flow and the same rise in peripheral resistance.

Table 2. Hypertension associated with high cardiac output*

I.	Essential hypertension
	a) Borderline hypertension
	b) Subset of established severe hypertension with marked hyperkinetic circulation
II.	Secondary hypertension
	a) Renal arterial disease
	b) Primary aldosteronism
	c) Pheochromocytoma
III.	Hypertension associated with
	a) Anaemia (uremic hypertensives)
	b) Hyper-β-adrenergic state
IV.	Hypertension treated with vasodilators

* from Tarazi et al. [15].

Accurate analysis of cardiac factors in hypertension

This must take into account the relationship between total blood volume, cardiopulmonary volume (CPV) and cardiac output or stroke volume [9, 19]. The ratio of cardiopulmonary to total blood volume is an estimate of the distribution of blood between the peripheral and central circulation [25, 26]. A significant increase indicates a redistribution of blood into the central circulation because of diminished capacity of the capacitance vessels, whereas a significant decrease indicates an increased capacity, presumably due to venodilatation. Cardiac performance could in turn be evaluated from the relation between stroke volume (SV) and cardiac output [19, 27]: a significant decrease of the SV/CPV ratio suggests enhanced myocardial performance, as has been shown both in humans [18, 19, 28] and experimental studies [29].

An initial study in 1969 of cardiopulmonary volume in hypertensive patients revealed a significant correlation between the volume and cardiac output [25], suggesting that differences in output among subjects depended mainly on the extent of central distribution of intravascular volume. Similar results were obtained by Safar et al. [30] in borderline hypertension but not by Ellis and Julius [29], who related the increased output to increased contractility. That both mechanisms, intravascular volume distribution and increased cardiac performance, may be involved concurrently in borderline hypertension was shown in a study by Tarazi et al. [19]. Cardiac output was increased and correlated with CPV, but at any level of the latter cardiac output was higher or lower depending on the level of cardiac performance (Figure 1). Based on these principles, the high output often seen in borderline hypertension was related to an enhanced cardiac performance probably related to an increased cardioadrenergic drive [19, 31]. In contrast, the higher cardiac index in patients with renal arterial disease was associated with a slightly reduced total blood volume (TBV) but an increased cardiopulmonary volume and higher CPV/TBV ratio [19, 25]; similar findings were obtained in dogs with perinephritic hypertension [32]. This is not to deny a possible increase in contractility in renovascular hypertension [33, 34], but the weight of present evidence favors a peripheral rather than a cardiogenic mechanism in the genesis of its hemodynamic pattern [19]. In contrast, the usual pattern associated with borderline essential hypertension suggests a greater cardiac participation in the increased flow (Fig. 1).

Relation of cardiac output to hypertension

In the ananlysis of a possible role of the heart in the development of hypertension, it is not sufficient to define its participation in the increase of cardiac output; more relevant to the problem is the relation of the increased output to the high systemic pressure. The number of types of hypertension associated with high output is not

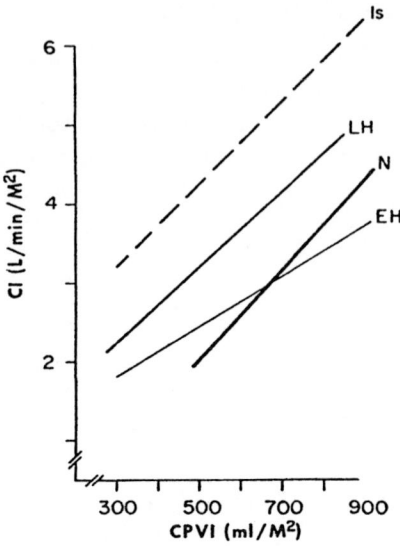

Figure 1. Regression lines defining the correlation between cardiac index (CI) and cardiopulmonary volume (CPV) in nine normotensive volunteers (N), 16 essential hypertensive patients (EH) and 11 patients with borderline (labile) hypertension (LVH); is defines the correlation obtained in 20 hypertensive patients given isoprenaline infusion ($0.03 \mu g \min^{-1} kg^{-1}$). The shift of the line to the left in LH as compared with EH was similar to that produced by isoprenaline. (From Tarazi et al. [19] and reproduced by permission from the American Heart Association).

negligible (Table 2) but this does not necessarily mean that blood pressure is maintained by the increased output. In fact, it has been repeatedly shown that in none of the 'high output types' is the increased flow a sufficient explanation for the maintenance of hypertension. In primary aldosteronism, cardiac output was inversely related to the level of arterial pressure [35]. Reducing output acutely with propranolol in labile, essential or renovascular hypertension did not lower arterial pressure [36], nor did the normalization of output by correcting anemia in end-stage kidney disease [37]. Reversal of high output hypertension was associated predominantly with changes in peripheral resistance rather than in output. This was documented with renal arterial disease [38] and in the reversal of experimental perinephritic hypertension [19].

These observations, however, do not mean that a high output might not have played a crucial role in the development of some types of clinical and experimental hypertension in which a phase of high output antedated the more persistent high resistance stage [9]. This well known hemodynamic sequence from high output to high resistance has been ascribed to total body autoregulation; a full discussion of this concept is outside the scope of this review. The doubts raised about its universality and role in the evolution of hypertension have been discussed in detail previously [18]. More pertinent to cardiogenic hypertension are those examples where the initiation of the rise in systemic pressure was induced by primary increases in cardiac inotropism.

Hypertension initiated by increased cardiac action

Electrical stimulation of the stellate ganglion in conscious dogs was shown by Liard et al. [39] to produce sustained hypertension for as long as the stimulation was maintained. After a transient increase in output, the increase in blood pressure was maintained by a rise in systemic vascular resistance (Figure 2); at no time was there any demonstrable volume expansion. Essentially similar results were later obtained by Liard [40] from continuous (7 days) infusion of dobut- amine into the left coronary artery in conscious dogs. In both instances it appeared that an increase in cardiac output unrelated to fluid load could lead to a hypertension characterized by increased peripheral resistance.

This experimental evidence raises two important questions. The first is related to the persistence of hypertension contrasting apparently with the concept that an increase in arterial pressure without a change in renal function will promote increased diuresis, returning arterial pressure to control values [41]. It is con- ceivable, however, that a shift of renal function curves relating pressure to diuresis may, in some conditions, be a consequence rather than a cause of the rise in arterial pressure. Omvik et al. [42] provided suggestive evidence for an adaptation of renal function to increased perfusion pressure, possibly in response

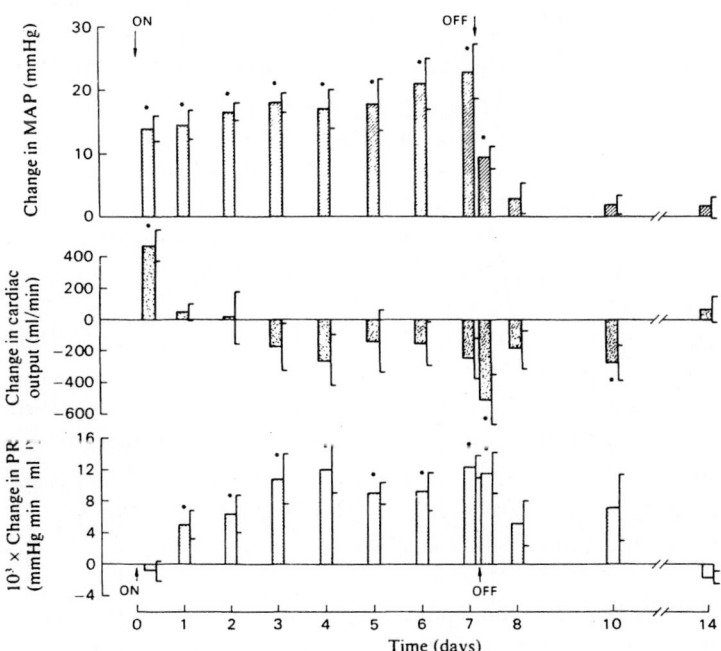

Figure 2. Changes ± SEM in mean arterial blood pressure (MAP), cardiac output and peripheral resistance (PR) in six dogs between 6 h (ON) and 7 days of continuous left stellate ganglion stimulation (OFF) and 2 h and 1, 3 and 7 days after discontinuation of the stimulation. * Significant difference. (From Liard et al. [39], with permission).

to threatened or actual fluid depletion. Whatever the mechanism, and others may be suggested [40], the observations stand of hypertension related primarily to increased cardiac inotropism.

The second question concerns the observation that cardiogenic hypertension was regularly associated with changes in peripheral resistance. Their hemo-dynamic pattern could be viewed as the result of a widespread adrenergic stimulation of both the heart and vessels, but it is conceivable that cardiac reflexes could participate in initiating or perpetuating the peripheral vasoconstriction [43]. A quieting of the heart might be one of the mechanisms by which beta-adrenoceptor blockers, such as the hydrophilic cardioselective drugs, could help lower arterial pressure [44]. The experiments of Cooper et al. [45] are significant in that regard; they showed that cardiac denervation prevented the pressor responses to hypo-thalamic stimulation.

Pressor reflexes from the heart

a) Clinical expressions of pressor reflexes from the cardiac area. For a long time it has been known that anginal attacks may be preceded by a rise in arterial pressure and that myocardial infarction may be accompanied by transient hyper-tension [46]. More recently, paroxysmal hypertension has been recognized as a frequent occurrence in the early hours after an aortic-coronary bypass graft [47] (Figure 3). The rise in arterial pressure was related to an increase in peripheral resistance with little or no change in cardiac output and no correlation with plasma renin activity [48, 49]. Unilateral infiltration of either stellate ganglion with novocaine led to rapid and sustained return of arterial pressure to normal in up to 75% of the cases associated with a fall in peripheral resistance and no significant change in output (Table 3). This form of hypertension was, therefore, interpreted to result from afferent pressor reflexes from the heart and/or great vessels, the human counterpart to the experiments of Liard et al. with unilateral stellate stimulation in dogs [39]. In that same context, Malliani et al. [50] have convincingly demonstrated the potential importance of pressor reflexes arising from distension of the aorta, such as could occur with dissecting aortic aneurysm.

All these might legitimately be called 'cardiogenic hypertension' in that they are an expression of powerful pressor reflexes from the heart. These can be triggered from distension of coronary vessels [51, 52], myocardial ischemia [53], or specific chemoreceptors [54], as well as from rhythmic stretch of the aortic wall [50]. Of particular interest is the reduction in baroceptor sensitivity produced by activation of the aortic pressor reflex [50, 55]. The clinical picture is that of a paroxysmal hypertension of varying severity; some of these are so impressive with marked tachycardia and intense vasoconstriction as to have been termed 'vasomotor storms'.

283

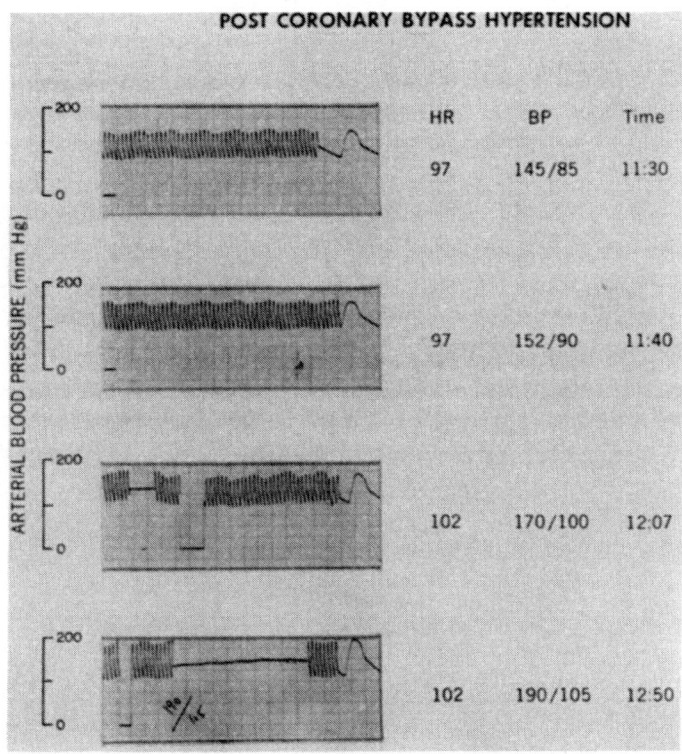

Figure 3. Hypertension developing after coronary bypass surgery despite sedation and analgesia. BP = blood pressure; HR = heart rate. (From Estafanous and Tarazi [47], with permission).

b) Pathophysiological considerations. These clinical observations have dramatically underscored the importance of the heart and large vessels as sources of blood pressure regulatory mechanisms; they have also shown that a cardiogenic hypertension could be marked by high resistance and intense vasoconstriction instead of an increased flow. Numerous studies in the past few years have reviewed the role of cardiopulmonary afferent stimuli in blood pressure regulation [56, 57]. Brown (3) has pointed out that the heart differs from other cardiovascular reflexogenic structures in that it has two prominent inputs into the central nervous system. One input is spinal and is mediated by afferent cardiac sympathetic nerve fibers; the other is medullary and mediated by afferent vagal fibers. The number of fibers projecting centrally appears to be similar in the two systems. The reflex effects produced by excitation of the two inputs are complicated and can be either pressor or depressor. The resulting picture can therefore, be quite complex; tachycardia with relatively little change in blood pressure [58], bradycardia and hypertension [59] and tachycardia and hypertension [43, 49]. Of

Table 3. * *

	Development of hypertension (n = 10)		Control by stellate block (n = 9)	
	Postsurgery	Hypertension	Hypertension	Stellate block
SBP	123 ± 4.0	173 ± 5.9*	168 ± 5.5	119 ± 3.9*
DBP	78 ± 1.5	101 ± 2.4*	99 ± 2.8	75 ± 2.2*
HR (min⁻¹)	102 ± 3.7	103 ± 3.0	94 ± 4.9	87 ± 5.1*
CO (1/min)	4.60 ± 0.4	4.72 ± 0.3	4.01 ± 0.4	3.49 ± 0.4
TPR	38 ± 2.5	47 ± 2.9*	66 ± 8.5	53 ± 6.4

The rise in blood pressure was related to an increase in peripheral resistance and its fall after unilateral right stellate block was related to a fall in resistance. SBP = systolic blood pressure; DBP = diastolic blood pressure, HR = heart rate; CO = cardiac output; TPR = total peripheral resistance.
* $p < 0.001$ at least.
** (From Fouad et al.]49]).

particular importance in the pressor reflexes from the myocardium, coronary vessels or aorta is the unstable, potentially dangerous positive feedback state that they can induce [50]. In the more familiar baroceptor reflexes, a rise in pressure reflexly leads to reduction in pressure (stabilizing negative feedback); with these pressor reflexes, vascular distension or distortion of myocardial receptors by increased pressure or increased cardiac action can lead to further rise in pressure and cardiac stimulation, generating a dangerous vicious circle.

Hypertension that could be directly related to cardiogenic pressor reflexes has been paroxysmal in type. However, the richness of cardiac innervation [3, 58], and particularly the tonic restricting influence of ventricular atrial and pulmonary receptors on the cardiovascular centers [56], raise important questions regarding a possible role of the heart in chronic hypertension. Of particular importance in that regard are the marked influences of atrial and cardiopulmonary receptors on blood volume regulation [60], renal hemodynamics [61], and renin release [62]. Reflexes from cardiopulmonary receptors interact with and can significantly alter the effect of arterial baroceptors and somatic reflexes [57]. There is admittedly no firm evidence for a cardiac role in long-term hypertension although the hypertension produced by cardiac stimulation in conscious dogs did persist unabated for 7 days [39].

In this context, it is possible that the usual animal models might not be the most pertinent for human hypertension. The situation in man appears different, first in that the cardiopulmonary receptors have a much greater influence on muscle flow than do the arterial baroceptors [56]. A reduction in cardiopulmonary volume by lower body subatmospheric pressure is associated with more marked increases in forearm vascular resistance in borderline hypertensive subjects than in normal subjects [63]. The normally upright position of man is bound to be associated with a greater influence of cardiopulmonary reflexes on cardiovascular homeostasis than would be the case in quadrupeds. Clinically, there are many instances of predominantly orthostatic hypertension in patients with near normal blood pressure at rest.

HEART IN CHRONIC HYPERTENSION

Cardiac hypertrophy is the usual response to prolonged or repeated increases in afterload. Contrary, however, to impressions derived from such indirect signs as the electrocardiogram, recent evidence both in man [64] and animals [65, 66] indicates that cardial hypertrophy can occur quite early in hypertension. In fact, the rate at which the heart can adapt its design to changes in pressure load was found to be rapid enough [65, 67–70] to suggest that its structural alterations must be taken into account as participants in the evolution of hypertension.

A detailed discussion of cardiac responses to increased afterload is outside the scope of this review (for references, see [71]). Studies from many centers have demonstred that hypertensive left ventricular hypertrophy is not a stereotyped concentric increase in wall thickness, slowly advancing to ventricular dilation and failure. The advent of echocardiography has introduced a new dimension in this domain as regards both the distribution of ventricular hypertrophy and its appropriateness to the cardiac load. The subject has been recently discussed extensively (Am Heart J 75 (Suppl 3A), 1983).

Asymmetric septal hypertrophy was reported to occur [72], particularly in early hypertension [73], not necessarily due to a genetically transmitted cardiomyopathy but secondary to left ventricular pressure overload [74]. The ratio of LV mass to volume or of LV wall thickness to radius were found to differ widely among patients, altering significantly the level of myocardial stress and of cardiac performance even among subjects with equal levels of arterial pressure. Grossman, Gaasch and their collaborators as well as Strauer and Fouad, have clearly demonstrated the dependence of left ventricular function on these ratios both in hypertensive [75, 76] and non-hypertensive conditions [77, 78]. Whatever the index of function used, the velocity of circumferential fiber shortening or the ejection fraction, the findings have been remarkably consistent; the greater the dilatation of the heart's cavity in relation to the thickening of its wall, the more marked the depression of its function.

Influence of myocardial hypertrophy on hypertensive mechanisms

The full impact of cardiac hypertrophy on the evolution of hemodynamic patterns in hypertension has yet to be completely defined. The change from high to low cardiac output with persistence of the disease may well be related among other factors to alterations in myocardial compliance [15, 79]. These have been documented even in early hypertension by Fouad et al. [80], who described a reduced filling rate of the left ventricle at a stage when ejection function was still well maintained. The restricted ability of even young hypertensive patients to increase stroke volume with exercise could well be related to this altered compliance [8].

At an even more fundamental level, ventricular hypertrophy may influence the resetting of autonomic nervous activity to ensure adequate cardiac filling and performance [6, 81, 82]. In a sequence of impressive studies, Hallback and her collaborators [81] have shown that the performance of the hypertrophied ventricle of the spontaneously hypertensive rat (SHR) varies in comparison with that of normal controls, depending on both filling pressure and afterload conditions. At high cardiac filling pressures, when the full resources of the hypertrophied ventricle are mobilized, cardiac performance was superior in SHR than in controls. The need to maintain this high filling pressure is associated with a greater splanchnic venoconstriction [81] and a central location of intravascular volume, a phenomenon which has been observed in many human and experimental hypertension [18]. Left artrial pressure was maintained at higher levels in SHR than in controls, whereas the left atrial C fibers were reset to a higher stimulation threshold [82].

This resetting of atrial reflexes in SHR was associated only with a change in stimulation threshold; the nerve fibers maintained their brisk respons to volume expansion [82]. This was in marked contrast with the resetting of atrial receptors observed during experimental heart failure dogs, which become very insensitive to pressure changes, possibly owing to degeneration of the receptor endings [83]. In spontaneously hypertensive rats, however, the maximal atrial receptor discharge is normal and there is no evidence that their cardiac hypertrophy is of a degenerative nature [82]. Instead, the resetting of their receptors is likely to be due to a structural adaptation of the left atrial wall. One might speculate whether the transition from hypertensive left ventricular hypertrophy to hypertensive heart failure might not be associated with some degenerative changes in cardiac receptors, reducing natriuresis and allowing fluid overload.

Other consequences of ventricular hypertrophy such as reduction of adrenergic responsiveness of the myocardium and of its contractile reserve [84], or encroachment on coronary vascular reserve [85], have recently been reviewed; they belong more properly to a discussion of the effects of hypertension on the heart rather than of the influence of the heart on the disease.

Reduced cardiac performance and arterial pressures

One of the strongest pieces of evidence in favor of an important role of the heart in the maintenance of hypertension is also paradoxically one of the weakest. I refer to the significant and sustained reduction of arterial pressure that follows the development of heart failure or the occurrence of a myocardial infarct [86]. The strength of the argument derives from its representing the counterpart to the development of hypertension when cardiac inotropism is increased. Its weakness is the relative 'softness of the data', most of which are based on clinical evidence, with its unavoidable limitations. Fishberg's description in 1954 remains particularly apt; the drop in blood pressure with the advent of heart failure affects the systolic more than the diastolic, but the latter may also be markedly lowered to normal or near-normal pressures. When cardiac failure in other than moribund patients is accompanied by sudden and marked falls in pressure, the cause is often a myocardial infarct.

Only recently have these observations been reproduced experimentally [87]; the reduction of arterial pressure by myocardial infarction in spontaneously hypertensive rats was roughly proportional to the infarct size. The fall in pressure appears to be a reduction of vascular resistance or at least an inability of total peripheral resistance to compensate for the reduction in cardiac output. The data of Fletcher et al. leave little doubt about the reduction in cardiac power after the experimental infarct and the heart's inability to maintain stroke volume in the face of an increased pressure load. The lack of rise in total peripheral resistance to compensate for any reduction of output by heart failure is surprising in view of the fact that the peripheral vessels apparently retain their capacity to vasoconstrict, as suggested clinically by the unchanged or even increased blood pressure seen in cases of cardiac failure [88] and as shown experimentally by their unaltered response to methoxamine [87]. Obviously the reduced pumping ability of the infarcted or failing heart must somehow be sensed and translated into an adjustment of peripheral resistance. The responsible mechanism(s) can only be guessed at, and the reasons for their absence in some cases are not evident.

ROLE OF THE HEART IN ANTIHYPERTENSIVE THERAPY

Cardiac complications used to head the list of causes of death from hypertension. The incidence of heart failure fell dramatically with the introduction of the first effective antihypertensive drug [89], but myocardial infarction has proven more difficult to prevent. Most available antihypertensive agents have important cardiac actions either because of fluid retention increasing preload, or of reflex cardiac stimulation stressing the myocardium and increasing its oxygen demands or by interference with adrenergic support to the heart. It is obvious, therefore, that the cardiac status of a patient will influence the indications, urgency and choice of therapy [90].

The factors dictating these therapeutic decisions are well known. More relevant to our purpose are those instances in which consideration of the role of the heart in hypertension might help reshape our approach to therapy. Antihypertensive treatment has been largely dictated by one goal, reduction of diastolic pressures with the minimum of side effects. Attention to the heart has raised some fundamental questions in that regard. These include the adequacy of diastolic pressure alone as a guide to treatment [71] and the advisability of defining additional goals beyond blood pressure control. The latter refers to the possibility of inducing reversal (and not simply arrest or prevention) or cardiac and vascular hypertrophy by some antihypertensive measures [91].

Importance of systolic blood pressure in guiding treatment

Hypertension has traditionally been defined in terms of diastolic blood pressures; however, cardiac work is related to systolic pressure. There are admittedly many problems in the correct definition of cardiac afterload [71]. Clinically, however, all studies correlating cardiac complications with arterial pressures have demonstrated that the systolic rather than the diastolic pressure is the value most closely predicting the incidence of cardiac complications [92]. The step-care therapy approach has been based on diastolic pressures; it is probably time to reexamine the postulates of that approach and to define, at least for cardiac patients, a specific role for systolic arterial pressure in directing antihypertensive therapy [93].

Cardiac stimulation as a cause of resistance to antihypertensive treatment

Reflex cardiac stimulation by vasodilators was shown to be a common and potent cause of resistance to treatment [94]. The increase in cardiac output secondary to arteriolar vasodilatation may help maintain a high arterial pressure despite the normalization of peripheral vascular resistance. More recently, pulmonary hypertension was described in response to hydralazine, diazoxide and minoxidil [90]. Two hemodynamic patterns could underlie that rise in pulmonary artery pressure. The first 'congestive pulmonary hypertension', seemed to reflect diminished cardiac efficiency, probably secondary to marked fluid retention and increased preload. The second pattern was a 'hyperkinetic pulmonary hypertension' characterized by a marked increase in cardiac output. In contrast with the first pattern, which indicated the need for more adequate volume depletion, the second type was usually responsive to more effective balance between the vasodilator and beta-receptor-blocker therapy. These observations underline the need for careful cardiac hemodynamic studies in the adjustment of therapy in resistant cases.

Reversal of cardiac hypertrophy

One of the more significant observations in the past few years has been the demonstration of the wide spectrum of changes in ventricular weight resulting from apparently equipotent antihypertensive drugs (Table 4) [68, 91]. The reversibility of hypertrophy by medical therapy and the various factors modulating cardiac structural responses to alterations in systemic arterial pressure have been reviewed in detail recently [91]. The dissociation between degree of blood pressure control and magnitude of regression of cardiac hypertrophy entails important clinical and theoretical implications. It has also pointed out the role of hormonal and neural factors in the modulation of hypertrophic responses to hypertension, a role that was easily overshadowed by the obvious hemodynamic effect of the increased pressure load. In practice, the present body of evidence suggests that antihypertensive drugs that reduce adrenergic activity, or at least do not stimulate it, are more effective in reversing the cardiovascular structural changes associated with hypertension.

The demonstration that cardiac hypertrophy can be reserved by medical antihypertensive therapy is lending urgency to the question of whether cardiac hypertrophy is advantageous or whether it represents the first step to failure. There have been few reported studies of ventricular function after reversal of cardiac hypertrophy by antihypertensive measures. On balance, it would appear as if regression of hypertrophy did not seriously harm the heart, but the results available are still incomplete. It is particularly important to differentiate the effects of blood pressure control from those of reversal of hypertrophy; Fouad et al. [95] have partly answered the question by utilizing the relationship between LV fractional shortening and end-systolic stress, which takes into account changes in afterload. No change was found following regression of LVH by enalapril. Papillary muscle studies can help in that respect, but since a reduction in cardiac mass may alter its geometry, the final effects of reversal on cardiac dynamics might differ from its effects on isolated muscles. It bears pointing out that determination of cardiac function only at rest is not sufficient to assess adequately cardiac reserve; the response of regressed hearts to sudden increases in load or to exercise still needs to be examined [91].

At more basic levels, LVH has been associated with reduction in inotropic responses to catecholamines [96] and in coronary vascular reserve [97]. Both may

Table 4. Antihypertensive therapy and cardiac hypertrophy in spontaneously hypertensive rats (SHR)

Group	Blood pressure (mmHg)	Ventricular weight (mg/g)
NORMAL	120	2·6
UNTREATED SHR	188	3·4
TREATED SHR		
Methyldopa	149	2·7
Hydralazine	123	3·4
Minoxidil	130	3·8

Results of antihypertensive therapy indicate that reversal of cardiac hypertrophy is not dependent on blood pressure control alone. (Data reproduced with permission: Sen et al. [65]).

290

play a role in the evolution or heart disease; their responses to therapy still need further definition. A wide spectrum of alterations at various points in the adenylate cyclase system has been described in the myocardium of hypertensive rats; progressive reduction of inotropic response to activators of that system may rob the hypertrophied ventricle of adrenergic support and play a role in the eventual progression from hypertrophy to failure. Early reports suggest that some of those abnormalities may be connected with regression of LVH. Reduction in coronary flow reserve is seen in severe hypertrophy. Of particular interest as regards blood pressure control and changes in LV mass is the balance present between coronary perfusion pressure and myocardial mass. A reduction in blood pressure without concomitant reduction in hypertrophy can upset this balance and interfere with coronary flow reserve [98]. If confirmed, these observations might have important clinical implications.

Finally, the regression of cardiac hypertrophy must be judged in relation to structural changes in the peripheral vessels, which bear the brunt of hypertension and contribute to its progress. It would be most important to define whether the response of cardiac hypertrophy mirrors or differs from the structural responses of both the central and pripheral arteries. A close relationship between alterations, reversal in cardiac mass and reduction of protein synthesis in the mesenteric arteries of SHR [99]. The same conclusions regarding the role of the neural influences on hypertrophic responses to hypertension seemed to apply to the vessels and the heart. Recent reports from Hallback et al. described a parallel regression in cardiac mass and in indices of thickening of the resistance vessels following antihypetensive treatment in SHR [100].

This discussion has both theoretical and practical implications; the importance of identifying factors modulating cardiac and vascular smooth muscle hypertrophy hardly needs stressing. As more is learned, one is tempted to speculate that antihypertensive therapy may be eventually guided by more than its effects on blood pressure alone.

ACKNOWLEDGMENTS

These studies were supported in part from grants from the National Institutes of Health (NHLBI-6835), the Hartford Foundation, Whitaker Foundation and the American Heart Association, Northeast Ohio Affiliate.

REFERENCES

1. Pickering G: The nature of essential hypertension. J and A Churchill, England, 1961, pp 1–151
2. Raab W, Lepeschkin E: Biochemical versus hemodynamic factors in the origin of hypertensive heart disease. Acta Med Scand 138: 81–93, 1950

3. Brown AM: Coronary pressor reflexes. Am J Cardiol 44: 849–851, 1979
4. Braunwald E: The autonomic nervous system in heart failure in the myocardium: failure and infarction. HP Publishing Co, New York, 1974, pp 59–69
5. Dustan HP, Tarazi RC: Cardiogenic hypertension. Ann Rev Med 29: 485–493, 1978
6. Folkow B: Cardiovascular structural adaptation: its role in the initiation and maintenance of primary hypertension. Clin Sci Mol Med 55 (Suppl 4): 3s–22s, 1978
7. Freis ED: Hemodynamics of hypertension. Phys Rev 40: 27–54, 1960
8. Lund-Johansen P: Hemodynamics in essential hypertension. Clin Sci 59 (Suppl 6): 343s–354s, 1980
9. Tarazi RC, Conway J: Hemodynamics of hypertension. In: Genest J, Kuchel O, Hamet P, Cantin M (eds), Hypertension, 2nd edition. McGraw-Hill, Inc, New York, 1983, pp 15–42
10. Frohlich ED, Kozul VJ, Tarazi RC, Dustan HP: Physiological comparison of labile and essential hypertension. Circ Res 26 27 (Suppl I): 55–69, 1970
11. Widimsky J, Fejfarova MH, Fejfar Z: Changes of cardiac output in hypertensive disease. Cardiologia 31: 381–389, 1957
12. Julius S, Conway J: Hemodynamic studies in patients with borderline blood pressure elevation. Circulation 38: 282–288, 1968
13. Safar ME, Weiss YA, Levenson JA, London GM, Mliiez PI: Hemodynamic study of 85 patients with borderline hypertension. Am J Cardiol 31: 315–319, 1973
14. Ledingham JM, Cohen RD: Role of the heart in the pathogenesis of renal hypertension. Lancet ii: 979–981, 1963
15. Tarazi RC, Ferrario CM, Dustan HP: The heart in hypertension. In: Genest J, Koiw E, Kuchel O (eds), Hypertension, physiopathology and treatment. McGraw-Hill, Inc, 1977, pp 738–754
16. Guyton AC, Jones CE, Coleman TG: Introduction the regulation of cardiac output. In: Circulatory physiology: cardiac output and its regulation. WB Saunders, Philadelphia, 1973, pp 137–146
17. Tarazi RC, Fouad FM, Ferrario CM: Can the heart initiate some forms of hypertension? Fed Proc 42: 2692–2697, 1983
18. Tarazi RC: Hemodynamic role of extracellular fluid in hypertension. Circ Res 38 (Suppl II): II-72–II-83, 1976
19. Tarazi RC, Ibrahim MM, Dustan HP, Ferrario CM: Cardiac factors in hypertension. Circ Res 34 (Suppl I): I-213–I-221, 1974
20. Julius S, Randall OS, Esler MD, Kashima T, Ellis C, Bennett J: Altered cardiac responsiveness and regulation in the normal cardiac output type of borderline hypertension. Circ Res 36 37 (Suppl I): I-199–I-207, 1975
21. Ibrahim MM, Tarazi RC, Dustan HP, Bravo EL: Cardioadrenergic factors in essential hypertension. Am Heart J 88: 724–732, 1974
22. Haddy FJ, Scott JB, Emerson TE, Overbeck HW, Daugherty RM Jr: Effects of generalized changes in plasma electrolyte concentration and osmalarith in blood pressure in the anesthetized dog. Circ Res 24 and 25 (Suppl I): I-54–I-74, 1969
23. Luetscher JA, Boyers DG, Cuthbertson JG, McMahon DF: A model of the human circulation: regulation by autonomic nervous system and renin-angiotensin system and influence of blood volume on cardiac output and blood pressure. Circ Res 32 and 33 (Suppl I): I-84–I-98, 1973
24. Laragh J: Vasoconstriction-volume analysis for understanding and treating hypertension: the use of renin and aldosterone profiles. Am J Med 55: 261–274, 1973
25. Ulrych M, Frohlich E, Tarazi RC, Dustan HP, Page IH: Cardiac output and distribution of blood volume in central and peripheral circulations in hypertensive and normotensive man. Brit Heart J 31: 570–564, 1969
26. Fouad FM, MacIntyre WJ, Tarazi RC: Noninvasive measurement of cardiopulmon-

ary blood volume. Evaluation of the centroid method. J Nuc Med 22: 204–211, 1981
27. Levinson GE, Pacifico AD, Frank MJ: Studies of cardiopulmonary blood volume. Measurement of total cardiopulmonary blood volume in normal human subjects at rest and during exercise. Circulation 33: 347–356, 1966
28. Ellis C, Julius S: Role of central blood volume in hyperkinetic borderline hypertension. Brit Heart J 35: 450–455, 1973
29. Van der Walt JJ, Van Rooyen JM, Cilliers GD, Van Ryssen JCJ, Van Aarde MN: Ratio of cardiopulmonary blood volume to stroke volume as an index of cardiac function in animals and in man. Cardiovasc Res 15: 580–587, 1981
30. Safar M, Weiss YA, London GM, Frackowiak RF, Milliez PL: Cardiolpulmonary blood volume in borderline hypertension. Clin Sci Mol Med 4: 152–164, 1974
31. Julius S, Essler M: Autonomic nervous cardiovascular regulation in borderline hypertension. Am J Cardiol 36: 685–696, 1975
32. Ferrario CM, Page IH, McCubbin JW: Increased cardiac output as a contributory factor in experimental renal hypertension in dogs. Circ Res 27: 799–810, 1970.
33. Hawthorne EW, Hinds EJ, Crawford WJ, Tearney RJ: Left ventricular myocardial contractility during the first week of renal hypertension in conscious instrumented dogs. Circ Res 34 (Suppl I): I-233–I-234, 1974
34. Pool PE, Piggott WJ, Seagrenb SC, Skelton CL: Augmented right ventricular function in systemic hypertension induced hypertrophy. Cardiovasc Res 10: 124–128, 1976
35. Tarazi RC, Ibrahim MM, Bravo EL, Dustan HP: Hemodynamic characteristics of primary aldosteronism. N Engl J Med 289: 1330–1335, 1973
36. Ulrych M, Frohlich ED, Dustan HP, Page IH: Immediate hemodynamic effects of beta-adrenergic blockade with propranolol in normotensive and hypertensive man. Circulation 37: 411–416, 1968
37. Neff MS, Kim KE, Persott M, Onesti G, Swartz C: Hemodynamics of uremic anemia. Circulation 43: 876–883, 1971
38. Tarazi RC, Frohlich ED, Dustan HP: Contribution of output to renovascular hypertension in man. Relation to surgical treatment. Am J Cardiol 31: 600–605, 1973
39. Liard JF, Tarazi RC, Ferrario CM, Manger WM: Hemodynamic and humoral characteristics of hypertension induced by prolonged stellate stimulation in conscious dogs. Circ Res 36: 455–464, 1975
40. Liard JF: Hypertension induced by prolonged intracoronary administration of dobutamine in conscious dogs. Clin Sci Mol Med 54: 153–160, 1978
41. Guyton AC, Granger JH, Coleman TG: Autoregulation of the total systemic circulation and its relation to control of cardiac output and arterial pressure. Circ Res 28: 93–97, 1971
42. Omvik P, Tarazi RC, Bravo EL: Regulation of sodium balance in hypertension. Hypertension 2: 515–523, 1980
43. James TN, Hageman GR, Urthaler F: Anatomic and physiologic considerations of a cardiogenic hypertensive chemoreflex. Am J Cardiol 44: 852–859, 1979
44. Tarazi RC: Antihypertensive effect of beta-blockade: relation of its hemodynamic components to other mechanisms. In: Braunwald E (ed), Beta-adrenergic blockade: a new era in cardiovascular medicine. Excerpta Medica/Elsevier, New York, 1978, pp 210–224
45. Cooper T, Peiss VN, Williams VL, Randall WC: A cardiac factor in hypertensive responses: delineation by transplantation of the heart. Circ Res 18 and 19 (Suppl I): I-85–I-95, 1966
46. Horwitz D, Sjoerdsma A: Proceedings of the Council for high blood pressure research, Am Heart Assoc 13: 39–44, 1965
47. Estafanous FG, Tarazi RC: Systemic arterial hypertension associated with cardiac surgery. Am J Cardiol 46: 685–694, 1980

48. Fouad FM, Estafanous FG, Tarazi RC: Hemodynamics of postmyocardial revascularization hypertension. Am J Cardiol 41: 564–569, 1978
49. Fouad FM, Estafanous FG, Bravo EL, Iyer KA, Maydak JH, Tarazi RC: Possible role of cardioaortic reflexes in post-coronary bypass hypertension. Am J Cardiol 44: 866–872, 1979
50. Malliani A, Pagani M, Bergamashi M: Positive feedback sympathetic reflexes and hypertension. Am J Cardiol 44: 860–865, 1979
51. Brown AM: Excitation of afferent cardiac sympathetic nerve fibers during myocardial ischaemia. J Physiol (Lond) 190: 35–53, 1967
52. Malliani A, Brown AM: Reflexes arising from coronary receptors. Brain Res 24: 352–355, 1970
53. Kent KM, Cooper T: Editorial: Cardiovascular reflexes. Circulation 52: 177–178, 1975
54. James TN, Isobe JH, Urthaler F: Analyses of components in a cardiogenic hypertensive chemoreflex. Circulation 52: 179–192, 1975
55. Schwartz PJ, Pagani M, Lombardi F, Malliani A, Brown AM: A cardio-cardiac sympathovagal reflex in the cat. Circ Res 32: 215–220, 1973
56. Donald DE, Shepherd JT: Cardiac receptors: normal and disturbed function. Am J Cardiol 44: 873–878, 1979
57. Abboud FM: Integration of reflex responses in the control of blood pressure and vascular resistance. Am J Cardio 14 4: 903–911, 1979
58. Linden RJ: Reflexes from the heart. Prog Cardiovasc Dis 18: 201–221, 1975
59. Oberg B, Thoren P: Circulatory responses to stimulation of left ventricular receptors in the cat. Acta Physiologica Scand 88: 8–22, 1973
60. Gauer OH, Henry JP: Circulatory basis of fluid volume control. Physiol Ref 43: 423–481, 1963
61. Linden RJ: Atrial reflexes and renal function. Am J Cardiol 44: 879–883, 1979
62. Zanchetti A: Overview of cardiovascular reflexes in hypertension. Am J Cardiol 44: 912–918, 1979
63. Mark AL, Kerber RE: Augmentation of cardiopulmonary baroreflex control of forearm vascular resistance in borderline hypertension. Hypertension 4: 39–46, 1982
64. Schichken RM, Clarke WR, Lauer WR: Left ventricular hypertrophy in children with blood pressures in the upper quintile of the distribution; the Muscatine study. Hypertension 3: 669–675, 1981
65. Sen S, Tarazi RC, Khairallah PA, Bumpus FM: Cardiac hypertrophy in spontaneously hypertensive rats. Circ Res 35: 775–781, 1974
66. Yamori Y, Mori C, Nishio T, Ooshima A, Horie R, Ohtaka M, Seda T, Saito M, Abe K, Nara Y, Nakao Y, Kihara M: Cardiac hypertrophy in early hypertension. Am J Cardiol 44: 964–969, 1979
67. Weiss L: Aspects of the relation between functional and structural cardiovascular factors in primary hypertension. Experimental studies in spontaneously hypertensive rats. Acta Physiol Scand, Suppl. 409, 1–58, 1974
68. Sen S, Tarazi RC, Bumpus FM: Biochemical changes associated with development and reversal of cardiac hypertrophy in spontaneously hypertensive rats. Cardiovasc Res 10: 254–261, 1976
69. Yamori Y, Tarazi RC, Ooshima A: Effect of beta-receptor blocking agents on cardiovascular structural changes in spontaneous and noradrenaline-induced hypertension in rats. Clin Sci 59 (Suppl 6): 457s–460s, 1980
70. Fouad FM, Nakashima Y, Tarazi RC, Salcedo E: Reversal of left ventricular hypertrophy in hypertensive patients treated with methyldopa. Lack of association with blood pressure control. Am J Cardiol 49L 795–801, 1982
71. Tarazi RC, Levy MN: Cardiac responses to increased afterload. Hypertension 4

294

(Suppl II): II-8–II-18, 1982
72. Von Bibra H, Richardson PJ: Left ventricular hypertrophy in patients with moderate essential hypertension: an echocardiographic study. In: Robertson JIS, Caldwell ADS (eds), Left ventricular hypertrophy in hypertension. Royal Society of Medicine international congress and symposium series, No. 9. The Royal Society of Medicine (Lond), Academic Press (Lond), Grune Stratton (New York), 1979, pp 55–66
73. Safar ME, Lehner JP, Vincent MI, Plainfosse MT, Simon AC: Echocardiographic dimensions in borderline and essential hypertension. AM J Cardiol 44: 930–935, 1979
74. Maron BJ, Edwards JE, Epstein SE: Disproportionate ventricular septal thickening in patients with systemic hypertension. Chest 73: 466–469, 1978
75. Strauer BE: Ventricular function and coronary hemodynamics in hypertensive heart disease. Am J Cardiol 44: 999–1006, 1979
76. Abi-Samra F, Fouad FM, Tarazi RC, Bravo EL: Determinants of left ventricular hypertrophy and function in hypertensive patients. Am J Med 75 (Suppl 3A): 26–33, 1983
77. Gaasch WH: Left ventricular radius to wall thickness ratio. Am J Cardiol 43: 1189–1194, 1979
78. Grossman W, Jones D, McLauern HP: Wall stress and patterns of hypertrophy in the human left ventricle. J Clin Invest 56: 56, 1975 (abstract)
79. Korner P: Mechanisms of hypertension. The sixth Volhard lecture. Clin Sci 63 (Suppl 8): 269–283, 1982.85
80. Fouad FM, Tarazi RC, Gallagher JH, MacIntyre WJ, Cook SA: Abnormal left ventricular relaxation in hypertensive patients. Clin Sci 59 (Suppl 6): 411s–414s, 1980
81. Hallback-Nordlander M, Noresson E, Thoren P: Hemodynamic consequences of left ventricular hypertrophy in spontaneously hypertensive rats. Am J Cardiol 44: 986–993, 1979
82. Thoren P, Noresson, Rickstein SE: Cardiac reflexes in normotensive and spontaneously hypertensive rats. Am J Cardiol 44: 884–888, 1979
83. Zucker IH, Earle AM, Gilmore JP: The mechanism of adaptation of left atrial stretch receptors in dogs with chronic congestive heart failure. J Clin Invest 60: 323–331, 1977
84. Saragoca M, Tarazi RC: Impaired cardiac contractile response to isoproterenol in the spontaneously hypertensive rat. Hypertension 3: 380–385, 1981
85. Wicker P, Tarazi RC: Coronary blood flow in left ventricular hypertrophy: a review of experimental data. Eur Heart J 3: 111–118, 1982
86. Fishberg AM: Hypertension and Nephritis. Balliere, Tindal and Cox, London, 1954, pp 788–789
87. Flectcher PL, Pfeffer JM, Pfeffer MA, Braunwald E: Myocardial function in experimental hypertension in rats: mechanism of the reduction in blood pressure. Clin Sci 59 (Suppl 6): 385s–387s, 1980
88. Franciosa JA, Heckel R, Limas C, Cohn JN: Progressive myocardial dysfunction associated with increased vascular resistance. Am J Physiol 239: H477–H482, 1980
89. Pickering G: High Blood Pressure. Grune and Stratton, New York, 1968, pp 422–425
90. Fouad FM, Tarazi RC: Cardiac factors in response to antihypertensive treatment. Hypertension 5 (Suppl III): III-43–III-48, 1983
91. Tarazi RC, Sen S, Fouad FM, Wicker P: Regression of myocardial hypertrophy: conditions and sequelae of reversal in hypertensive heart disease. In: Alpert NR (ed), Perspectives in cardiovascular research, Vol 7, Myocardial hypertrophy and failure. Raven Press, New York, 1983, pp 637–652
92. Kannel WB: Role of blood pressure in cardiovascular morbidity and mortality. Prog Cardiovas Dis 17: 5–24, 1974

93. Tarazi RC, Gifford RW Jr.: Systemic arterial pressure. In: Sodeman WA, Sodeman WA Jr (eds), Pathologic physiology. W.B. Saunders, Philadelphia, 1974, pp 177–205

94. Dustan HP, Tarazi RC, Bravo EL: False tolerance to antihypertensive drugs. In: Sambhi MP (ed), Systemic effects of antihypertensive agents. Stratton Intercontinental Medical Book Company, New York, 1976, pp 51–67

95. Fouad FM, Tarazi RC, Bravo EL: Cardiac and haemodynamic effects of enalapril. J Hypertension 1 (Suppl I): 135–142, 1983

96. Ayobe MH, Tarazi RC: Beta-receptors and contractile reserve in left ventricular hypertrophy. Hypertension 5 (Suppl I): I-192–I-197, 1983

97. Marcus ML, Mueller TM, Gascho JA, Kerber RE: Effects of cardiac hypertrophy secondary to hypertension on the coronary circulation. Am J Cardiol 49: 1023–1028, 1979

98. Wicker P, Tarazi RC, Kobayashi K: Coronary blood flow during the development and regression of left ventricular hypertrophy in renovascular hypertensive rats. Am J Cardiol 51: 1744–1749, 1983

99. Yamori Y, Nakada T, Lovenberg W: Effect of antihypertensive therapy on lysine incorproation into vascular protein in the spontaneously hypertensive rat. Eur J Pharmacol 38: 349–355, 1976

100. Hallback-Nordlander M: Functional consequences of structural adaptation of the heart in hypertension. Hypertension (in press)

22. STRUCTURAL CHANGE IN THE BLOOD VESSEL WALL
The fundamental self-perpetuating process in primary hypertension

ROSEMARY D. BEVAN, JOHN A. BEVAN

INTRODUCTION

The structural hypothesis for the mechanism of development and maintenance of primary hypertension may be stated as follows (see Figure 1). Factors stressful to the vasculature, particularly during its growth and maturation, which may be of intrinsic or extrinsic origin, cause a vascular load which is associated with a rise in arterial and/or venous pressures. The factors may originate from different sources for example, neurogenic, renal, endocrine or dietary and although there may be quantitative differences in the regional distribution, magnitude and duration of their effects, they initiate a qualitatively similar response of the vascular wall. A crucial element in the structural hypothesis is that the induced changes are additive and that initially at any rate the wall changes exaggerate the response to subsequent stimuli, thus accelerating the change. By this means, the structural change becomes self-perpetuating and over a prolonged period of time leads to manifest alteration in the circulation. This hypothesis has received its greatest elaboration, particularly in relation to studies of the spontaneously hypertensive rat in a review by Folkow [12].

There are several components of the responses of the blood vessel wall to such a pressure load. An increase occurs in the amount of vascular smooth muscle, either in the number of cells or their size or both, resulting in an increase in the ability of the vascular wall to develop tone and thus to constrict to appropriate stimuli (see for example, Sivertsson [26]. Another effect is an increase in the synthesis of extracellular material, from vascular smooth muscle cells in the media and fibroblasts in the adventitia (see for example, Wolinsky [32]. This results in a wall that is stiffer, i.e., which exhibits decreased compliance. In addition, changes may occur in the sympathetic innervation of the blood vessel secondary to the rise in intravascular pressure (see for example, Bevan et al. [1, 5]. All the above changes might be expected to have a number of physiological sequelae, including an increase in peripheral resistance, a decrease in peripheral venous compliance, and a blunting of the homeostatic reflex vascular control.

Alteration in the size and physical characteristics of the vascular wall that occur during growth and aging arise in response to changes in stretch, volume load, neurohumoral agents, local modulators and in the tissues supplied by a change in

Sambhi, M.P. (ed.) Fundamental fault in hypertension
© *1984, Martinus Nijhoff Publishers. Boston/The Hague/Dordrecht/Lancaster.*
ISBN 978-94-010-9006-3

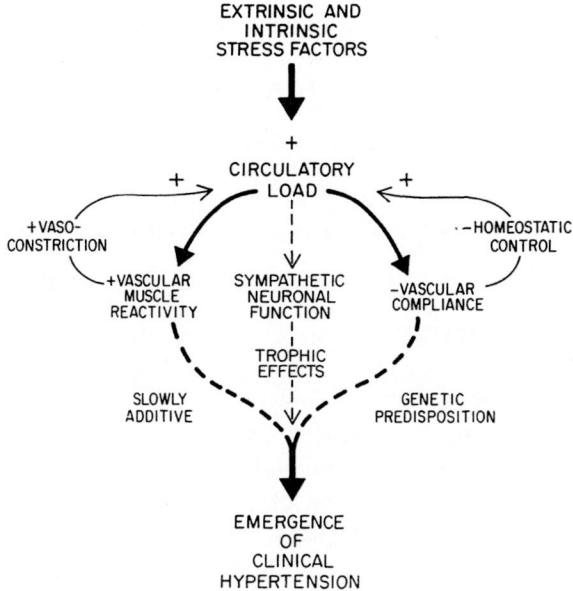

Figure 1. Diagramatic representation of the Structural Hypothesis of Hypertension.

metabolism of the component cells of the wall. An implication of the structural hypothesis is that either the stimuli or the responses, or both are exaggerated in magnitude and/or duration in some individuals resulting in an inappropriately large vascular change. Exaggerated responses may depend in part upon a genetic predisposition but require a suitable stimulus for expression.

During growth the interaction between the principle regulator of neurogenic vascular tone, the peripheral adrenergic neurons, and the smooth muscle are complex and deviations in normal maturation of either could lead to permanent changes in neuroeffector relationships. This area has not been adequately explored. Early changes would occur in the vasculature without overt alteration in arterial pressure. Evidence of such alterations could be detected only for example as an altered response to stress, e.g. exercise [19]. Eventually, due to the additive consequences of repeated vascular adaptation, hypertension would become established. The emergence of this state would be facilitated by blunting of homeostatic reflexes as a consequence of structural change in reflexogenic zones. The resetting of the baroreceptors would however in part offset this effect.

An adaptive response of the blood vessel wall to an elevation in tangential stress (intramural pressure) is common to all forms of chronic hypertension. In addition, based upon animal studies [33, 34, 6] there is a possibility that the sympathetic nervous system exerts a positive trophic influence on the blood vessel wall affecting vascular smooth muscle and extracellular tissue content. Increased sympathetic discharge is a component of the response to many forms of stress. It should be emphasized that this possible mechanism is a special trophic influence resulting from neural activity *per se*, mediated by the neurotransmitter or an as yet, unidentified substance(s) released at the same time, independent of any associated change in arterial pressure. Humoral substances could have a similar action.

CHANGES IN THE VASCULAR WALL CONSEQUENT UPON AN INCREASE IN TANGENTIAL STRESS

In studies of the rabbit after partial abdominal aortic constriction (PAAC), a model of hypertension that allows a simultaneous analysis of changes in neuroeffector mechanism of both arteries and veins and to some degree the nature of the cause, hyperplasia associated with an increase in smooth muscle mass was observed [2]. This occurred exclusively in blood vessels of all sizes found in that part of the arterial tree exposed to an elevation in pressure. Hypertrophy of smooth muscle cells would also be expected to be a component of the increased mass but stereologic measurements were not made. As the changes did not occur in vessels in the posterior normotensive compartment except in the collateral development around the constriction, nor in the veins, this change is associated presumably with the increased pressure not with any generalized stimulus [4]. An alternate or additional possibility is that increased pressure changes the permeability of the blood vessel wall and consequently the environment of the component cells exposing them to an increase in growth factor. It may be argued that if a circulating substance was responsible for these changes, it would influence all blood vessels, or at least all arteries. It was observed that hyperplasia appeared to be inversely proportional to the caliber of the arterial vessel down to the arteriolar level and could occur in the absence of any damage to the vessel wall detectable by light microscopy.

A positive correlation was established between vessel DNA content in a large and middle-sized artery, the level of mean arterial pressure and also the maximum developed force to norepinephrine [1]. In addition, there were alterations in the physical characteristics of the vessel wall which became stiffer and in certain functional parameters of the sympathetic nerve terminal plexus. There was no measurable alteration in vascular internal diameter of these large arteries.

Detailed morphometric study of the wall dimension of small mesenteric arteries of lumen diameter about 150 μm from the spontaneously hypertensive rat has shown that the increase in media size is contributed to by both an increase in cell size and number – although the increase in size as determined by an increase in cell cross-sectional area was not significant [30]. The data was consistent with increases in extracellular material leading to increased stiffness as determined by steeper passive stress-strain curves. The exact cause of change in the vasculature of this hypertensive model is not established. There is conflicting evidence concerning an early increase in neurogenic tone [18, 28]. Changes in some of the membrane characteristics of the vascular smooth muscle cells have been confirmed by a number of investigators [17,14,13]. Thus, these changes cannot be considered as exclusively passive alterations in the vessel wall. There is functional evidence that the changes that occur in the resistance vessels of the spontaneously hypertensive rat result in some encroachment on the vessel lumen and alteration in the sympathetic neuronal and extraneuronal function [11, 22, 29].

CHANGES IN THE SYMPATHETIC MECHANISM: THEIR POSSIBLE SIGNIFICANCE

The alpha-adrenoceptor mediated response of blood vessels can be influenced in a number of ways by preceding conditions [24]. Because of this, it may be questioned whether the experimental observation of the change in responsiveness in experimental hypertension is necessarily of etiological significance. It has been shown experimentally that the response to a catecholamine is dependent upon the prior short and long-term level of sympathetic activity [25]. This level is dictated *in vivo* by many factors, external and environmental, genetic and internal.

In addition, contractility is affected by preceding levels of muscular activity independent of their cause. Neuronal function also depends upon the preceding levels of tonic discharge, adding yet more complexity to the analysis [31]. Thus, observed changes in the characteristics of the adrenergic neuroeffector mechanism in experimental hypertension are not necessarily of primary etiological significance. To achieve such a designation, a change must be shown not to be secondary to other effects. Thus it is the onus and responsibility of the experimenter to determine which changes in adrenergic parameters are primary and which are secondary. Such an analysis has not been effectively achieved to date.

INFLUENCE OF SYMPATHETIC INNERVATION ON VASCULAR WALL STRUCTURE

Interruption of the tonic sympathetic drive to an artery in the rabbit ear by post-ganglionic sympathectomy, particularly in the growing animal, resulted in a number of changes in its wall substance – both adventitial and medial and its reactivity [33]. Similar changes also resulted from pre-ganglionic sympathetic nerve section [36]. There was diminished muscle mass in the growing animal associated with a reduction in the capacity of the vascular wall to develop tone and at the same time a change in the extracellular matrix resulting in an increased stiffness of the vessel. The magnitude and also the quality of the change was dependent on the age at which sympathetic nerve influence was removed. Arterial wall structure and function in this vascular bed was shown to be dependent on nerve impulses [7]. Sympathetic nerves also influenced the pattern of the microcirculation during growth in the rabbit ear [33].

300

EXPERIMENTAL EVIDENCE IN SUPPORT OF THE STRUCTURAL HYPOTHESIS:

Some of the necessary conditions of the structural hypothesis revolve around the relative rate of induction and resolution of the structural change (see Figure 2). Structural response should occur as a result of a perturbation in arterial pressure of a size and duration not infrequently found in the circulation. The resolution of induced structural change should be slow in comparison to the rate of their establishment. The refinement of such considerations is not feasible without additional experimental information. However, it is self-evident that if the vasculature is to be the respository of the consequences of repeated vascular load, then resolution must be slower than rates of induction otherwise accumulation of effective change would never take place. The following is offered as supporting (but not definitive) evidence for the structural hypothesis.

Rates of onset of structural change

(a) In the PAAC rabbit there is a similarity in the time course of rise in arterial pressure and two indices of the vascular muscle change – the mitotic index and the ^{3}H-thymidine labeling index (Figure 3). Within the framework of resolution of the periodic observations, there is no evidence of a significant lag of cellular response behind pressure rise nor do these evidences of active vascular change persist once arterial pressure has stabilized at a new equilibrium level. The evidence suggests a fairly close dynamic equilibrium between the changes in pressure and response.

(b) Experimentally determined changes in blood vessels from the anterior compartment of the PAAC rabbit, for example, the capacity to develop tone, to take up precursors of new cellular structure and the increase in vascular wall mass, positively correlate with the level of arterial pressure of each experimental animal. Regression lines between such changes ad the level of pressure can be extended to include changes observed in normotensive controls [4]. This implies a continuous relationship between vascular wall change in hypertension and these parameters in normotensive animals.

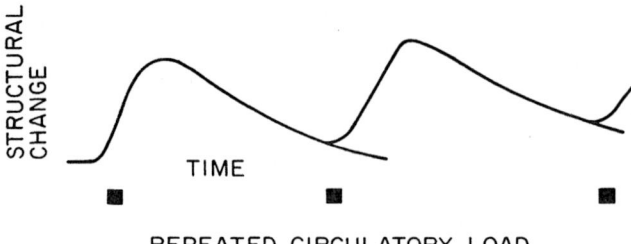

Figure 2. Time course of structural change consequent upon repeated circulatory load.

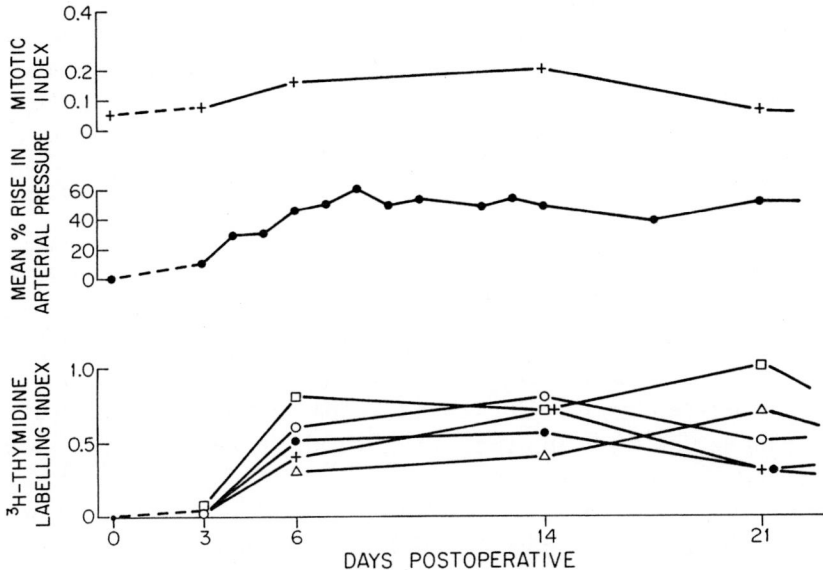

Figure 3. Time course of changes in mitotic index in splenic artery, in H-thymidine labeling index in ○ splenic artery, □ post-gastric artery, + common carotid artery, △ ear artery, ● proximal thoracic aorta, and in the arterial pressure from the anterior hypertensive vascular segment of rabbit after partial abdominal aortic constriction.

(c) Preliminary studies in the sino-aortic denervated rabbits where there is little change in the mean arterial pressure, only its lability show, after only 4 days, a significant increase in the uptake of labeled amino acid precursors in the wall of a muscular artery [21]. The relative importance of increased pressure and the increased sympathetic activity that undoubtedly occurs in this model in causing such changes has not been determined.

(d) An increased tension applied to an isolated artery *in vitro* results in an increase in amino acid and thymidine uptake after a latency of 4 days [16]. The level of uptake is related to the amount of applied force.

Rates of resolution of structural change

(a) The structural change in the vessel wall observed only a short time after the arterial pressure has reached a new equilibrium tends to persist. After 8 months of sustained elevated pressure, such characteristics of the vessel wall, such as mass, thickness, capacity to develop tone etc., have changed very little [3]. This suggests that the amount of structural adaptation was set by the absolute level of pressure in this model.

(b) After 8 months of elevated pressure the circumference of the lumen of some vessels e.g. the basilar artery showed a positive correlation with the pressure of the donor animal. Thus the basilar artery of hypertensive animals had a greater

302

internal circumference than the normotensive – a change which was not observed after 2 months of hypertension. As this increase probably reflects an alteration in the collagen skeleton or matrix of the blood vessel, it is an indication of the slow rate of vascular wall remodeling. This in turn reflects the slow rate of turnover of the more stable elements in the blood vessel wall.

EVIDENCE SUPPORTIVE OF THE STRUCTURAL HYPOTHESIS FROM HUMAN PRIMARY HYPERTENSION

Because convincing evidence can only be derived from the study of early or initial events when no secondary pathological changes have intervened, evidence from humans is limited. What support there is must ideally be obtained from borderline or early hypertensive patients.

Increased muscle mass. All investigators who have studied this problem agree that there is an increase in thickness of the wall of arteries from hypertensive patients. That this increase in arterial thickness includes an increase in contractility may be deduced from the observation that the vasoconstriction that follows intra-arterial sympathomimetics is greater in the hypertensive than the normotensive patient [26].

Decrease in vascular wall compliance. A 10-year follow up of mild hypertensives has shown that arterial pressure levels had not significantly altered during that period of time and no overt complications had occurred. However, cardiovascular parameters, particularly those of central hemodynamics, had deteriorated more than might be expected from age alone. The systolic index had decreased and total peripheral resistance increased. The capacity of resistance vessels to dilate during exercise had also diminished. It may be argued that these changes reflect slowly progressive structural alterations not only in resistance vessels but in the heart and possibly the great veins as well [20].

A number of studies has suggested decreased distensibility of peripheral veins in borderline hypertensives. Only part of this decrease was reversed by acute blockade of tonic activity of the sympathetic nervous system. It was concluded that most of the decrease was due to nonadrenergic mechanisms [27]. Possible bases for the alteration in vein properties is a structural change consequent upon repeated intermittent increases in load, or a change in neurohumoral trophic influences.

SUBNORMAL RESPONSIVENESS OF CAROTID BAROFLEX:

In borderline hypertension, although baroreceptor sensitivity was shifted to function at the patients usual arterial pressure, i.e. resetting occurred, their responsiveness to an increment in pressure change was altered. There was a gradient of responsiveness related to arterial pressure level. In those with an average systolic arterial pressure greater than 140 mmHg, the reflex was consistently subnormal. The consequence was suboptimal baroreceptor buffering [10]. One of the possible bases for this change is a structural alteration in the physical characteristics of the carotid sinus wall.

INCREASED SYMPATHETIC EFFERENT ACTIVITY

Despite problems in selecting control subjects and in utilizing plasma cate-cholamine levels as an index of sympathetic drive, clinical studies strongly suggest the existence of a subset of patients with hypertension associated with evidence of increased sympathetic tone [23, 9]. Although an increased sympathetic drive is not a prerequisite of the structural theory, and structural adaptation is probably a consequence of increased blood pressure irrespective of its cause, an intrinsic part of our hypothesis is that increased sympathetic drive contributes an added trophic component to the changes in the blood vessel wall, that may be occurring in response to a pressure increase. The trophic action on vascular structure is most important during body growth.

FAILURE OF CHRONIC SYMPATHETIC STIMULATION TO ESTABLISH
HYPERTENSION

Perhaps the strongest argument put forward against the initiation of structural change by neurogenic activity is the consistent failure of experimental chronic sympathetic stimulation to initiate maintained hypertension. In general, however, experiments have not realistically tested the hypothesis and the age factor has not been taken into account. In some studies utilizing chronically implanted electrodes in the brain, local tissue damage was shown to occur [8]. Thus the consistent effectiveness of stimuli to produce prolonged increases in sympathetic drive must be demonstrated. A major prerequisite or condition in testing the theory is the duration of stimulation: the rate of resolution of vascular wall elements is not known with precision but probably is measured in terms of weeks or months. A stimulation period which is some multiple of the half time of regression of the slowest and most stable element would be needed for an effective test. Finally, as noted above, initial structural changes may occur in the vasculature which are not reflected in an alteration in overt blood pressure because of the efficient homeostatic capacity of animals. Measurements of greater sensitivity and precision than arterial pressure must be utilized to test for early structural change.

The demonstration by Henry et al. [15] that social stress in mice can lead to establishment of a hypertensive state, although indirect, is strongly supportive of the efficacy of repetitive vascular stress in leading to permanent circulatory alteration.

SUMMARY

Central to the structural hypothesis is the requirement that repeated circulatory loads lead to increased muscle and extracellular material in the vessel wall and that the rate of formation of these new elements is considerably faster than their rate of resolution. This latter process must be sufficiently slow to allow additive change in the vessel wall which, over a prolonged period of time, leads to overt hypertension. Tonic activity of the sympathetic nervous system may play an additive and even initiating role in this process. Thus the ascular wall becomes the repository of repeated, additive, circulatory and neural insults which exaggerate its response to subsequent stress. These changes are thus self-perpetuating and in time become apparent to our relatively insensitive means of observation and assessment. The most important site of vascular change with respect to primary hypertension may be in the kidney.

ACKNOWLEDGEMENT

Some of the research included in this paper was supported by U.S.P.H.S. Grant HL 20581

POST SCRIPT

This manuscript was written in 1979 for the Workshop 'The Fundamental Fault in Hypertension'. It has been left essentially unchanged for we feel the hypothesis is still valid. Since 1979 much important and relevant information has accumulated and the reader should refer to the recent review by Professor Bjorn Folkow. The reference is Physiological Reviews 62(2): 347–504. 1982

REFERENCES

1. Bevan JA, Bevan RD, Chang PC, Pegram BL, Purdy RE, Su C: Analysis of changes in reactivity of rabbit arteries and veins two weeks after induction of hypertension by coarctation of the abdominal aorta. Circ Res 37: 183–190, 1975
2. Bevan RD: An autoradiographic and pathological study of cellular proliferation in rabbit arteries correlated with changes in arterial pressure. Blood Vessels 13: 100–124, 1976
3. Bevan RD, Eggena P, Hume WR, Lais LT, Van Marthens E, Bevan JA: An 8-month

longitudinal study of changes in elastic and muscular arteries and veins of the rabbit with sustained hypertension after abdominal aorta constriction. Clin Sci 57 (Suppl 5): 7s–9s, 1980

4. Bevan RD, Hume WR, Bevan JA: The response of the arterial wall to a rise in intravascular pressure. In: Spontaneous hypertension: its pathogenesis and complications. Proceedings of the second international symposium on the spontaneously hypertensive rat. DHEW Publication No. (NIH) 77–1179, Newport Beach California, 1976

5. Bevan RD, Purdy RE, Su C, Bevan JA: Evidence for an increase in adrenergic nerve function in blood vessels from experimental hypertensive rabbits. Circ Res 37: 503–508, 1975

6. Bevan RD, Tsuru H: Functional and structural changes in the rabbit ear artery following sympathetic denervation. Circ Res 49: 478–485, 1981

7. Bevan RD, Tsuru H: Long-term influence of the sympathetic nervous system on arterial structure and reactivity: possible factor in hypertension. In: Abboud FM, Fozzard HA, Gilmore JP Reis DJ (eds), Disturbances in neurogenic control of the circulation. Clinical Physiology Series. Bethesda, Am Physiol Soc pp 153–160, 1981

8. Bunag R, Riley E: Chronic hypothalamic stimulation in awake rats fails to induce hypertension. Hypertension 1: 498–507, 1979

9. de Champlain Jacques: The sympathetic system in hypertension. Clin in Endocrin and Metab 6: 633–655, 1977

10. Eckberg Dwain L: Carotid baroflex function in young men with borderline blood pressure elevation. Circ 59: 632–636, 1979

11. Folkow Bjorn: Structural changes in the vascular bed.[1] In: Vascular neuroeffector mechanisms. Second international symposium on vascular neuroeffector mechanisms, Odense, pp 170–181, 1976

12. Folkow, Bjorn: The fourth Volhard lecture: Cardiovascular structural adaptation; its role in the initiation and maintenance of primary hypertension. Clin Sci and Mol Med 55: 3s–22s, 1978

13. Friedman SM: Arterial contractility and reactivity. In: Genest J, Koiw E, Kuchel O, (eds), Hypertension. McGraw Hill, New York, pp 470–485, 1977

14. Hansen TR, Abrams GD, Bohr DF: Role of pressure in structural and functional changes in arteries of hypertensive rats. Circ Res 34 (Suppl. 1): 101–107, 1974

15. Henry JP, Stephens PM, Santisteban GA: A model of psychosocial hypertension showing reversibility and progression of cardiovascular complications. Circ Res 36: 156–164, 1975

16. Hume WR, Bevan JA, Bevan RD: Wall tension and blood vessel structure *in vitro*. American Heart Association's 52nd Scientific Sessions, Anaheim. Circulation 59 & 60 (Suppl. II) 10, 1979

17. Jones AW: Altered ion transport in vascular smooth muscle from spontaneously hypertensive rats. Circ Res 33: 563–572, 1973

18. Judy WV, Murphy WR, Watanabe AM, Besch Jr HR, Henry DP, Yu PL: Sympathetic nerve activity in spontaneously hypertensive rats. In: Spontaneous hypertension: its pathogenesis and complications. Proceedings of the second international symposium on the spontaneously hypertensive rat. DHEW No. 77–1179, pp 223–236, 1976

19. Lund-Johanson P: Hemodynamics in essential hypertension. Clin Sci 59: 343s–354s, 1980

20. Lund-Johansen Per: Hemodynamic trends in untreated essential hypertension. Acta Medica Scand 620: 68–76, 1976

21. MacLean AG, Bevan RD, Hume WR, Ransome RW, Bevan JA: Vascular changes in sino-aortic denervated rats. Fed Proc 39: 963, 1980

22. Nagatsu T, Ikuta K, Numata Y (Sudo), Kato T, Sano M: Vascular and brain dopamine beta-hydroxylase activity in young spontaneously hypertensive rats. Science 191: 290–291, 1976
23. DeQuattro V, Miura Y: Neurogenic factors in human hypertension: mechanism or myth? Amer J of Med 55: 632–678, 1973
24. Rapoport R, Bevan JA: Acute stress reduces the sensitivity of the vasculature to sympathetic control.[1] Experientia 35: 1609–1610, 1979
25. Rapoport R: Compared to effects of various procedures causing vascular smooth muscle contraction on a subsequent responsiveness. Ph D Thesis, University of California, 1980
26. Sivertsson Ramon: The hemodynamic importance of structural vascular changes in essential hypertension. Acta Physiol Scand Supplementum 343: 3–56, 1970
27. Takeshita A, Mark AL: Decreased venous distensibility in borderline hypertension. Hypertension 1: 202–206, 1979
28. Touw KB, Haywood JR, Shaffer RA, Brody MJ: Contribution of the sympathetic nervous system to vascular resistance in conscious young and adult spontaneously hypertensive rats. Hypertension 2: 408–418, 1980.
29. Trajkov T, Berkowitz BA, Spector S: Catechol-O-methyltransferase and dopamine-β-hydroxylase activity in the blood vessels of hypertensive rats. Blood Vessels 11: 101–109, 1974
30. Warshaw David M, Mulvany MJ, Halpern W: Mechanical and morphological properties of arterial resistance vessels in young and old spontaneously hypertensive rats. Circ Res 45: 250–259, 1979
31. Weiner N, Cloutier G, Bjur R, Pfeffer RI: Modification of norepinephrine synthesis in intact tissue by drugs and during short-term adrenergic nerve stimulation. Pharmacol Rev 25: 203–221, 1972
32. Wolinsky H: Long-term effects of hypertension on the rat aortic wall and their relation to concurrent aging changes. Circ Res 30: 301–309, 1972
33. Morris JL, Bevan RD: Proliferation of arterio-venous anastomoses after denervation of the young rabbit ear. Fed Proc 1983; 42: 485
34. Abel PW, Hermsmeyer K: Sympathetic cross-innervation of SHR and genetic controls suggests a trophic influence on vascular muscle membranes. Circ Res 1981; 49: 1311–18
35. Aprigliano O, Hermsmeyer K: Trophic influence of the sympathetic nervous system on the rat portal vein. Circ Res 1977; 41: 198–206

VIII. HOW IS THE RENIN SYSTEM INVOLVED?

23.   IS THERE A FAULT IN THE RENIN-ANGIOTENSIN SYSTEM IN
       ESSENTIAL HYPERTENSION?

John D. Swales

I should admit, first of all, that the concept of a 'fault' in any system in essential
hypertension worries me. Recognition of a fault implies that some individuals
have that fault and others do not. This seems to be dangerously close to the heresy
that held that hypertension was a discrete disease – a view so thoroughly refuted
by Pickering [22]. Elevated blood pressure is like tallness, obesity, and an
extrovert personality – a quantitative deviation from the norm. We are no more
successful in finding a cause for high blood pressure in most hypertensive patients
than we are in discovering a cause for a particular body stature or personality. In
each case we are observing a constitutional quality that is determined multifactorially; we are particularly interested in hypertension because that quality is
harmful to health and survival. If it were not, I strongly suspect that most of us
would accept high blood pressure as part of a biological spectrum. Because
hypertension has discrete consequences – strokes and heart attacks – we er-
roneously think of it as a discrete disease.

The systems that control blood pressure are only partially understood. I will
take one of these, the renin-angiotensin system, and examine the case for its
involvement in the pathogenesis of essential hypertension. Although my conclusions are largely negative, I hope that a consideration of the possible role of
one of the most intensively studied systems may throw some light on the problems
involved in searching for a 'fault' in essential hypertension, problems that are
often conceptual rather than technical.

THE PROBLEM

The most commonly employed means of assessing activity of the renin-angiotensin system is the measurement of plasma renin or angiotensin II. The results of
each assay are closely correlated in essential hypertension [31], so that I will
simply show ambulant plasma renin activity (PRA) in a group of consecutively
referred hypertensive patients in whom there was no evidence for secondary
hypertension. Plasma renin among such patients is distributed in a smooth
unimodal but skewed fashion [35]. The distribution is very similar to that observed in normotensive subjects, except that 10–15% of patients with essential

Sambhi, M.P. (ed.) Fundamental fault in hypertension
© *1984, Martinus Nijhoff Publishers. Boston/The Hague/Dordrecht/Lancaster.*
ISBN 978-94-010-9006-3

310

hypertension have plasma renin levels above the range of the normotensives. The majority of hypertensive patients, therefore, have a 'normal' plasma renin, although it is possible, by means of stimulation tests, to distinguish a further subgroup of patients whose plasma renin is relatively unresponsive to stimuli that would normally cause hyper-reninemia [7]. If we compare plasma renin in essential hypertension with plasma renin values obtained under similar conditions from patients with renovascular hypertension subsequently corrected by surgery (Figure 1), we find an almost exact mirror image, i.e., plasma renin values above the normal range in most cases, although a minority of patients have a 'normal' plasma renin. It seems unlikely, even in such renovascular hypertension, that the renin-angiotensin system performs more than a partial role in the maintenance of blood pressure [4, 28]. At face value, therefore, the view that the renin-angiotensin system is at fault in essential hypertension would seem to lack support.

POSSIBLE SOLUTIONS

There are three possible ways in which the renin-angiotensin system could maintain blood pressure despite apparently normal renin levels; each possibility has been advocated in the last few years. These are increased vascular responsiveness to angiotensin II; inappropriate renin secretion; and increased renin concen-

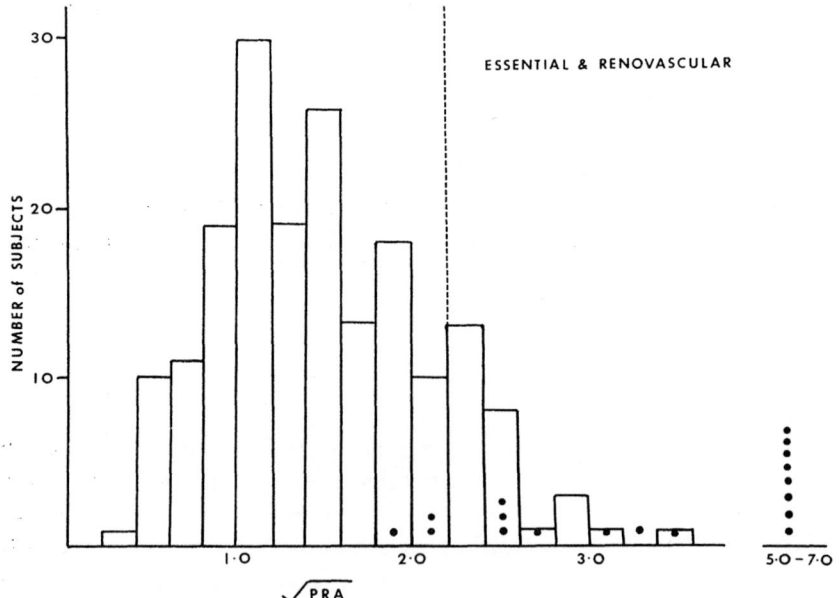

Figure 1. Distribution of plasma renin activity (PRA) among 183 untreated patients with essential hypertension attending hospital out-patient services. Dots show PRA in patients with renovascular hypertension that responded to surgery.

tration at a critical site, e.g., the resistance vessel wall and the central nervous system.

Increased vascular responsiveness

The response of the cardiovascular system to a pressor agent depends upon both the concentration of that agent at the receptor site and the subsequent chemo-mechanical events. A change in the latter will therefore produce a modified response even in the absence of changes in pressor hormone concentration. Although such altered responsiveness is regularly observed in essential hypertension [6, 19], cause and effect need to be distinguished. Resistance vessel wall hypertrophy with an increased wall-to-lumen ratio gives rise to non-specifically enhanced responsiveness to vasoconstrictor agents [8]. This, of course, is a consequence and not a cause of hypertension. Changes in specific hypersensitivity to angiotensin II can also be the result of the mechanisms that give rise to hypertension. Thus, one of the most important determinants of the pressor response to angiotensin II infusion is the degree of occupancy of vascular angiotensin II receptors by angiotensin II generated by endogenous renin [33]. High renin levels lead to occupation of relatively more available receptors, and so produce specific depression in angiotensin II responsiveness. Likewise, reduction in occupancy leads to increased responsiveness. Receptor occupancy is an important factor in the hyper-responsiveness to angiotensin II that can be demonstrated in experimental steroid hypertension (a low renin model) and in the depression of the responsiveness observed in Goldblatt 2-kidney hypertension (a high renin model). Thus, when endogenous angiotensin II formation is inhibited by converting enzyme blockade, pressor responsiveness to angiotensin II is enhanced in the Goldblatt model to a level that barely falls short of that observed in DOC hypertension [18]. It would be difficult to implicate such changes in responsiveness in the pathogenesis of hypertension.

Fewer studies of receptor affinity and number have been carried out in experimental hypertension, and none in essential hypertension although receptor number is probably dependent upon circulating angiotensin II levels [13]. In one study, however, receptor numbers were unchanged in Goldblatt 2-kidney hypertension, and reduced in Gldblatt 1-kidney and DOC saline hypertension [5]. An increase in vascular angiotensin II receptors has not so far been demonstrated in experimental or clinical hypertension. There is other indirect evidence that hypertension is not in general mediated by a specific increase in vascular angiotensin responsiveness. Thus, blockade of the renin-angiotensin system by the competitive angiotensin II antagonist sarcosine-1-alanine-8 angiotensin II (saralasin) produces a fall in blood pressure within minutes, closely correlated to circulating plasma renin or angiotensin II levels [26]. The consistent deviation from this pattern that would be predicted if enhanced sensitivity were of patho-

312

genetic importance has not been found in any clinical or experimental form of hypertension.

Inappropriate renin secretion

It has been argued that 'volume' and 'vasoconstrictor' factors (of which renin is the most important) perform complementary roles in hypertension [16], so that, when the 'volume' component is eliminated by salt depletion, blood pressure is maintained by renin [10, 11]. Thus, it is argued that renin levels are 'inappropriately' high in relation to sodium status [24, 14, 38, 3]. It could equally well be argued that plasma renin is inappropriately high for the blood pressure in essential hypertension, as a high renal perfusion pressure would normally suppress renin secretion. It is worthwhile to examine this concept a little more closely. The cardinal example of inappropriate hormone secretion is the syndrome of inappropriate secretion of ADH (SISADH) [25]; here the concept of 'inappropriateness' is straightforward. Antidiuretic hormone secretion is normally stimulated by two factors-increased plasmo osmolality and decreased extracellular fluid volume (Figure 2). Inappropriate secretion of ADH was postulated by the Schwartz group because neither factor was operating, i.e., plasma osmolality was low and extracellular fluid volume was expanded by water retention. The term 'inappropriate secretion' can only be applied to situations where secretion of a hormone is occurring that is demonstrably out of proportion to the normal regulatory stimuli for that hormone. The difficulty in applying this idea to renin secretion is apparent from the complexity of the physiological control mechanisms (Figure 3): any one stimulus may be producing hyperreninemia and is impossible to detect without knowing the precise state of each

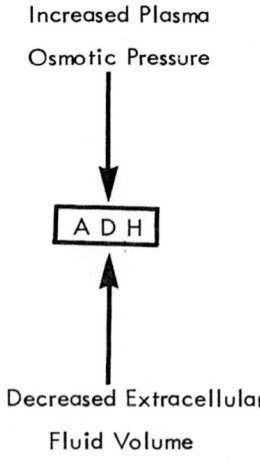

Increased Plasma

Osmotic Pressure

A D H

Decreased Extracellular

Fluid Volume

Figure 2. Factors controlling ADH release.

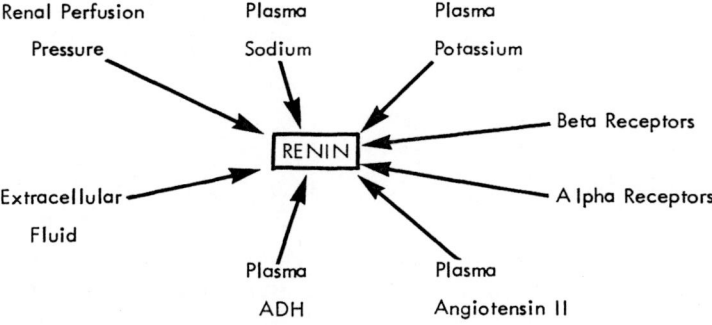

Figure 3. Factors controlling renin release

control mechanism appropriateness or otherwise. In addition, it is of course necessary to know how these factors interact, as none is an independent agent in controlling renin release. Thus, a raised plasma renin may be inappropriate to high blood pressure level, yet appropriate to a state of extracellular fluid volume depletion in forms of hypertension where perfusion pressure natriuresis occurs (e.g., the Goldblatt 2-kidney one-clip model; Swales et al. [32]. Diazoxide produces increased plasma renin and angiotensin II despite simultaneous expansion of the extracellular fluid [15]. Plasma renin might well be regarded as being inappropriately high' in relation to sodium balance; nevertheless, it could also be regarded as an entirely appropriate response to the fall in blood pressure or sympathetic nervous system activation that occur at the same time. When hormonal secretion is under the control of multiple factors, it becomes increasingly difficult to predict the net result in one particular situation. Therefore, while apparent abnormalities of renin secretion can be demonstrated in hypertension, it is unjustified to use the tem 'inappropriate' without a complete analysis of all the relevant factors and their interaction – an impossibility in view of the mechanisms that control renin secretion [27]. The analogy with tumor secretion of ADH would seem far-fetched.

Increased tissue renin

Renin could accumulate at a strategic site as a result of either local synthesis or selective uptake from plasma. Two such sites have been widely discussed in relation to blood pressure control: the central nervous system and the peripheral blood vessels. Although an important role has been attributed to the former (e.g., Ganten et al. [9]), its nature and physiological existence are still in doubt [23], and certainly there is no convincing evidence of any abnormality of this postulated system in hypertension.

Two postulates have to be met for vascular renin to maintain blood pressure despite a normal plasma renin: first, renin within the vessel wall has to generate

314

angiotensin II, which binds the vascular angiotensin receptors in resistance vessels; second, the components of the vessel wall renin-angiotensin system have to be increased despite normal plasma concentration. Aortic wall homogenate contains proteolytic enzymes that generate angiotensin I at most pH values [34]. Although some of these acid proteases probably have no role in renin-angiotensin system activity in vivo, the measurement of aortic renin activity using an incubation pH of 6.5 (the optimum for rat plasma renin) shows changes in aortic renin that parallel changes in plasma renin i.e., aortic renin is elevated in salt depletion and reduced by salt loading [34]. This effect could of course be physiologically important, or aortic renin-like activity could simply reflect renin taken up passively from the plasma and having no physiological role.

To assess the role of arterial renin we have to examine the possible effect of changes in vascular renin upon blood pressure control. If large amounts of local renin generate angiotensin II, the activation of vascular receptors by angiotensin II will have two effects: firstly blood pressure will be elevated, and second, increased occupation of receptors will reduce the specific response to exogenous angiotensin II, as the number of receptors available to bind exogenous angiotensin will be reduced. Both these effects can be reversed by converting enzyme inhibition, which lowers blood pressure and increases the pressor sensitivity to angiotensin II [36, 18]. Therefore, if we can find a situation where plasma and aortic renin activities diverge, we can perhaps identify the role of vascular renin. One such situation is found after bilateral nephrectomy in rats with Goldblatt 2-kidney hypertension [37] (Figure 4). Plasma renin concentration falls rapidly, with a half-life of 10–15 min, while aortic renin-like activity (measured with an incubation pH of 6.5) shows a much slower decline. Indeed, there is little change over the first two hours. If we look at the blood pressure fall produced by converting enzyme inhibitor, an excellent response is seen at one and two hours, to be lost only at 6 and 24 hr. This effect can be blocked with saralasin, and is therefore due to renin-angiotensin blockade rather than to any additional vasodepressor action of our inhibitor. Pressor sensitivity to angiotensin II, which, as we saw, is partly determined by endogenous angiotensin II, is scarcely changed until 6 hr after bilateral nephrectomy [30]. This sort of evidence has suggested that vascular renin-like activity does perform a role [27, 12, 1, 2]. Further, the delayed decline after bilateral nephrectomy suggests that it is of renal origin. More recently we have confirmed this observation by demonstrating that renin injected into nephrectomised rats is taken up by the aortic wall and results in prolonged elevation of blood pressure despite the return of plasma renin to normal [17]. Is it possible therefore that disproportionately high vascular renin levels maintain blood pressure when plasma renin is normal? I think this is unlikely. For one thing, we do not see the specific impairment in pressor responsiveness to angiotensin II that characterizes high receptor occupancy states. In addition, in all the steady-state conditions we have examined, plasma and aortic renin are closely related: they diverge only in non-steady-state conditions such as

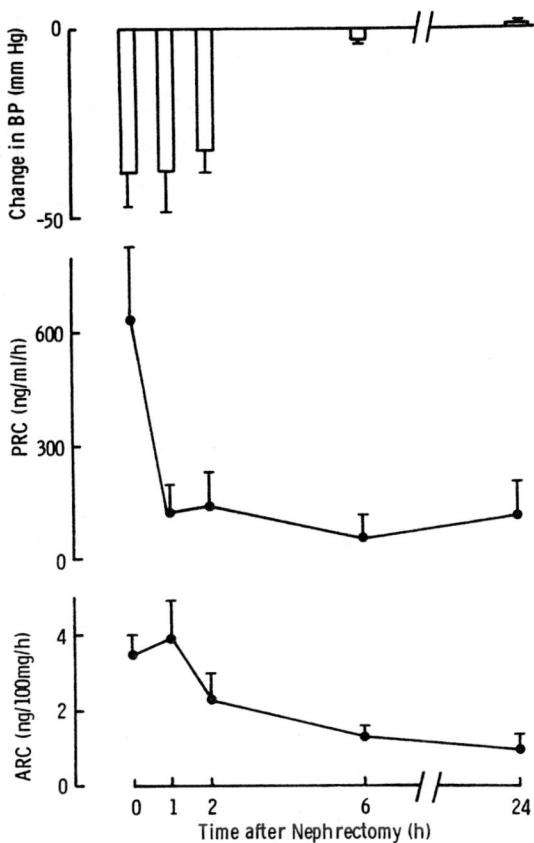

Figure 4. Changes in blood pressure induced by the converting enzyme inhibitor teprotide in rats with Goldblatt 2-kidney 1-clip hypertension after bilateral nephrectomy. A blood pressure response is seen even after plasma renin (PRA) has reached its nadir. Responsiveness is much better correlated with aortic renin (ARC).

after bilateral nephrectomy or after renin injection. Other groups, however, have observed a divergence produced by antihypertensive drug treatment in animals [1]; this is an area we have not ourselves studied. I feel, nevertheless, that the relationship between plasma renin (or angiotensin II) and the blood pressure fall produced by saralasin argue more persuasively against a selective increase in vascular renin in hypertension. If the saralasin molecule were competing at the receptor site with concentrations of angiotensin II that bear no overall relation to plasma angiotensin II, the relationship would not have been observed. I would only like to point out that the plasma concentration of saralasin needed to produce these effects is 100–100 times the simultaneous concentrations of angiotensin II in plasma [21], despite the fact that in vitro activity of saralasin can be detected with equimolar doses of saralasin and angiotensin II [20]. This suggests that saralasin is competing with much higher local concentrations of angiotensin II than those observed in the plasma, and supports our interpretation of the data presented.

CONCLUSIONS

While this evidence suggests that we should perhaps rethink our ideas of the mode of action of the renin-angiotensin system, I must regretfully conclude that I do not think that local generation of angiotensin II in the blood vessel wall provides a mechanism whereby the renin-angiotensin system can maintain blood pressure in the absence of elevated plasma renin levels. It seems to me much more likely that the renin-angiotensin system plays little or no role in blood pressure maintenance where plasma renin is normal, and it seems equally likely that the observed abnormalities of the renin-angiotensin system in patients with essential hypertension are secondary. The distribution of plasma renin in essential hyper-tension is reminiscent of the distribution of blood pressure in the community, and suggests that renin is, like blood pressure, a multifactorially determined variable. We have no evidence for an etiologically separate subgroup of patients in whom the renin-angiotensin system is a pathogenetic factor, neither is there evidence that the renin-angiotensin system is responsible for blood pressure maintenance through either hyper-reactivity of 'inappropriate' secretion of renin. Abnor-malities in plasma renin observed in patients with essential hypertension are more likely to be an effect rather than a cause of the condition.

REFERENCES

1. Barrett JD, Eggena P, Sambhi MP: Partial characterisation of aortic renin in the spontaneously hypertensive rat and its interrelationship with plasma renin, blood pressure and sodium balance. Clin Sci & Mol Med 55: 261–270, 1978
2. Bing J, Nielson K: Cause of the prolonged pressor action of renin in nephrectomised rats. Acta Path et Microbiol A 81: 247–253, 1973
3. Brunner HR, Wauters JP, McKinstry D, Waeber B, Turini G, Gavras H: Inappropri-ate renin secretion unmasked by captopril (SQ14225) in hypertension of chronic renal failure. Lancet ii: 704–707, 1978
4. Davis JO: The pathogenesis of chronic renovascular hypertension. Circ Res 40: 439–444, 1977
5. Devynck MA, Pernollet MG, MacDonald GJ, Matthews PG, Raisman RS, Meyer P: Alterations of adrenal and uterine angiotensin II receptors during variations of so-dium intake and/or experimental hypertension. Clin Sci Mol Med 55: 4: 171s–174s, 1978
6. Doyle AE: Vascular reactivity in human hypertension. New Zealand Med J 67: 295–303, 1968
7. Dunn MJ, Tannen RL: Low-renin hypertension. Kidney Int 5: 317–325, 1974
8. Folkow B, Hallback M, Lundgren Y, Sivertsson R, Weiss L: Importance of adaptive changes in vascular design for establishment of primary hypertension studied in man and in spontaneously hypertensive rats. Cir Res (32)1: 2–16, 1973
9. Ganten D, Schelling P, Vecsei P, Ganten U: Iso-renin of extrarenal origin. Am J Med 60: 760–772, 1976
10. Gavras H, Brunner HR, Thurston H, Laragh JH: Reciprocation of renin dependency with sodium volume dependency in renal hypertension. Science 188: 1316–1317, 1975

11. Gavras H, Brunner HR, Vaughan ED, Laragh JH: Angiotensin-sodium interaction in blood pressure maintenance of renal hypertensive and normotensive rats. Science 180: 1369–1372, 1973
12. Gould AB, Skeggs LT, Kahn JR: Presence of renin activity in blood vessel walls. J Exp Med 119: 389–399, 1964
13. Gunther S, Gimbrone MA, Alexander RW: Regulation by angiotensin II of its receptors in resistance blood vessels. Nature 287: 230–232, 1980
14. Helmchen U, Kneissler U, Peters G: Disturbance of the control renin secretion in chronic one-kidney Goldblatt hypertension in the rat. Pflugers Arch 348: 197–204, 1974
15. Kuchel O, Fishman LM, Liddle GW, Michelakis A: Effect of diazoxide on plasma renin activity in hypertensive patients. Ann Intern Med 67: 791–799, 1967
16. Laragh JH: Vasoconstriction-volume analysis for understanding and treating hypertension: the use of renin and aldosterone properties. Am J Med 55: 261–274, 1973
17. Loudon M, Bing RF, Swales JD, Thurston H: Changes in blood pressure in relation to vascular and plasma renin after renin injection in rats. Clinical Science 63: 153s–156s, 1982
18. Marks ES, Russell GI, Thurston H, Bing RF, Swales JD: Responsiveness to pressor agents in experimental and steroid hypertension. Hypertension 4: 238–244, 1982
19. Mendlowitz M: Vascular reactivity in systemic arterial hypertension. Amer Heart J 85: 252–259, 1973
20. Pals DT, Masucci FD, Denning GS, Sipos F, Fessler DC: Role of the pressor action of angiotensin II in experimental hypertension. Circ Res 29: 673–681, 1971
21. Pettinger WA, Keeton K, Tanaka K: Radioimmunoassay and pharmacokinetics of saralasin in the rat and hypertensive patients. Clin Pharmacol Ther 17: 140–158, 1975
22. Pickering GW: High Blood Pressur. J and A Churchill, London, 1968
23. Reid IA: Is there a brain renin-angiotensin system? Circ Res 41: 147–153, 1977
24. Schalekamp MA, Beevers DG, Briggs JD, Brown JJ, Davies DL, Fraser R, Lebel M, Lever AF, Medina A, Morton JL, Robertson JIS, Tree M: Hypertension in chronic renal failure: an abnormal relation between sodium and the renin-angiotensin system. Am J Med 55: 379–390, 1973
25. Schwartz WB, Bennett W, Curelop S, Bartter FC: A syndrome of renal sodium loss and hyponatremia probably resulting from inappropriate secretion of antidiuretic hormone. Am J Med 23: 529–542, 1957
26. Streeten DHP, Anderson GH, Freiberg JM, Dalakos TG: Use of an angiotensin II antagonist (saralasin) in the recognition of 'angiotensinogenic' hypertension. N Engl J Med 292: 657–662, 1975
27. Swales JD: On the inappropriate in hypertension research. Lancet ii: 702–704, 1977
28. Swales JD: Renin-angiotensin system in hypertension. Pharmac Ther 7: 173–201, 1979
29. Swales JD: Arterial wall or plasma renin in hypertension. Clin Sci 56: 293 298, 1979
30. Swales JD, Tange JD, Thurston H: Vascular angiotensin II receptors and sodium balance in rats. Role of kidneys and vascular renin activity. Circ Res 37: 96–100, 1975
31. Swales JD, Thurston H: Plasma renin and angiotensin II measurement in hypertensive and normotensive subjects: correlation of basal and stimulated states. J Clin Endocrinol Metab 45: 159–163, 1977
32. Swales JD, Thurston H, Querioz FP, Medina A: Sodium balance during the development of experimental hypertension. J Lab Clin Med 80: 539–547, 1972
33. Thurston H: Vascular angiotensin receptors and their role in blood pressure control. Am J Med 61: 768–778, 1976
34. Thurston H, Bing RF, Hurst B, Swales JD: Role of persistent vascular renin after bilateral nephrectomy in Goldblatt two-kidney hypertension. Clin Sci Mol Med 55: 4: 23s–26s, 1978

35. Thurston H, Bing RF, Pohl JEF, Swales JD: Renin sub-groups in essential hypertension: an analysis and critique. Quart J Med 47: 325–337, 1978
36. Thurston H, Laragh JH: Prior receptor occupancy as a determinant of the pressor activity of infused angiotensin II in the rat. Cir Res 36: 113–117, 1975
37. Thurston H, Swales JD, Bing RF, Hurst BC, Marks ES: Vascular renin like activity and blood pressure maintenance in the rat: studies of the effect of changes in sodium balance, hypertension and nephrectomy. Hypertension 1: 643–649, 1979
38. Weidmann P, Maxwell MH: The renin angiotensin aldosterone system in terminal renal failure. Kidney Int 8: 5: 219s–234s, 1975

24. BIOLOGICAL SIGNIFICANCE OF ACTIVE AND INACTIVE RENIN IN HYPERTENSIVE PATIENTS

P. Lijnen, R. Fagard, J. Staessen, L. Verschueren, A. Amery

SUMMARY

The biological significance of active and inactive renin was investigated by comparison of in vitro assays of active, total and inactive plasma renin concentration (APRC, TPRC, IPRC), plasma renin activity (PRA), plasma angiotensin I and II concentration (PA I, PA II), with in vivo changes in mean arterial pressure (MAP) produced by angiotensin antagonism with saralasin and by angiotensin converting enzyme blockade with captopril. Significant relationships between the changes in MAP during saralasin and captopril administration with the pretreatment levels of PRA, APRC, TPRC, and PA II were found; the preexisting level of inactive renin was not a predictor for the hypotensive effects of saralasin and captopril. During captopril and saralasin treatment significant increases in PRA, PA I, TPRC, and APRC were found, with no change in IPRC.

INTRODUCTION

Inactive forms of renin in human plasma can be converted in vitro into active renin by acidification of plasma [1, 4, 7, 16, 18, 27], by trypsin treatment [2], by cold treatment [23, 24], or by kallikrein [3, 17, 19, 20, 21]. Many in vitro studies have investigated the proportions in human plasma of active and inactive renin and the correlations between angiotensin II and both forms of renin [8, 15].

As no direct, in vivo evidence of the relative biological significance of (in)active renin is available, however, we investigated the in vitro measurement of active, inactive, and total renin concentration, angiotensin I and II concentration, and plasma renin activity with an 'in vivo' change in mean arterial pressure produced by angiotensin antagonism with saralasin and by angiotensin converting enzyme blockade with captopril.

SUBJECTS

Twelve hypertensive patients (eight males) with an average age of 39.9 ± 3.1,

Sambhi, M.P. (ed.) Fundamental fault in hypertension
© *1984, Martinus Nijhoff Publishers. Boston/The Hague/Dordrecht/Lancaster.*
ISBN 978-94-010-9006-3

weighing 71.0 ± 2.7 kg were studied; six had essential hypertension, and six hypertension with renal artery stenosis. The severity of hypertension was assessed by the criteria of the World Health Organization; six were stage I, five stage II, and one stage III because of an eye fundus grade 3.

The study complied with the WHO code of ethics for human experimentation (Declaration of Helsinki). During an initial run-in period on placebo, laboratory studies were performed, including hemogram, urinalysis, fasting blood sugar, serum creatinine, electrolytes, bilirubin, plasma renin, urinary catecholamines, electrocardiogram, pulmonary function tests, and chest X-ray. All patients had previously had an intravenous pyelogram, and some a renal arteriogram if indicated.

Patients with any of the following were excluded: signs of heart failure; history or signs of bronchospasm; hematological, hepatic, or non-hypertensive cardiac disease; possibility of pregnancy by history; a recent cerebrovascular accident; a creatinine clearance below 30 ml per minute; insulin-requiring diabetes mellitus.

STUDY PROTOCOL

The patients were followed on an outpatient basis for about a month on three placebo tablets a day, and were instructed to observe a low sodium diet; four of these patients were also treated with chlorthalidone, 50 mg a day. The 24-hour urinary sodium excretion in the patients not on chlorthalidone averaged 72 mEq. In two patients with rather high pressures, the run-in period was shortened to one week because it was considered unethical to keep these patients off treatment. Informed consent was obtained.

The patients were studied in the recumbent position, in the morning, after a light breakfast, in the laboratory (room temperature, 18–22°C; humidity, 40–60%). A small catheter (Vygon, 115.09) was introduced into the brachial artery for sampling of blood and for recording intra-arterial pressure using an Elema Schonander EMT pressure transducer; pressure was continuously recorded on a Mingograph 81 recorder, and mean arterial pressure (MAP) was obtained by electrical damping every 5 min.

After the technical procedures, including insertion of a needle into an arm vein, a control period of 30 min was observed while glucose 5% was given intravenously. Saralasin was infused at a ratio of 10 μg/kg/min for 45 min. After an interruption of the drug infusion, a wash-out period of 90 min was observed. Then the patient received one 25 mg tablet of captopril, and blood pressure was followed for another 75 min. Arterial blood was drawn before and at the end of the saralasin infusion, and also before captopril administration and at the end of the observation period.

METHODS

Plasma renin activity

Plasma renin activity (PRA) was measured by radioimmunoassay of the angiotensin I generated during a 1-hour incubation of the plasma samples with the endogenous renin substrate at pH 6.0 and 37° C, according to the method of [5].

Plasma renin concentration

The 'total' plasma renin concentration (TPRC) was measured as the rate of angiotensin I generated during a 1-hour incubation with renin substrate from a bilaterally nephrectomized sheep at pH 7.4 under zero order kinetic conditions, according to the method of Skinner [26], adapted for radioimmunoassay [11]. This assay consists first of a denaturation of endogenous substrate by dialysis against a 0.05 M glycine buffer, pH 3.3, containing 5 mM EDTA and 90 mM NaCl, and of an inactivation of the angiotensinases by heating at 32° C for 1 hour. Then the samples are dialysed against a 0.17 M phosphate buffer, pH 7.4. The pH 3.3 dialysis partially activates inactive renin.

The 'active' plasma renin concentration (ARPC) was determined after dialysing the plasma against a 0.05 M aminoacetic buffer, pH 4.5, and after heating the dialysate at 32° C for 1 hour to obtain an adequate inhibition of the angiotensinases. Incubation was performed with an excess of sheep renin substrate at pH 7.4, during 1 hour. The influence of pH on the assayed plasma renin concentration is shown in Figure 1 [9]. The difference (TPRC–APRC) will be presented as the 'inactive' plasma renin concentration (IPRC).

Assay of plasma angiotensin I and II, and of converting enzyme

A radioimmunoassay method was used for the measurement of plasma angiotensin I and II concentration (PA I, PA II), as previously described [12, 14]. Plasma angiotensin converting enzyme (kininase II) activity (ACE) was measured spectrophotometrically as described before [10].

Statistical analysis

The statistical methods used were regression analysis and Student's two tailed t-test for paired data. The dispersion of the data is given by the standard error of the mean (SEM). Except for ACE activity, the biochemicall parameters were transformed to their logarithms, as only their log distribution was Gaussian.

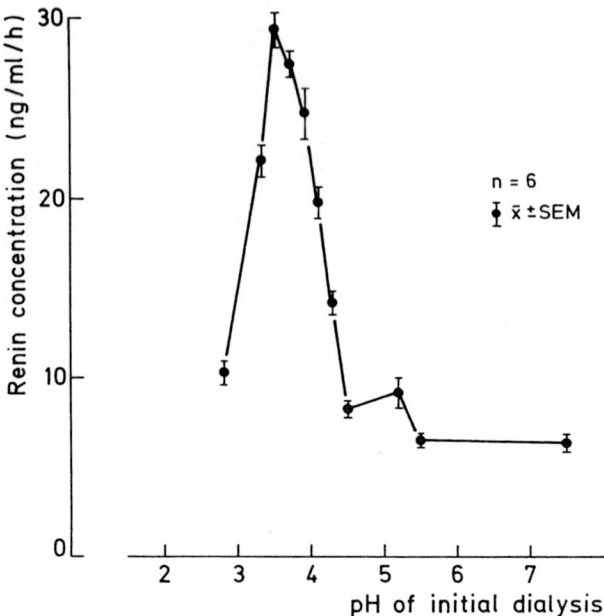

Figure 1. Influence of the dialysis pH on the assayed plasma renin concentration.

Blood sampling

All the blood samples were withdrawn from the brachial artery into an inhibitor solution (0.16 M EDTA and 0.025 M o-phenantrolin) and processed as described in the methodology of the assays [12, 14, 10].

RESULTS

Specificity of anti-angiotensin II serum

Figure 2 shows the standard curve of [1]Asp-[5]Ile-angiotensin II and the cross-reactions of [1]Asp-[5]Ile-angiotensin I, sheep renin substrate, [1]Sar-[8]Ala-angiotensin II, and human renin with the antiserum to [1]Asp-[5]Ile-angiotensin II. The percentage of cross-reactivity was calculated from the relative amounts of [1]Asp-[5]Ile-angiotensin II (32 pg/100 μl) and the test compound, to reduce the initial binding of angiotensin II (5-L-Isoleucine) (Tyrosyl-^{125}I) monoiodinated by 50%. The cross-reaction percentages were 0.33% for [1]Asp-[5]Ile-angiotensin I, 0.0064% for renin substrate , 0.0025% for [1]Sar-[8]Ala-angiotensin II, and nil for human renin. Displacement from the 100% bound starts from a concentration of 1000 pg/100 μl for [1]Asp-[5]Ile-angiotensin I, and from 100,000 pg/100 μl for [1]Sar-[8]Ala-angiotensin II. Thus, angiotensin I starts to interfere in the assay of angiotensin II above a

323

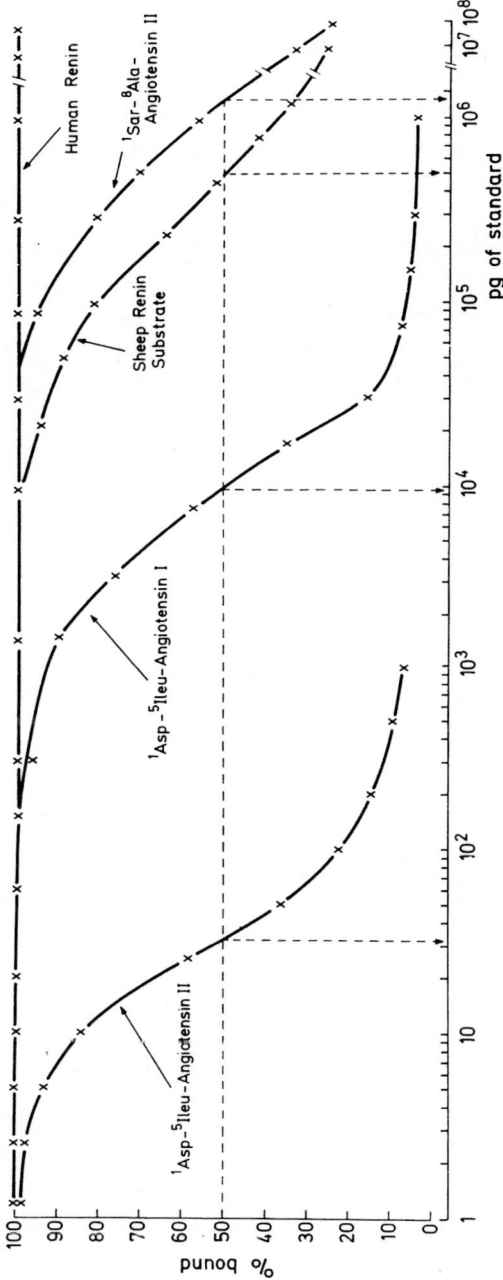

% Cross-Reaction of ^{1}Asp-^{5}Ileu-Angiotensin I $\frac{32 \times 100}{9600} = 0.33\%$; Sheep Renin Substrate $\frac{32 \times 100}{5 \cdot 10^5} = 0.0064$; ^{1}Sar-^{8}Ala-Angiotensin II $\frac{32 \times 100}{1.3 \cdot 10^6} = 0.0025\%$; Human Renin nihil

Figure 2. Cross-reactivity of human angiotensin I, sheep renin substrate, saralasin, and human renin in the radioimmunoassay of human angiotensin II.

plasma concentration of 10,000 pg/ml. The highest plasma angiotensin I concentration found in the present study after captopril treatment was only 6330 pg/ml. In the study of Semple et al. [25], a higher (0.6%) cross-reaction of the angiotensin II antiserum with angiotensin I was noted.

Acute changes in the plasma renin-angiotensin system during treatment with saralasin and captopril

As shown in Table 1, saralasin and captopril produced significant ($p < 0.001$) two- to threefold increases in PRA, PA I, TPRC, and APRC, and no change in IPRC. Plasma angiotensin II increased significantly with saralasin, while it dropped ($p < 0.001$) with captopril. No significant change was found in ACE activity during saralasin infusion, while with captopril ACE activity was reduced significantly ($p < 0.001$).

Table 1. Acute changes in renin, angiotensin I and II, and converting enzyme before and during treatment with saralasin and captopril

	Saralasin		Captopril	
	Before	During	Before	During
log PRA (log ng/ml/h)	0.31 ± 0.18	$0.67 \pm 0.25^*$	0.35 ± 0.21	$0.91 \pm 0.22^{**}$
Antilog of mean	2.04	4.68	2.24	8.13
log PA I (log pg/ml)	2.19 ± 0.16	$2.63 \pm 0.22^{***}$	2.22 ± 0.17	$2.82 \pm 0.19^{***}$
Antilog of mean	156	431	167	666
log PA II (log pg/ml)	1.61 ± 0.11	$1.96 \pm 0.18^{***}$	1.66 ± 0.11	$1.21 \pm 0.10^{***}$
Antilog of mean	41.0	90.6	45.6	16.3
log TPRC (log ng/ml/h)	1.66 ± 0.11	$1.86 \pm 0.16^*$	1.74 ± 0.12	$1.98 \pm 0.15^{***}$
Antilog of mean	45.7	72.4	55.0	95.5
log APRC (log ng/ml/h)	1.26 ± 0.16	$1.49 \pm 0.22^*$	1.34 ± 0.17	$1.70 \pm 0.20^{***}$
Antilog of mean	18.2	30.9	21.9	50.1
log IPRC (log ng/ml/h)	1.26 ± 0.28	1.48 ± 0.11	1.38 ± 0.13	1.47 ± 0.14
Antilog of mean	18.2	30.2	24.0	29.5
ACE activity (U/ml)	32.3 ± 2.9	32.4 ± 3.3	32.7 ± 3.4	$18.1 \pm 2.8^{***}$

n = 12 for all determinations; the mean ± SE is given
* $0.01 < p < 0.05$ when compared to the value respectively before saralasin and captopril
** $0.001 < p < 0.01$
*** $p < 0.001$.

Table 2. Correlations between plasma angiotensin II and active, inactive, and total renin, plasma angiotensin I, and ACE activity (y = A + Bx) (n = 34)

Y	X	A	B	r	p
log PA II	log PRA	1.5027	0.5091	0.79	<0.001
	log TPRC	0.0428	0.9546	0.92	<0.001
	log APRC	0.7970	0.6676	0.88	<0.001
	log IPRC	0.8153	0.6699	0.55	<0.001
	log PA II	0.2163	0.6662	0.91	<0.001
	ACE	1.6585	0.0005	0.01	>0.10

Arterial blood samples were withdrawn before and after saralasin infusions. Results obtained after captopril administration are not included.

Relationship between plasmia angiotensin II and the other biochemical variables during glucose and saralasin infusion

Plasma angiotensin II was significantly (p<0.001) related to simultaneously determined PRA, TPRC, APRC, and PA I (Table 2). The correlation coefficients were of the same magnitude (between 0.79 and 0.92), except for IPRC, where a small coefficient was noted (r = 0.55). No relation between PA II and ACE activity was found (r = 0.01; p>0.10).

Relationship of the acute changes in MAP to pre-existing PRA, PA II, APRC, TPRC, and IPRC

The change in MAP during saralasin treatment was closely related to the logs of PRA, PA II, TPRC, and APRC before its infusion (Figures 3–6), but not to log IPRC (Figure 7). In addition, the captopril-provoked changes in MAP were significantly related to the logs of PRA, PA II, TPRC, and APRC before its ingestion, but not to log IPRC (Figures 3–7).

DISCUSSION

Human plasma contains at least two types of renin. One is enzymatically active at neutral pH, and is known as active renin [27]. The other, called inactive renin, is not enzymatically active in its native form, but has renin-like activiy after in vitro exposure to low pH [27], to proteolytic enzymes [18] or to the cold [23].

An optimal acid activation of plasma renin is obtained at pH 3.3–3.5 [9, 27]. The greatest cryoactivation of inactive renin is obtained between pH 7 and 9; no activation has been found in the frozen state [23]. Exogenous trypsin activates inactive renin in plasma at normal pH and at 4°, 23°, or 37° C, proving that neither low pH nor cold are essential [2].

326

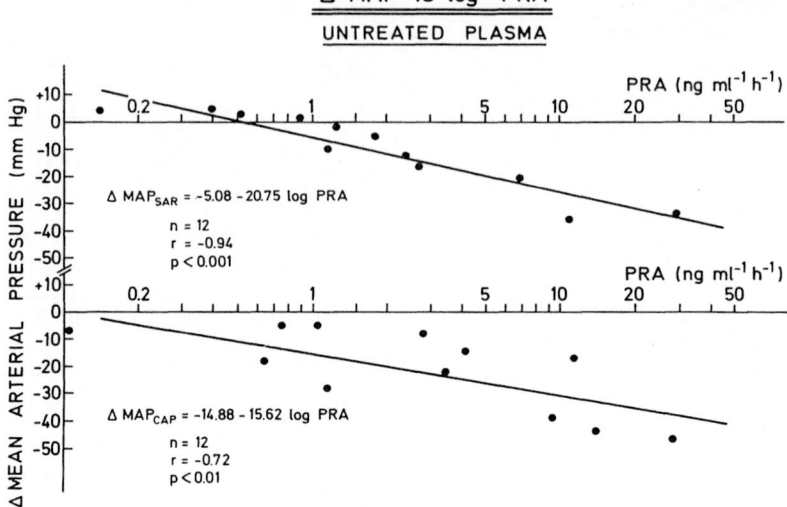

Figure 3. Relationship of △ mean arterial (△ MAP) during treatment with saralasin (above, SAR) and captopril (below, CAP) with control log plasma renin activity (PRA).

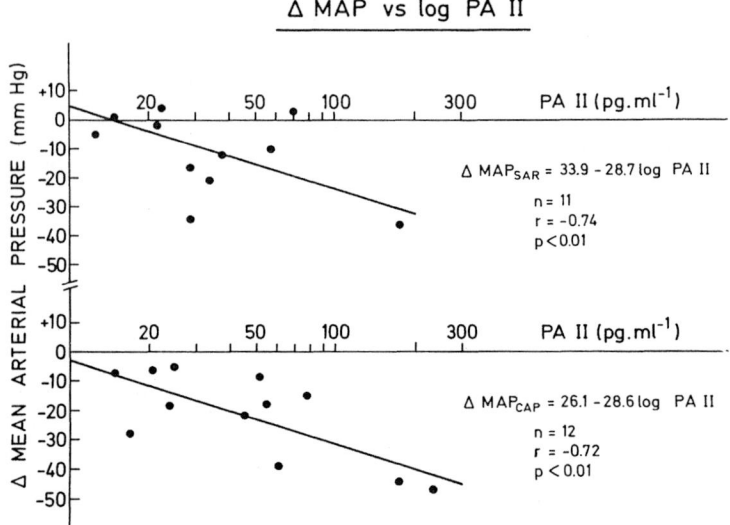

Figure 4. Relationship of △ MAP during treatment with saralasin (above, SAR) and captopril (below, CAP) with control log plasma angiotensin II (PA II).

Two thirds of the total renin in normal human plasma consist of an inactive, acid-activable form [27]. In normal human plasma Lijnen et al. [15] found on average 34% of total renin to be in the active form. According to Leckie et al. [8], the percentage of inactive renin varied from 36 to 71% of the total renin concentration in normal subjects on an unrestricted diet. Boyd [1] also reported active renin as about 50% of the total renin concentration, and found inactive renin present in all subjects. Inactive renin comprises a larger fraction [6] of total renin

Δ MAP vs TPRC

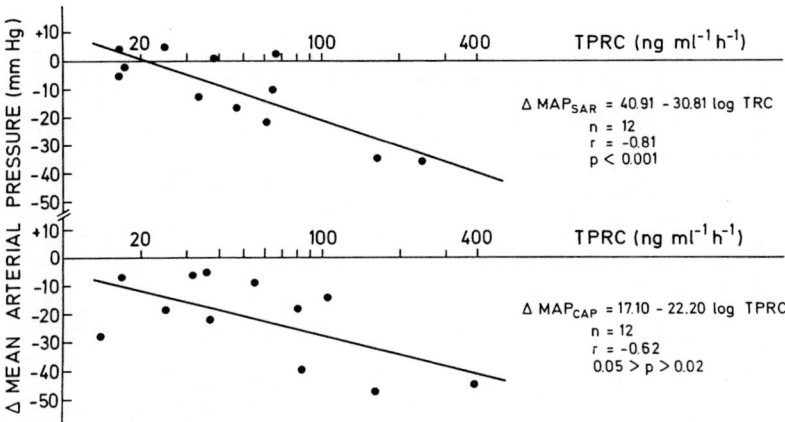

Figure 5. Relationship of Δ MAP during treatment with saralasin (above, SAR) and captopril (below, CAP) with control log total plasma renin concentration (TPRC).

Δ MAP vs APRC

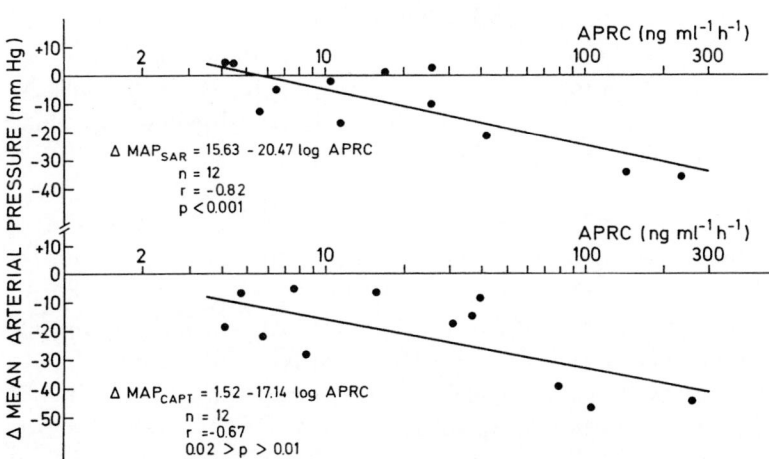

Figure 6 Relationship of Δ MAP during treatment with saralasin (above, SAR) and captopril (below, CAP) with control log active plasma renin concentration (APRC).

in plasma of salt-loaded healthy subjects (82%) than of salt-depleted subjects (62%).

The in vivo activation of inactive renin is not yet fully understood, although a link between renin and kallikrein-kinin has been proposed [22]. Derckx et al. [4] found that in Fletcher plasma (which is prekallikrein deficient), only a small amount of inactive renin was activated by acid, thus indicating that the acid activation of renin appears to be prekallikrein-dependent.

On the other hand, Millar et al. [17] found appreciable acid activation of

Δ MAP vs IPRC

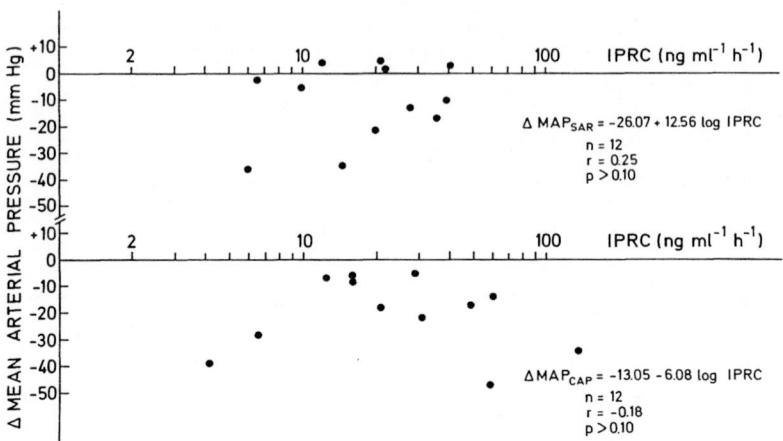

Figure 7. Relationship of Δ MAP during treatment with saralasin (above, SAR) and captopril (below, CAP) with control log inactive plasm renin concentration (IPRC).

inactive renin in plasma from two patients with inherited deficiency of Fletcher factor (prekallikrein) and suggested therefore that plasma kallikrein is not the activator of renin in vitro. Osmond et al. [19] also reported that inactive renin consists of an above-normal proportion of total renin in Fletcher plasma, whether estimated by cryoactivation (93.3%) or by tryptic activation (95.6%), whereas a low basal PRA (active renin) was found. This suggests that endogenous plasma prekallikrein-kallikrein is required for a normal active renin level and a normal ratio of active to inactive renin, but not necessarily for cryoactivation, tryptic activation, or acid activation of inactive renin.

Our in vitro studies with saralasin show no change in inactive renin and a two- to threefold increase in active renin (PRA or APRC), PA II, and PA I (Table 1). During converting enzyme blockade with captopril, no change in IPRC, an increase in active renin and PA I, and a reduction in PA II and ACE activity were observed. These in vitro results clearly show a distinction between the active and inactive renin response during saralasin infusion and captopril administration. Looking to the correlation studies between simultaneously determined angiotensin II and inactive or active renin levels, however, a significant correlation between inactive renin and PA II was found, indicating that a pure, in vitro comparison can be misleading, especially in correlation studies where the range is very important. Restricting the range to normal subjects on an unrestricted diet, Lijnen et al. [13] found no significant correlation between IPRC and PA II, whereas PA II was significantly related to active renin (APRC or PRA). Similar results were reported by Leckie et al. [8], who suggested that inactive renin does not produce angiotensin II in vivo. It is difficult to draw such a conclusion from in vitro comparisons, however.

In addition to these in vitro studies, another approach was used to investigate the physiological significance of the various forms of renin: we studied the correlation between in vitro measurements of (in)active renin and in vivo-determined changes in MAP. The changes in MAP during angiotensin antagonism with saralasin and converting enzyme blockade with captopril were closely related to active renin (PRA or APRC), to PA II, and to TPRC, but not to inactive renin (IPRC). These results also indicate that inactive renin is not a predictor of the in vivo hypotensive effect of saralasin and captopril.

ACKNOWLEDGMENTS

The authors gratefully acknowledge the technical assistance of Miss G. Lommelen, Miss S. Taelemand, Mrs. K. Van Hoorenbeeck-Bijttebier, Mr. L. Cockx, Mr. J. Huysecom, and the secretarial help of Mrs. M. Cober-Stinissen.

We thank Norwich Pharmacal Co. and the Squibb Institute for Medical Research for the generous supply of drugs.

This study was supported by a grant from the National Fund for Medical Research (NFWO) of Belgium.

REFERENCES

1. Boyd GW: An inactive higher-molecular weight renin in normal subjects and hypertensive patients. Lancet i: 215–218, 1977
2. Cooper RM, Murlay GE, Osmond DH: Trypsin induced activation of renin precursor in plasma of normal and anephric man. Circ Res 40, Suppl I: 171–179, 1977
3. Derckx FHM, Man in 't Veld AJ, Schalekamp MADH: Prekallikrein (Fletcher factor)-dependent pathway for activating inactive renin. IRMC Med Sci 7: 135, 1979
4. Derckx FHM, Wenting GJ, Man in 't Veld AJ, Verhoeven RP, Schalekamp MADH: Control of enzymatically inactive renin in man under various pathological conditions: implications for the interpretation of renin measurements in peripheral and renal venous plasma. Clin Sci Mol Med 54: 529–538, 1978
5. Fyhrquist F, Puutula L: Faster radioimmunoassay of angiotensin I at 37° C. Clin Chem 24: 115–118, 1978
6. Hsueh WA, Luetscher JA, Carlson EJ, Grislis G: Big renin in plasma of healthy subjects on high sodium intake. Lance i: 1281–1284, 1978
7. Leckie BJ, McConnell A: A renin inhibitor from rabbit kidney. Conversion of a large inactie renin to smaller active enzyme. Circ Res 36: 513–519, 1975
8. Leckie BJ, McConnell A, Grant J, Morton J, Tree M, Brown JJ: An inactive renin in human plasma. Circ Res 40, Suppl I: 46–51, 1977
9. Lijnen P, Amery A: Influence of acid treatment of plasma on the renin concentration. Arch Int Physiol Biochim 85: 183–184, 1977
10. Lijnen P, Amery A: Spectrophotometric assay of plasma kininase II activity. Arch Int Physiol Biochim 86: 436–437, 1978
11. Lijnen P, Amery A, Fagard R: Comparison between a biological and a radioimmunological assay of plasma renin concentration. FEBS Lett 61: 32–33, 1976
12. Lijnen P, Amery A, Fagard R: Endogenous angiotensin I in human plasma. J Lab

Clin Med 92: 353–362, 1978

13. Lijnen P, Amery A, Fagard R: Active and inactive renin in normal human plasma. Comparison between acid activation and cryoactivation. Clin Chim Acta 95: 227–234, 1979
14. Lijnen P, Amery A, Fagard R, Katz F: Radioimmunoassay of angiotensin II in unextracted plasma. Clin Chim Acta 88: 403–412, 1978
15. Lijnen P, Amery A, Fagard R, Reybrouck T, Moerman E, De Schaepdryver A: The effects of beta-adrenoceptor blockade on renin, angiotensin, aldosterone and catecholamines at rest and during exercise. Br J Clin Pharmacol 7: 175–181, 1979
16. Lumbers ER: Activation of renin in human amniotic fluid by low pH. Enzymologia 40: 321–326, 1971
17. Millar JA, Clappison BH, Johnston CI: Kallikrein and plasmin as activators of inactive renin. Lancet i: 1376, 1978
18. Morris BJ, Lumbers ER: The activation of renin in human amniotic fluid by proteolytic enzymes. Biochem Biophys Acta 289: 385–391, 1972
19. Osmond DH, Lo EK, Loh AY, Zingy EA, Hedlin AH: Kallikrein and plasmin as activators of inactive renin. Lancet i: 1375, 1978
20. Rumpf KW, Lankisch PG, Koop H, Becker K, Schmidt S, Scheler F: Endogenous proteases and the activation of pro-renin. (Abstract 178:30), 13th Annual meeting of the European society of clinical investigation, March 22–24, Cambridge, England, 1979
21. Sealey JE, Atlas SA, Laragh JH: Human urinary kallikrein converts inactive to active renin and is a possible physiological activator of renin. Nature 275: 144, 1978
22. Sealey JE, Atlas SA, Laragh JH: Linking the kallikrein and renin systems via activation of inactive renin. New data and hypothesis. Am J Med 65: 994–1000, 1978
23. Sealey JE, Moon C, Laragh JH, Alderman M: Plasma prorenin: cryoactivation and relationship to renin substrate in normal subjects. Am J Med 61: 731–737, 1976
24. Sealey JE, Moon C, Laragh JH, Atlas SA: Plasma prorenin in normal, hypertensive and anephric subjects and its effect on renin measurements. Circ Res 40, Suppl I: 41–45, 1977
25. Semple PF, Boyd AS, Dawes PM, Morton JJ: Angiotensin II and its heptapeptide (2–8), hexapeptide (3–8), and pentapeptide (4–8) metabolites in arterial and venous blood of man. Circ Res 39: 671–678, 1976
26. Skinner SL: Improved assay methods for renin concentration and activity in human plasma. Circ Res 20: 391–402, 1967
27. Skinner SL, Cran EJ, Gibson R, Taylor R, Walters WAW, Catt KJ: Angiotensins I and II, active and inactive renin, renin substrate, renin activity and angiotensinase in human liquor and plasma. Am J Obstet Gynecol 121: 626–630, 1975

25. THE RELATION OF PLASMA RENIN SUBSTRATE TO BLOOD PRESSURE IN ESSENTIAL HYPERTENSION

W. Gordon Walker, Hiroshi Saito

Physiologic data provide abundant documentation for the blood pressure regulatory role of the renin-angiotensin system to be exercised through its capacity for altering the levels of circulating angiotensin II [22, 7, 13]. Although angiotensin II is the only product of this system that has a direct vasoconstrictor effect and should correlate directly with blood pressure readings, its measurement is more difficult than the measurement of renin activity, and hence data on that correlation are limited [22, 4, 2]. Plasma renin activity is the variable component of this regulatory system most often measured, and from this single determination inferences are made about the physiologic state of the renin-angiotensin system and indirectly about the level of circulating angiotensin II [3, 25, 8]. In fact, several components of the renin-angiotensin system may exert an important and variable influence upon the rate of angiotensin II production and upon plasma angiotensin II concentrations.

In addition to the concentration of renin in the circulating plasma, the rate of production and plasma concentration of angiotensin II may be influenced by the plasma concentrations of substrate and angiotensin I (particularly the concentration of angiotensin I in the pulmonary artery blood), as well as the quantity and location of converting enzyme at different sites within the vascular bed. The interrelationships of these constituents are shown in Figure 1. Under appropriate circumstances, any of the illustrated constituents in the reaction sequence prior to the production of angiotensin II could exert a major or dominant influence in the control of the rate of production of angiotensin II. Thus, a physiologic mechanism for regulating the levels of activity or availability of converting enzyme could, if present, produce a major alteration in the rate of production of angiotensin II and hence in its plasma concentration. The pharmacologic counterpart of this control is well recognized, and has resulted in the production of agents that show great promise as antihypertensive drugs [12]. Similarly, it is easy to imagine circumstances in which the concentration of angiotensin I could also exert a controlling influence. Both the renin concentration and the substrate concentration are potential controlling points for the production of angiotensin I. If all other components of the reaction remain unchanged, the concentration of angiotensin II would be determined by changes in the product of the concentrations of enzyme and substrate. Complete definition of the mechanism whereby the renin-

Sambhi, M.P. (ed.) Fundamental fault in hypertension
© *1984, Martinus Nijhoff Publishers. Boston/The Hague/Dordrecht/Lancaster.*
ISBN 978-94-010-9006-3

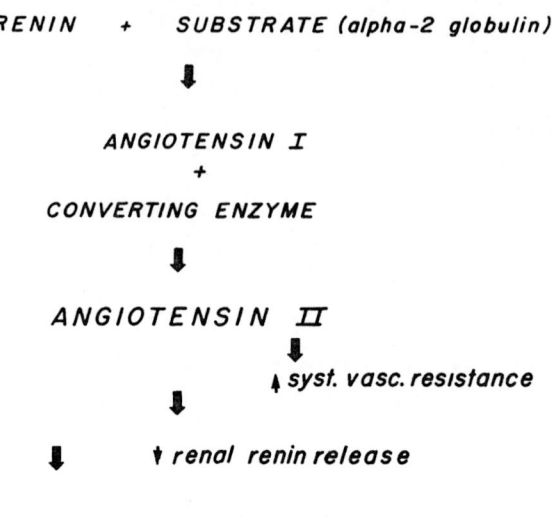

Figure 1. Scheme of the reaction sequence of the renin-angiotensin-aldosterone system.

angiotensin system participates in the control of blood pressure would require a careful characterization of the physiologic influence of each of the steps in the reaction sequence shown in Figure 1. This presentation examines only the potential role of renin substrate upon blood pressure and reviews some data from our laboratory that suggest that it may be quite significant. The approach we have used in examining this role is presented below [24].

THE ROLE OF SUBSTRATE IN THE PHYSIOLOGIC REGULATION OF ANGIOTENSIN II

Several investigators have presented contradictory views on the role of substrate in influencing the renin-renin substrate reaction and, by inference, in influencing the rate of production of angiotensin II [26, 5]. Different investigators have reported a range of values for the Km of the renin-renin substrate reaction when the reaction velocity is measured in vitro; on the basis of such in vitro studies, inferences have been made regarding the behavior of the system in vivo [26, 5, 6, 15]. Some investigators propose that the level of substrate in the plasma is sufficiently above the Km value of the pure renin-renin substrate reaction for the substrate to play no role in regulating the production of angiotensin II. Others have expressed contrary views, based upon different Km values measured under different experimental conditions. In fact, the data required to support or negate such views must include measurement of the Km under conditions identical to those existing in circulating plasma. Not only are the plasma concentrations of both renin and renin substrate important, but possible inhibitors or accelerators, if such exist in circulating plasma, must also be present in the same concentration [16, 9, 10]. No Km measurements have been made under such conditions. Unless it is shown that the Km measured under those conditions is less than 10% of the average substrate concentration in the plasma, it may be safely asserted that the system is at least partially responsive to fluctuations in circulating levels of renin substrate [17].

As the renin-angiotensin system in intact man cannot be isolated in any way that permits in vivo observation of the consequences of systematic variation of the concentration of renin substrate while other components are held constant, an alternate approach is necessary for the evaluation of the physiologic role of substrate concentration. We have reported an alternate approach that yielded evidence of a significant physiologic role for substrate in blood pressure regulation [24]. As in most biologic systems where individual reaction sequences cannot be isolated and controlled, a search for correlations between various reactants within the system may provide insights into the behavior of the system and the relative importance of each of its component parts. Thus, if one postulates that the blood pressure is directly controlled by circulating levels of renin the plasma, it should be possible to demonstrate a significant correlation (positive) between the concentration of renin and the simultaneously determined blood pressure. Alternately, hypertension attributable to excess aldosterone production sustained by some stimulus other than the renin-angiotensin system should yield a correlation between plasma aldosterone concentration and blood pressure. The sodium retention engendered by this excess steroid might be expected to suppress renin release, and thus also lead to a negative correlation between blood pressure changes and levels of plasma renin. While correlations do not prove causality, such information is essential to an accurate description of the physiologic behavior of the system and is of value in subsequent experimental design.

RELATION BETWEEN PLASMA RENIN SUBSTRATE AND BLOOD PRESSURE

We have looked for significant correlations in studying the relationship between blood pressure and the constituents of the renin-angiotensin system in 574 subjects. Observations were made with the subjects ambulatory and before any dietary manipulation had been attempted; this avoided any possible artifactual alteration of any of the components of the renin-angiotensin system. Measurements of plasma renin activity, plasma aldosterone, renin substrate, angiotensin II, and urinary sodium and potassium were recorded. Details of subject selection and analytic methods have been presented elsewhere [20, 21, 22, 24]. The study was designed to examine the relation between blood pressure and the constituents of the renin-angiotensin system and electrolyte excretion as independent variables. Some of the findings are presented in Table 1, which summarizes some

Table 1.

	Diast. BP >90	Diast. BP ≤	Total group
n	115	199	314
Age	32.38 ± .73	31.44 ± .48	31.9 ± .40
Rec. Syst. BP	151.05 ± 1.883	126.87 ± .95	135.68 ± 1.12
Rec. Diast. BP	104.57 ± 1.09	80.29 ± .56	89.1 ± .85
Pl. Ren. Act.	0.284 ± .022	.31 ± .01	.299 ± .011
Pl. Ren. Subst.	2203.35 ± 54.1	1668.95 ± 27.9	1864.74 ± 30.25
Pl. Aldosterone	12.25 ± .775	16.9 ± .85	15.21 ± .624
Urine Na/K	3.196 ± .258	2.00 ± .16	2.64 ± .1075

of the data from 314 subjects in whom renin substrate measurements were completed. The table presents mean values ($\pm$ SEM) for age, plasma renin activity, renin substrate, and urinary sodium: potassium ratio. Also included are the corresponding mean values ($\pm$SEM) when the total population is divided into subgroups according to blood pressure, comparing subjects with diastolic pressure equal to or less than 90 mmHg (n = 119) with those with diastolic blood pressure above 90 mmHg (n = 115). The substrate concentrations are significantly greater in the subgroup with the elevated blood pressure (normotensive subjects, 1673 ± 28 ng/ml versus 2188 ± 53 ng/ml for hypertensive subjects; p<0.001). The ages of the two groups did not differ significantly (Table 1), and there was no evidence that these findings were a spurious result of a maldistribution of the sexes in the two groups. To examine this more critically, all females were excluded and only the data of the males in the study were compared. When this was done and normotensive males were compared with hypertensive males, the significant difference persisted (1611 ± 25 SEM, n = 176 for those whose blood pressures equaled or were less than 90 mmHg, versus 2045 ± 65; n = 79 ng/ml, for those with diastolic blood pressures greater than 90 mmHg; p<0.001). Thus, the difference could not be accounted for by a difference in the sex ratio; indeed, significant differences could also be demonstrated between diastolic blood pressure and plasma renin substrate in the female subjects when grouped according to blood pressure (BP≦90 mmHg, n = 24, substrate = 2122 ± 110; BP>90 mmHg, n = 34, substrate = 2519± 64; p<0.005).

A highly significant positive correlation was demonstrated between recumbent diastolic blood pressure and renin substrate for all subjects. This relationship, between recumbent diastolic blood pressure obtained just prior to the venipuncture for renin sampling and substrate measurement yielded a correlation coefficient equal to r = + 0.54; p<<0.001 for all 314 subjects (Table 2). The correlation for the mean arterial blood pressure and renin substrate was virtually identical (r = 0.52; p<<0.001). This positive correlation was demonstrated in both groups after dividing the subjects into the two subsets according to blood pressure as described above (Table 1). This remarkably strong positive correlation between plasma renin substrate and blood pressure stood in sharp contrast to the much

Table 2. Relation between blood pressure and renin angiotensin system*

Bivariate correlations	Corr. coeff.	95% Conf. interval	Signif.
Mean art. press. sitting vs. renin substrate	+.459	+.367→+.542	<.0001
Mean art. press. rec. vs. renin substrate	+.517	+.431→+.594	<.0001
Rec. diastolic press. vs. renin substrate	+.541	+.457→+.615	<.0001
Rec. diastolic pressure vs. plasma renin act.	−.132	−.021→−.240	<.02
Rec. diastolic pressure vs. aldosterone	−.160	−.05→−.27	<.005
Plasma renin substrate vs. plasma ren. act.	−.006	–	NS

* n = 314

weaker negative correlation identified between plasma renin activity and blood pressure ($r = -0.12$; $p < 0.05$; $n = 314$).

PLASMA RENIN ACTIVITY

As confirmation of the finding of elevated substrate levels in the subjects with higher blood pressure, we also measured and compared the plasma renin reactivity in samplings of the subjects with higher and lower blood pressure [14]. The test measures the initial reaction velocity after a constant amount of renin is added to the plasma and thus provides a reaction rate proportional to substrate concentration. This assay yielded results that were consistent with the substrate measurements summarized above. Thus, after addition of 1×10^{-4} Goldblatt units of human renin to the plasma samples, the 26 hypertensive subjects yielded an initial reaction rate that was substantially higher than that of the subjects whose blood pressures were below 90 mmHg (759 ± 26 vs. 631 ± 19 pg/ml/hr respectively; $p < 0.001$). Moreover, in the 50 subjects whose plasma renin reactivity (PRR) was measured, examination of the relationship between this PRR and the previously measured substrate yielded a significant correlation ($r = +0.50$; $p < 0.01$). This represents further evidence that the difference in renin reactivity is related to differences in substrate concentration. No significant relationship could be established between plasma renin substrate and age in this study.

POSSIBLE SIGNIFICANCE OF RELATION BETWEEN SUBSTRATE AND BLOOD PRESSURE

The presence of significantly greater substrate concentrations in subjects with elevated blood pressure and the relationship between blood pressure and substrate raise a question about a potential primary role for substrate in the regulation of blood pressure. Among the questions that require answers are: a) What is the mechanism responsible for this increase with increasing blood pressure? b) What is the effect of this higher substrate concentration upon the physiologic behavior of the renin-angiotensin system? c) What pathogenetic or pathophysiologic significance can be attributed to this substrate elevation? The prognostic and therapeutic implications of this association between renin substrate and the arterial blood pressure require examination.

The controlling factors responsible for the regulation of plasma renin substrate levels have not been adequately studied. The influences of steroid excess are well established [11]. There are no adequate data available on the behavior of substrate levels in response to fluctuations over time in the renin-angiotensin system. The liver removes most of the angiotensin II reaching it, but it is not clear whether either angiotensin II or the plasma renin concentration may serve as a feedback stimulus to angiotensinogen or substrate production [1, 18]. A possible explanation for the present findings may be that the suppressed renin levels in hypertensive patients result in decreased substrate consumption, with attendant substrate accumulation serving to increase the concentration. This explanation is difficult to reconcile with the fact that a much weaker correlation was demonstrated between blood pressure and plasma renin activity than between blood pressure and substrate. Moreover, this proposal, which offers an explanation for the relationship of events occurring only in subjects with elevated blood pressure, fails to account for the demonstrated correlation between substrate and blood pressure in subjects with diastolic blood pressures of 90 mmHg or below. Thus, the possibility at least exists that the relationship between substrate and blood pressure is a primary one, rather than one mediated through alterations in plasma renin concentration associated with sluggish response to increasing levels of circulating substrate.

Possible consequences of reduced substrate consumption in hypertensive subjects can be explored if one assumes that production of angiotensin I is the initial step in the sequence of reactions leading to the degradation of renin substrate, and that this is the only mechanism by which substrate can be degraded. Although there is no evidence for or against the latter part of this assumption, the first part is inherent in our methodology for measuring plasma renin substrate. As we measured substrate by total conversion to angiotensin I, we do not include in our measurement any substrate moiety from which angiotensin I was previously cleaved. We previously reported that angiotensin I was converted to angiotensin II at the rate of 10 ng/min. by the pulmonary vascular bed [20]. If this is taken as the rate of degradation of plasma renin substrate, then, based upon the assumptions above, this would correspond to a plasma half-life for substrate of 231 days. There are no comparable data available for conversion of angiotensin I to angiotension II in the pulmonary vascular bed of hypertensive subjects, but we reported previously that the mean value for plasma angiotensin II concentration in hypertensive subjects is less than one third the value obtained in normal subjects [24]. If this reflects reduced production of angiotensin I and consequent reduced conversion to angiotensin II, this reduced consumption of substrate would lead to a lengthening of the half-life of circulating substrate by more than a factor of 3. These very long half-lives are quite improbable, according to our present knowledge about other half-life values of the various plasma protein constituents, and hence the assumptions upon which these calculations are made are suspect [23]. The estimates do underscore the potential importance of substrate metabolism in regulating the kinetics of the renin-angiotensin system, however, and thereby stress the importance of more critical study of substrate metabolism in hypertension.

The contribution made by this increased substrate to higher levels of angiotensin II in the circulating plasma depends both upon the concentration of renin in plasma and upon its Km value in vivo. Km values have been reported ranging between 303 ng/ml in a partially purified system to 1712 ng/ml [5, 6, 15, 26]. Most measurements were made in partially purified systems; few data are available defining Km under physiologic conditions in the plasma. The renin substrate reaction is strongly influenced by proteins and there is, in addition, good evidence of the presence of inhibitors of the renin substrate reaction in plasma; thus, the Km of the system in plasma in vivo is not known. Knowledge on this point is crucial to accurate assessment of the significance of alterations in substrate concentration on the renin-angiotensin reaction. Unless the lower values obtained in the group with diastolic blood pressure $\leqq 90$ mmHg are tenfold greater than the in vivo Km value, the higher levels observed in the hypertensive subjects can be expected to increase the velocity of the renin-renin substrate reaction significantly. Under such circumstances, two effects may be expected. First, any level of renin in the plasma would produce a greater quantity of circulating angiotensin II at the higher level of circulating substrate. Second, surges or rapid release of renin may be expected to produce sudden and acute increases in angiotensin II. Either of these events could have undesirable consequences in the hypertensive patient. Thus, at the least, these elevated substrate levels possess significant potential for aggravating or accelerating the hypertension, regardless of the underlying cause of the elevated blood pressure.

Perhaps the strongest argument favoring a primary contribution of substrate to the elevated blood pressure can be made from the data in Table 2. Substrate is the only constituent of the renin-angiotensin system that correlates positively with arterial blood pressure. More importantly, even though there is a weak negative correlation between plasma renin activity and blood pressure that could be used as evidence for decreased substrate consumption in hypertension, no correlation can be demonstrated between renin substrate concentration and renin activity. It thus seems highly unlikely that the elevated substrate levels seen in these hypertensive subjects were a direct consequence of the modest renin suppression demonstrated in subjects with elevated blood pressure. Furthermore, the individuals with higher blood pressure had lower levels of plasma angiotensin II. Hence, if it is proposed that at least one initiating event leading to essential hypertension is elevation of plasma renin substrate leading to an increase in circulating levels of angiotensin II, the observed lower levels of angiotensin II in the hypertensive subjects require the postulation of some modulating or inhibitory influence that suppresses conversion to angiotensin II relatively early in the development of essential hypertension.

It is evident that additional information is needed, including definition of the time-course of the increase in substrate concentration in relation to the increase in blood pressure. An increase in substrate levels and angiotensin II levels that precede the development of significant elevation in blood pressure would obviously be more important etiologically than an elevation occurring after the blood pressure rises, but the difficulties in acquiring such data in large numbers of subjects are evident.

SUMMARY

These observations, made in both normal subjects and in subjects with untreated essential hypertension, demonstrate that plasma renin substrate is the only constituent of the renin-angiotensin system that correlates positively with blood pressure. This finding suggests that renin substrate may play a significant role in the pathogenesis of high blood pressure in essential hypertension, but more information about the physiologicval behavior and metabolism of substrate is necessary before the role of substrate can be clarified.

ACKNOWLEDGMENTS

Supported in parts by USPHS Grants#HL3303, RR0035, RR00722; the O'Neill Endowment Fund of the Good Samaritan Hospital; and a grant from The Jane Hilder Harris Foundation.

REFERENCES

1. Beckerhoff R, Luetscher JA, Wilkinson R, Gonzales C, Nokes GW: Plasma renin concentration, activity and substrate in hypertension induced by oral contraceptives. J Clin Endocrinol Metab 34: 1067, 1972
2. Brown JJ, Lever AF, Morton JJ, Frazer R, Love DR, Robertson JIS: Raised plasma angiotensin II and aldosterone during dietary sodium restriction in man. Lancet 2: 1106, 1972
3. Brunner HR, Laragh JH, Baer L, Newton MA, Goodwin FT, Krakoff LR, Bard RH,

Buhler FR: Essential hypertension: renin and aldosterone, heart attack and stroke. N Engl J Med 286: 441, 1972

4. Gocke DJ, Gerten J, Sherwood LN, Laragh JH: Physiological and pathological variations of plasma angiotensin II in man. Circ Res 24 (Suppl 1): 131, 1969

5. Gould AB, Green D: Kinetics of the human renin and human substrate reaction. Cardiovasc Res 5: 86, 1971

6. Gould AB, Skeggs LT, Joseph K: Measurement of renin and substrate concentration in human serum. Lab Invest 15: 1802, 1966

7. Haber E, Koerner T, Page LB, Kliman B, Purnod EA: Application of a radio-immunoassay for angiotensin I to the physiologic measurements of plasma renin activity in normal human subjects. J Clin Endocrinol Metab 29: 1349, 1969

8. Helmer OM: Renin activity in blood from patients with hypertension. Can Med Assoc J 90: 221, 1964

9. Kotchen TA, Talwalker RT, Kotchen JN, Miller MC, Welch WJ: Evidence for the existence of an acetone soluble inhibiting factor in normal human plasma. Circ Res 36/37 (Suppl I): 17, 1975

10. Kotchen TA, Talwalker RT, Miller MC, Welch WJ: Modification of renin reactivity by lipds extracted from normal, hypertensive and uremic plasma. J Clin Endocrinol Metab 43: 971, 1976

11. Krakoff LR: Plasma renin substrate: measurement by radioimmunoassay of angiotensin I concentration in syndromes associated with steroid excess. J Clin Endocrinol Metab 37: 110, 1973

12. Needleman P, Johnson EM Jr, Vine W, et al.: Pharmacology of antagonists of angiotensin I and II. Circ Res 31: 862, 1972

13. Peach MJ: Renin-angiotensin system: biochemistry and mechanisms of action. Physiol Rev 57: 313, 1977

14. Saito H, Hermann J, Walker WG: Kinetic studies of renin-angiotensin system in plasma from normotensive and hypertensive subjects. In: Abstracts of sixth scientific meeting of the International society of hypertension, Goteborg, Sweden, 1979

15. Sambhi MP: Renin substrate reaction. Circ Res 41 (Suppl II): 1, 1977

16. Sambhi MP, Eggena P, Barrett JD, Tuck M, Wiedeman CE, Thananopavarn C: A circulating renin activator in essential hypertension. Circ Res 36 (Suppl I): I–28, 1975

17. Segal IH: Enzyme kinetics: behavior and analysis of rapid equilibrium and steady state enzyme system. John Wiley and Sons, 1975

18. Skinner SL, Lumbers ER, Symonds EM: Alterations by oral contraceptives and of normal menstrual changes on plasma renin activity, concentration and substrate. Clin Sci 36: 67, 1967

19. Walker WG, Horvath JS, Moore MA, Russell RP: Some observations on arterial and venous levels of angiotensin II in man. Trans Am Clin Climat Assoc 85: 151, 1973

20. Walker WG, Horvath JS, Moore MA, Russell RP, Conti CR, Mitch WE: Pulmonary generation and peripheral uptake of endogenous angiotensin II in man. Trans Assoc Am Phys 86: 226, 1973

21. Walker WG, Horvath JS, Moore MA, Whelton PK, Russell RP: Relation between plasma renin activity and aldosterone in mild untreated hypertension. Circ Res 38: 470, 1976

22. Walker WG, Moore MA, Horvath JS, Whelton PK: Arterial and venous angiotensin II in normal subjects: relation to plasma renin activity and plasma aldosterone concentration, in response to posture and volume. Circ Res 38: 477, 1976

23. Walker WG, Ross RS, Hammond JDS: Study of the relationship between plasma volume and transcapillary protein exchange using ^{131}I labeled albumin and ^{125}I labeled globulin. Circ Res 8: 1028, 1960

24. Walker WG, Whelton PK, Saito H, Russell RP, Hermann J: Relation between blood pressure and renin, renin substrate, angiotensin II, aldosterone, urinary sodium and potassium in 574 subjects. Hypertension 1: 287, 1979
25. Woods JW, Pittman AW, Pulliam CC, Werk EE, Waider W, Allen CA: Renin profiling in hypertension and its use in treatment with propranolol and chlorthalidone. N Engl J Med 294: 1137, 1976
26. Workman RJ, McKown MM, Greggerman RI: Renin inhibition by protein and peptides. Biochemistry 13: 3029, 1974

26. ON RENIN SUBSTRATE AND HYPERTENSION
A hypothesis

MOHINDER P. SAMBHI

In essential hypertension, the renin angiotensin system as measured in the peripheral circulating blood has failed to qualify as one of the contenders for a primary 'fault' in hypertension. The question is ably discussed by Professor John Swales in this volume. Renin, the proteolytic enzyme responsible for generating the vasoactive angiotensin from angiotensinogen, has been traditionally regarded as the driving force for the entire system. In untreated patients with essential hypertension, measurements of plasma renin activity correlate well with measured levels of the active end product of the system; e.g., angiotensin II. The same is true if renin release is acutely stimulated or suppressed. Under most conditions, the activity of the renin angiotensin system in the periphery is presumably altered by changing the amount the enzyme renin released, as the levels of angiotensinogen in plasma are not altered, either, in essential hypertension or during acute stimulatory or suppressive responses of renin release. Furthermore, there is no good available evidence (Swales, this volume) that the activity of the peripheral renin angiotensin system in essential hypertension is dictated by an inappropriate metabolic fate or altered sensitivity to the generated angiotensin at the receptor sites on the blood vessels.

There are at least three other potential factors needing comment that may potentially alter the activity of the renin angiotensin system, independent of the measured levels of the concentration of the enzyme renin. The first of these factors is the possible interconversion of the enzyme renin into more or less active and inactive forms. Lijnen, Fagard, Staessen, Amery 1981 have provided data to mitigate the physiopathological importance of the phenomenon in the circulation. The second factor is the putative naturally occurring endogenous modifiers of renin-substrate reaction, activators or inhibitors that may influence angiotensin generation independently of the levels of renin or renin substrate. None of these factors has been clearly identified or characterized [14]. The third factor potentially capable of altering the activity of the renin angiotensin system in the periphery, or in the tissues, is angiotensinogen, which is the subject of this discussion.

Can angiotensinogen be one of the primary culprits in the genesis of hypertension? The correct answer to this question should be that the available evidence is insufficient to answer the question with a categorical 'yes' or 'no'. Let us phrase a

Sambhi, M.P. (ed.) Fundamental fault in hypertension
© *1984, Martinus Nijhoff Publishers. Boston/The Hague/Dordrecht/Lancaster.*
ISBN 978-94-010-9006-3

second question very differently: Is there enough circumstantial evidence that is capable of achieving the dignity of a postulate and can justify the asking of the first question? The following is presented in support of an affirmative answer.

PLASMA ANGIOTENSINOGEN LEVELS AS DETERMINANTS OF THE ACTIVITY OF THE RENIN SYSTEM

It has been recognized for several years that renin substrate concentration in plasma is rate limiting for the end product, angiotensin generation by the enzyme renin. In normal subjects and in patients with essential hypertension, the substrate concentration barely exceeds that required for half maximal velocity of the enzyme reaction (Km). In order to achieve maximal velocity or zero order reaction with respect to substrate, concentrations in excess of ten-fold the Km are needed. Figure 1 indicates that even the highest measured substrate concentrations in term pregnancy plasma are only 2.5-fold the Km value. The measured velocity of the reaction, in this case, approximated two-thirds of the calculated potential maximum [2]. These findings indicate that under all clinical conditions, renin alone cannot be considered as the sole driving force for the reaction, and the substrate concentrations, unless relatively constant, have an important influence on the generation rate of angiotensin, and hence on the activity of the system.

THE ROLE OF MULTIPLE FORMS OF ANGIOTENSINOGEN

Human plasma renin substrate was purified [3] and a direct radioimmunoassay was developed in our laboratory [4]. The direct radioimmunoassay of the protein angiotensinogen in most patients with essential hypertension correlated well, giving a 1:1 ratio with the indirect renin substrate concentrations measured by the radioimmunoassay of the peptide angiotensin I generated by the action of enzyme renin. The simultaneous availability of the two methods, direct and indirect, for the quantitation of renin substrate allowed us to distinguish abnormal forms of angiotensinogen that were capable of generating angiotensin; however, they did not cross-react with the antibody raised against the normal plasma angiotensinogen [5]. Two abnormal forms of angiotensinogen with different, albeit remarkably constant, rf values on polyacrylamide gel were seen in normotensive females on oral contraceptive pills. The same forms of this protein were also seen in male patients on estrogen therapy for prostatic cancer. The abnormal forms appeared only in those subjects in whom the levels of plasma renin substrate were stimulated in excess of 5 micrograms angiotensin I equivalents per ml. Glucocorticoid mediated stimulation of plasma renin substrate also showed one abnormal form, which, however, was different in its mobility on polyacrylamid gel Ph 8.6, as compared to the two forms observed in the plasma of estrogen treated subjects.

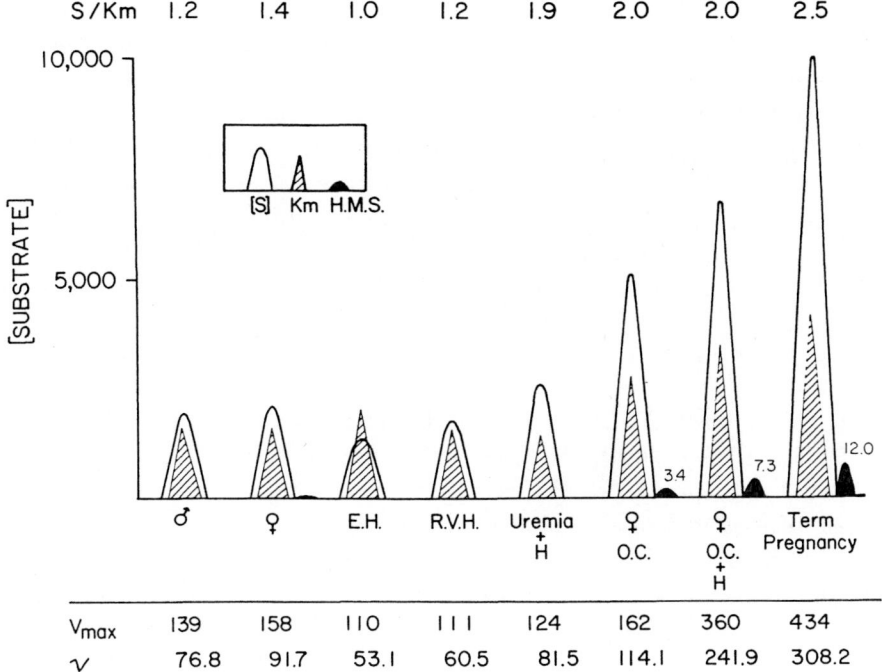

S/Km	1.2	1.4	1.0	1.2	1.9	2.0	2.0	2.5
	♂	♀	E.H.	R.V.H.	Uremia + H	♀ O.C.	♀ O.C. + H	Term Pregnancy
Vmax	139	158	110	111	124	162	360	434
V	76.8	91.7	53.1	60.5	81.5	114.1	241.9	308.2

Figure 1. Renin substrate concentration is expressed as ng angiotensin I equivalent per ml plasma.
(S) = Plasma renin substrate concentration
Km = Michaelis constant
H.M.S. = High molecular weight renin substrate. The numbers indicate percent of total.
S/Km = approximate ratio of renin substrate in plasma to its Michaelis constant (Km) determined through a lineveawer Burke Plot.
Vmax = Maximal velocity (Michaelis constant)
V = calculated initial velocity $= \dfrac{S. \, Vmax}{Km + S}$

♂ = Normal males n = 13
♀ = Normal females n = 18
EH = Essential hypertensive ♂ n = 12
R.V.H. = Renovascular hypertension n = 5
Uremia + hypertension n = 4
♀ o.c. = Normotensive females on oral contraceptives n = 20
♀ o.c. + H = Estrogenic hypertension n = 5
Term pregnancy = Pooled plasma n = 2

The estrogen mediated stimulation of plasma renin substrate was shown to be dose dependent and was more pronounced with the use of synthetic than the naturally occurring estrogens [6].

On further characterization, the abnormal forms of plasma angiotensinogen contained a high molecular weight angiotensinogen (several fold higher than normal plasma angiotensinogen) that was shown not to be an aggregate. The higher molecular weight angiotensinogen in preliminary experiments was shown to have a lower Km (higher affinity) with human renin. More interestingly, the relative proportion of the higher molecular weight plasma angiotensinogen, with respect to the total plasma renin substrate concentration, was more than two-fold higher in five women who became hypertensive on oral contraceptive therapy than those (n = 20) who remained normotensive. The greatest percent amount of higher molecular weight plasma angiotensinogen, however, was observed in females at term pregnancy [7]. The physiopathological role of the high molecular weight angiotensinogen remains to be further investigated. Nevertheless, its higher affinity with renin and its higher concentration in females on oral contraceptives developing hypertension is of great interest.

ANGIOTENSINOGEN IN THE CENTRAL NERVOUS SYSTEM

Angiotensinogen in human cerebrospinal fluid approaches 10% of the concentration of plasma angiotensinogen, whereas plasma proteins in general cross the barrier (blood-brain, or C.S.F.) only to the extent of less than 2% [8]. Local synthesis of angiotensinogen in the brain tissue was, therefore, considered a likely possibility. This suggestion was confirmed by the demonstration in our laboratory indicating that the direct radioimmunoassay of the protein angiotensinogen (developed with the antibody raised against human plasma angiotensinogen) in human C.S.F. from normal subjects or patients with essential hypertension measured less than 1% of the total concentration of angiotensinogen present in the C.S.F., as measurable by the indirect method of angiotensin generation with added human renin [10]. This degree of non-recognition of the C.S.F. angiotensinogen by the antibody raised against plasma angiotensinogen constituted a conclusive evidence in favor of the view that the angiotensinogen measurable in the C.S.F. originates from local synthesis.

A comparison of the physicochemical characteristics of human plasma vs. C.S.F. angiotensinogen indicated a similar molecular weight, as well as identical mobility on polyacrylamid gel electrophoresis; however, clear differences between the two proteins were apparent on isoelectric focusing. The plasma angiotensinogen was shown to have a single isoelectric point, whereas the C.S.F. angiotensinogen separated into three forms with different isoelectric points [10]. Different patterns of heterogeneity of angiotensinogen were further demonstrated in the rat comparing the renin substrate released in vitro from isolated rat hepatocytes with that extracted from rat brain tissue [11]. More importantly, the in vitro release of angiotensinogen from rat hepatocytes was shown to be clearly stimulated if the rats were previously subjected to estrogen treatment or bilateral nephrectomy. The content of angiotensinogen in the brain extracts of the same animals showed no changes. More recent experiments from our laboratory have compared in vitro release of renin substrate from rat liver and brain slices, and also compared the differential effects of various in vivo stimulatory procedures. The release of renin substrate from rat brain slices was substantial (exceeding 50% of that from rat liver slices) and in animals pretreated with dexamethasone showed a greater stimulation than the release from liver slices. Conversely, the stimulation of renin substrate release was much less marked after nephrectomy from brain than from liver slices. Estrogen treatment of animals, a consistent and pronounced stimulus for the release of renin substrate from liver slices, was without effect on brain slices, unless very high doses were used. The release of renin substrate from both liver and brain slices was shown to be depressed if general inhibitors of protein synthesis were added to the mediums [12]. These experiments support the existence, synthesis, and functional modulation of a distinct renin angiotensin system in the brain. The specific stimulatory effect of corticosteroids is most intriguing.

HYPOTHESIS

In peripheral plasma, acute and subacute alterations in the activity of the renin system are predominantly mediated through changes in renin release. Long-term sustained alterations in the activity of the system, however, can conceivably be mediated through availability of increased amounts of renin substrate, or in some cases, the occurrence of additional, more reactive forms of renin substrate. Walker et al., in this volume present statistical evidence in a larger population survey indicating that renin substrate, more than any other component of the renin system, correlated with the level of diastolic blood pressure. If such a mechanism is operative in essential hypertension, concrete evidence in support of this view remains to be elicited.

On the other hand, the presence of renin substrate in brain tissue, the demonstration of its local synthesis, and its release from brain slices, coupled with its modulation by corticosteroids, make it very plausible that the renin system in the brain has a functional role. Ganten, Printz, Unger and Lang [13] present compelling arguments in favor of this view. Renin is known to be present intracellularly in brain tissue, albeit in rather small amounts. The substantial quantities of angiotensinogen present in various parts of brain tissue make it highly probable that local angiotensin generation is controlled by the availability of renin substrate. A primary role of renin substrate in the genesis of essential hypertension, however, remains a hypothesis at this time.

REFERENCES

1. Lijnen P, Fagard R, Staessen J, Amery A: Comparison between active and inactive renin and angiotensin II in man. In: Heterogeneity of renin and renin substrate, Sambhi MP (ed), Elsevier, New York, 1981, pp 227–236
2. Eggena P, Barrett JD, Shionoiri H, Sambhi MP: Enzymatic studies with renin substrate. In: Topics on pathophysiology of hypertension, Villarreal H and Sambhi MP (eds), Martinus Nijhoff, The Hague, in press

346

3. Eggena P, Chu CL, Barrett JD, Sambhi MP: Purification and partial characterization of human angiotensinogen. Biochim Biophys Acta 427: 208–217, 1976
4. Eggena P, Barrett JD, Hidaka H, Chu CL, Thananopavarn C, Golub MS, Sambhi MP: A direct radioimmunoassay for human renin substrate and identification of multiple substrate types in plasma. Circ Res 41 (Suppl I): II-34-II-37, 1977
5. Eggena P, Hidaka H, Barrett JD, Sambhi MP: Multiple forms of human plasma renin substrate. J Clin Invest 62: 367–372, 1978
6. Eggena P, Barrett JD, Shionori H, Ito T, Mandel F, Judd H, Sambhi MP: The influence of estrogens on plasma renin substrate. In: Heterogeneity of renin and renin substrate, Sambhi MP (ed), Elsevier, New York, 1981, pp 255–260
7. Shionoiri H, Eggena P, Barrett JD, Thananopavarn C, Golub MS, Nakamura R, Judd HL, Sambhi MP: An increase in high molecular weight renin substrate associated with estrogenic hypertension. Biochem Med 29: 14–22, 1983
8. Printz MP, Gregory TJ: Brain angiotensinogen: Evidence for an independent and functional central angiotensin system. In: Buckley JP, Ferrario CM (eds), Central nervous system mechanisms in hypertension. Raven Press, New York, 1981, pp 311–326
9. Ito T, Eggena P, Barrett JD, Katz D, Metter J, Sambhi MP: Studies on angiotensinogen of plasma and cerebral spinal fluid in normal and hypertensive human subjects. Hypertension 2: 432–436, 1980
10. Ito T, Eggena P, Barrett JD, Sambhi MP: Angiotensinogen in human cerebral spinal fluid. In: Sambhi MP (ed), Heterogeneity of renin and renin substrate. Elsevier, 1981, pp 313–316
11. Murakami E, Eggena P, Barrett JD, Sambhi MP: Heterogeneity of renin substrate released from hepatocytes and in brain extracts. Life Sciences, Jan. 1984
12. Murakami E, Eggena P, Barrett JD, Sambhi MP: Release of renin substrate from rat liver and brain slices. Hypertension, in press
13. Ganten D, Printz M, Unger Th, Lang RE: The brain renin-angiotensin system: problems and answers. In: Villarreal H and Sambhi MP (eds), Topics on pathophysiology of hypertension, Martinus Nijhoff, The Hague, 1984
14. Sambhi MP: Prorenin and activators and inhibitors of renin. In: Genest J, Kuchel O, Hamet P, Cantin M (eds), Hypertension – physiopathology and treatment Mc Graw Hill. New York, 1983, pp 210–224